Imaging of Lung Cancer: Update on Staging and Therapy

Editors

JEREMY J. ERASMUS
MYLENE T. TRUONG

RADIOLOGIC CLINICS OF NORTH AMERICA

www.radiologic.theclinics.com

Consulting Editor
FRANK H. MILLER

May 2018 • Volume 56 • Number 3

ELSEVIER

1600 John F. Kennedy Boulevard ● Suite 1800 ● Philadelphia, Pennsylvania, 19103-2899

http://www.theclinics.com

RADIOLOGIC CLINICS OF NORTH AMERICA Volume 56, Number 3
May 2018 ISSN 0033-8389, ISBN 13: 978-0-323-58374-9

Editor: John Vassallo (j.vassallo@elsevier.com)
Developmental Editor: Donald Mumford

Radiologic Clinics of North America (ISSN 0033-8389) is published bimonthly by Elsevier Inc., 360 Park Avenue South, New York, NY 10010-1710. Months of issue are January, March, May, July, September, and November. Periodicals postage paid at New York, NY and additional mailing offices. Subscription prices are USD 493 per year for US individuals, USD 889 per year for US institutions, USD 100 per year for US students and residents, USD 573 per year for Canadian individuals, USD 1136 per year for Canadian institutions, USD 680 per year for international individuals, USD 1136 per year for international institutions, and USD 315 per year for Canadian and international students/residents. To receive student and resident rate, orders must be accompanied by name of affiliated institution, date of term and the signature of program/residency coordinatior on institution letterhead. Orders will be billed at individual rate until proof of status is received. Foreign air speed delivery is included in all *Clinics* subscription prices. All prices are subject to change without notice. **POSTMASTER:** Send address changes to *Radiologic Clinics of North America*, Elsevier Health Sciences Division, Subscription Customer Service, 3251 Riverport Lane, Maryland Heights, MO63043. **Customer Service: Telephone: 1-800-654-2452** (U.S. and Canada); **1-314-447-8871** (outside U.S. and Canada). **Fax: 1-314-447-8029. E-mail: journalscustomerservice-usa@ elsevier.com (for print support); journalsonlinesupport-usa@elsevier.com (for online support)**.

Reprints. For copies of 100 or more of articles in this publication, please contact the Commercial Reprints Department, Elsevier Inc., 360 Park Avenue South, New York, New York 10010-1710. Tel.: +1-212-633-3874; Fax: +1-212-633-3820; E-mail: reprints@elsevier.com.

Radiologic Clinics of North America also published in Greek Paschalidis Medical Publications, Athens, Greece.

Radiologic Clinics of North America is covered in *MEDLINE/PubMed (Index Medicus), EMBASE/Excerpta Medica, Current Contents/Life Sciences, Current Contents/Clinical Medicine, RSNA Index to Imaging Literature, BIOSIS, Science Citation Index,* and *ISI/BIOMED.*

Contributors

CONSULTING EDITOR

FRANK H. MILLER, MD
Chief, Body Imaging Section and Fellowship
Program, Medical Director of MRI, Professor,
Department of Radiology, Northwestern
University Feinberg School of Medicine,
Chicago, Illinois, USA

EDITORS

JEREMY J. ERASMUS, MD
Professor, Department of Diagnostic
Radiology, The University of Texas MD
Anderson Cancer Center, Houston, Texas,
USA

MYLENE T. TRUONG, MD
Professor, Department of Diagnostic
Radiology, The University of Texas MD
Anderson Cancer Center, Houston, Texas,
USA

AUTHORS

GERALD F. ABBOTT, MD
Thoracic Imaging and Interventions,
Massachusetts General Hospital, Boston,
Massachusetts, USA

JEFFREY B. ALPERT, MD
Department of Radiology, Thoracic Imaging,
NYU Langone Health, New York, New York,
USA

MARCELO F. BENVENISTE, MD
Department of Diagnostic Radiology, The
University of Texas MD Anderson Cancer
Center, Houston, Texas, USA

SONIA L. BETANCOURT CUELLAR, MD
Department of Diagnostic Radiology, The
University of Texas MD Anderson Cancer
Center, Houston, Texas, USA

SANJEEV BHALLA, MD
Mallinckrodt Institute of Radiology, St Louis,
Missouri, USA

BRETT W. CARTER, MD
Department of Diagnostic Radiology, The
University of Texas MD Anderson Cancer
Center, Houston, Texas, USA

MARIO CILIBERTO, MD
Division of Functional and Diagnostic Imaging
Research, Department of Radiology,
Advanced Biomedical Imaging Research
Center, Kobe University Graduate School of
Medicine, Kobe, Hyogo, Japan; Department of
Radiology, Catholic University of the Sacred
Heart, A. Gemelli Hospital, Roma, Rome, Italy

PATRICIA M. DE GROOT, MD
Associate Professor, Department of Diagnostic
Radiology, The University of Texas MD
Anderson Cancer Center, Houston, Texas,
USA

AHMED H. EL-SHERIEF, MD
Section of Thoracic Imaging, Department of
Diagnostic Radiology, VA Greater Los Angeles
Healthcare System, David Geffen School of
Medicine at UCLA, University of California,
Los Angeles, Los Angeles, California, USA

JEREMY J. ERASMUS, MD
Professor, Department of Diagnostic
Radiology, The University of Texas MD
Anderson Cancer Center, Houston, Texas,
USA

MATTHEW D. GILMAN, MD
Thoracic Imaging and Interventions,
Massachusetts General Hospital, Boston,
Massachusetts, USA

MYRNA C.B. GODOY, MD, PhD
Associate Professor, Department of Diagnostic
Radiology, The University of Texas MD
Anderson Cancer Center, Houston, Texas,
USA

RYDHWANA HOSSAIN, MD
Thoracic Imaging and Interventions,
Massachusetts General Hospital, Boston,
Massachusetts, USA

YUJI KISHIDA, MD
Division of Radiology, Department of
Radiology, Kobe University Graduate
School of Medicine, Kobe, Hyogo,
Japan

JANE P. KO, MD
Department of Radiology, Thoracic Imaging,
NYU Langone Health, New York, New York,
USA

CHARLES T. LAU, MD, MBA
Section of Cardiothoracic Imaging, Radiology
Service, VA Palo Alto Healthcare System,
Palo Alto, California, USA

EDITH M. MAROM, MD
Department of Diagnostic Radiology, The
University of Texas MD Anderson Cancer
Center, Houston, Texas, USA; Department of
Diagnostic Imaging, The Chaim Sheba Medical
Center, Affiliated with Tel Aviv University,
Tel Aviv, Ramat Gan, Israel

ERIKA G.L.C. ODISIO, MD
Cardiothoracic Fellow, Department of
Diagnostic Radiology, The University of Texas
MD Anderson Cancer Center, Houston, Texas,
USA

YOSHIHARU OHNO, MD, PhD
Division of Functional and Diagnostic Imaging
Research, Department of Radiology,
Advanced Biomedical Imaging Research
Center, Kobe University Graduate
School of Medicine, Kobe, Hyogo,
Japan

**VASSILIKI A. PAPADIMITRAKOPOULOU,
MD**
Department of Thoracic/Head and Neck
Medical Oncology, The University of Texas
MD Anderson Cancer Center, Houston, Texas,
USA

CONSTANTINE A. RAPTIS, MD
Mallinckrodt Institute of Radiology, St Louis,
Missouri, USA

CAROLINE L. ROBB, BS
Washington University School of Medicine in
St. Louis, St Louis, Missouri, USA

BRADLEY S. SABLOFF, MD
Department of Diagnostic Radiology, The
University of Texas MD Anderson Cancer
Center, Houston, Texas, USA

SHINICHIRO SEKI, MD, PhD
Division of Functional and Diagnostic Imaging
Research, Department of Radiology,
Advanced Biomedical Imaging Research
Center, Kobe University Graduate School of
Medicine, Kobe, Hyogo, Japan

AMITA SHARMA, MD
Assistant Professor, Department of Radiology,
Division of Thoracic Imaging and Intervention,
Massachusetts General Hospital, Boston,
Massachusetts, USA

JO-ANNE O. SHEPARD, MD
Professor, Department of Radiology, Director,
Division of Thoracic Imaging and Intervention,
Massachusetts General Hospital, Boston,
Massachusetts, USA

GIRISH S. SHROFF, MD
Associate Professor, Department of Diagnostic
Radiology, The University of Texas MD
Anderson Cancer Center, Houston, Texas,
USA

MYLENE T. TRUONG, MD
Professor, Department of Diagnostic
Radiology, The University of Texas MD
Anderson Cancer Center, Houston, Texas,
USA

CHITRA VISWANATHAN, MD
Department of Diagnostic Radiology, The
University of Texas MD Anderson Cancer
Center, Houston, Texas, USA

IOANNIS VLAHOS, BSc, MBBS, MRCP, FRCR
Department of Radiology, St. George's Medical School, University of London, St. James Wing, St. George's University Hospitals NHS Foundation Trust, London, United Kingdom

JAMES WELSH, MD
Department of Radiation Oncology, The University of Texas MD Anderson Cancer Center, Houston, Texas, USA

CAROL C. WU, MD
Department of Diagnostic Radiology, The University of Texas MD Anderson Cancer Center, Houston, Texas, USA

TAKESHI YOSHIKAWA, MD, PhD
Division of Functional and Diagnostic Imaging Research, Department of Radiology, Advanced Biomedical Imaging Research Center, Kobe University Graduate School of Medicine, Kobe, Hyogo, Japan

Contents

> Incidentally detected lung nodules are increasingly common in routine diagnostic computed tomography (CT) imaging. Formal management recommendations for incidental nodules, such as those outlined by the Fleischner Society, must therefore reflect a balance of malignancy risk and the clinical context in which nodules are discovered. Nodule size, attenuation, morphology, and location all influence the likelihood of malignancy and, thus, the necessity and timing of follow-up according to current Fleischner recommendations. As technologic advancements in CT imaging continue, there may be greater reliance on advanced computerized analysis of lung nodule features to help determine the risk of clinically significant disease.

> The number of screening-detected lung nodules is expected to increase as low-dose computed tomography screening is implemented nationally. Standardized guidelines for image acquisition, interpretation, and screen-detected nodule workup are essential to ensure a high standard of medical care and that lung cancer screening is implemented safely and cost-effectively. In this article, the authors review the current guidelines for pulmonary nodule management in the lung cancer screening setting.

> The chest radiograph is one of the most commonly used imaging studies and is the modality of choice for the initial evaluation of many common clinical scenarios. Over the last two decades, chest computed tomography has been increasingly used for a wide variety of indications, including respiratory illnesses, trauma, oncologic staging, and more recently lung cancer screening. Diagnostic radiologists should be familiar with the common causes of missed lung cancers on imaging studies to avoid detection and interpretation errors. Failure to detect these lesions can potentially have serious implications for both patients and the interpreting radiologist.

> Image-guided percutaneous transthoracic needle biopsy (PTNB) is a well-established and minimally invasive technique for evaluating pulmonary nodules. Implementation of a national lung screening program and increased use of chest

computed tomography have contributed to the frequent identification of indeterminate pulmonary nodules that may require tissue sampling. The advent of biomarker-driven lung cancer therapy has led to an increased use of repeat PTNB after diagnosis. Percutaneous insertion of markers for preoperative localization of small nodules can aid in minimally invasive surgery and radiation treatment planning. This article discusses PTNB, patient selection, and biopsy technique, including minimizing and managing complications.

Several important modifications have been proposed for the tumor (T) descriptor for lung cancers. New size cutoffs have been determined, and there are new T descriptors for adenocarcinoma in situ, minimally invasive adenocarcinoma, and part-solid adenocarcinomas with a solid component > 0.5 to 3 cm (T1a, T1b, T1c). There are also recommendations for multifocal adenocarcinoma, which are classified by the lesion with the highest level T descriptor, and the number of lesions is indicated. Knowledge of these changes is important in the appropriate clinical staging of patients with lung cancer.

This article reviews regional lymph node assessment in lung cancer. In the absence of a distant metastasis, the absence or location of lung cancer spread to a regional mediastinal lymph node affects treatment options and prognosis. Regional lymph node maps have been created to standardize the assessment of the N descriptor. The International Association for the Study of Lung Cancer lymph node map is used for the standardization of N descriptor assessment. Computed tomography (CT), PET/CT with fluorodeoxyglucose, endobronchial ultrasound–guided and/or esophageal ultrasound–guided biopsy, and mediastinoscopy are common modalities used to determine the N descriptor.

The updated eighth edition of the tumor, node, metastasis (TNM) classification for lung cancer includes revisions to T and M descriptors. In terms of the M descriptor, the classification of intrathoracic metastatic disease as M1a is unchanged from TNM-7. Extrathoracic metastatic disease, which was classified as M1b in TNM-7, is now subdivided into M1b (single metastasis, single organ) and M1c (multiple metastases in one or multiple organs) descriptors. In this article, the rationale for changes in the M descriptors, the utility of preoperative staging with PET/computed tomography, and the treatment options available for patients with oligometastatic disease are discussed.

The advent of the eighth edition of the lung cancer staging system reflects a further meticulous evidence-based advance in the stratification of the survival of patients with lung cancer. Although this edition addresses many limitations of earlier staging systems, several limitations in staging remain. This article reviews from a radiologic perspective the limitations of the current staging system, highlighting the process of TNM restructuring, the residual issues with regards to the assignment of T, N, M descriptors, and their associated stage groupings and how these dilemmas affect guidance of multidisciplinary teams taking care of patients with lung cancer.

Update of MR Imaging for Evaluation of Lung Cancer   437

Mario Ciliberto, Yuji Kishida, Shinichiro Seki, Takeshi Yoshikawa, and Yoshiharu Ohno

Since MR imaging was introduced for the assessment of thoracic and lung diseases, various limitations have hindered its widespread adoption in clinical practice. Since 2000, various techniques have been developed that have demonstrated the usefulness of MR imaging for lung cancer evaluation, and it is now reimbursed by health insurance companies in many countries. This article reviews recent advances in lung MR imaging, focusing on its use for lung cancer evaluation, especially with regard to pulmonary nodule detection, pulmonary nodule and mass assessment, lung cancer staging and detection of recurrence, postoperative lung function prediction, and therapeutic response evaluation and prediction.

Lung Cancer: Posttreatment Imaging: Radiation Therapy and Imaging Findings   471

Marcelo F. Benveniste, James Welsh, Chitra Viswanathan, Girish S. Shroff, Sonia L. Betancourt Cuellar, Brett W. Carter, and Edith M. Marom

This article discusses the different radiation delivery techniques available to treat non–small cell lung cancer, typical radiologic manifestations of conventional radiotherapy, and different patterns of lung injury and temporal evolution of the newer radiotherapy techniques. More sophisticated techniques include intensity-modulated radiotherapy, stereotactic body radiotherapy, proton therapy, and respiration-correlated computed tomography or 4-dimensional computed tomography for radiotherapy planning. Knowledge of the radiation treatment plan and technique, the completion date of radiotherapy, and the temporal evolution of radiation-induced lung injury is important to identify expected manifestations of radiation-induced lung injury and differentiate them from tumor recurrence or infection.

Targeted Therapy and Immunotherapy in the Treatment of Non–Small Cell Lung Cancer   485

Girish S. Shroff, Patricia M. de Groot, Vassiliki A. Papadimitrakopoulou, Mylene T. Truong, and Brett W. Carter

The treatment strategy in advanced non–small cell lung cancer (NSCLC) has evolved from empirical chemotherapy to a personalized approach based on histology and molecular markers of primary tumors. Targeted therapies are directed at the products of oncogenic driver mutations. Immunotherapy facilitates the recognition of cancer as foreign by the host immune system, stimulates the immune system, and alleviates the inhibition that allows the growth and spread of cancer cells. The authors describe the role of targeted therapy and immunotherapy in the treatment of NSCLC, patterns of disease present on imaging studies, and immune-related adverse events encountered with immunotherapy.

PROGRAM OBJECTIVE

The objective of the *Radiologic Clinics of North America* is to keep practicing radiologists and radiology residents up to date with current clinical practice in radiology by providing timely articles reviewing the state of the art in patient care.

TARGET AUDIENCE

Practicing radiologists, radiology residents, and other healthcare professionals who provide patient care utilizing radiologic findings.

LEARNING OBJECTIVES

Upon completion of this activity, participants will be able to:

1. Review current management strategy of incidental lung nodules.
2. Discuss staging lung cancer dilemmas, metastasis, and regional lymph node classification.
3. Recognize updates of MRI evaluation of lung cancer.

ACCREDITATION

The Elsevier Office of Continuing Medical Education (EOCME) is accredited by the Accreditation Council for Continuing Medical Education (ACCME) to provide continuing medical education for physicians.

The EOCME designates this enduring material for a maximum of 15 *AMA PRA Category 1 Credit*(s)™. Physicians should claim only the credit commensurate with the extent of their participation in the activity.

All other healthcare professionals requesting continuing education credit for this enduring material will be issued a certificate of participation.

DISCLOSURE OF CONFLICTS OF INTEREST

The EOCME assesses conflict of interest with its instructors, faculty, planners, and other individuals who are in a position to control the content of CME activities. All relevant conflicts of interest that are identified are thoroughly vetted by EOCME for fair balance, scientific objectivity, and patient care recommendations. EOCME is committed to providing its learners with CME activities that promote improvements or quality in healthcare and not a specific proprietary business or a commercial interest.

The planning committee, staff, authors and editors listed below have identified no financial relationships or relationships to products or devices they or their spouse/life partner have with commercial interest related to the content of this CME activity:

Gerald F. Abbott, MD; Jeffrey B. Alpert, MD; Marcelo F. Benveniste, MD; Sonia L. Betancourt Cuellar, MD; Sanjeev Bhalla, MD; Brett W. Carter, MD; Mario Ciliberto, MD; Patricia M. de Groot, MD; Ahmed H. El-Sherief, MD; Jeremy J. Erasmus, MD; Matthew D. Gilman, MD; Myrna C.B. Godoy, MD, PhD; Rydhwana Hossain, MD; Alison Kemp; Yuji Kishida, MD; Jane P. Ko, MD; Charles T. Lau, MD, MBA; Edith M. Marom, MD; Erika G.L.C. Odisio, MD; Constantine A. Raptis, MD; Caroline L. Robb, BS; Bradley S. Sabloff, MD; Amita Sharma, MD; Jo-Anne O. Shepard, MD; Girish S. Shroff, MD; Karthik Subramaniam; Mylene T. Truong, MD; John Vassallo; Chitra Viswanathan, MD; Ioannis Vlahos, BSc, MBBS, MRCP, FRCR; James Welsh, MD; Carol C. Wu, MD.

The planning committee, staff, authors and editors listed below have identified financial relationships or relationships to products or devices they or their spouse/life partner have with commercial interest related to the content of this CME activity:

Yoshiharu Ohno, MD, PhD: has received research support from Canon Medical Systems Corportion, Philips Electronics Japan, Ltd, Bayer AG, Guerbet Japan, Daiichi Sankyo Company, Ltd, and Fuji Pharma Co, Ltd.

Vassiliki A. Papadimitrakopoulou, MD: has been or is currently an advisor/consultant with Bristol-Myers Squibb, Merck & Co., F. Hoffmann-La Roche AG, Novartis, Loxo Oncology, Pfizer, AstraZeneca, Arrys Therapeuitics, Inc., and Eli Lilly and Company.

Shinichiro Seki, MD, PhD: has received research support from Canon Medical Systems Corportion.

Takeshi Yoshikawa, MD, PhD: receives research support from Canon Medical Solutions Corporation.

UNAPPROVED/OFF-LABEL USE DISCLOSURE

The EOCME requires CME faculty to disclose to the participants:

1. When products or procedures being discussed are off-label, unlabelled, experimental, and/or investigational (not US Food and Drug Administration [FDA] approved); and
2. Any limitations on the information presented, such as data that are preliminary or that represent ongoing research, interim analyses, and/or unsupported opinions. Faculty may discuss information about pharmaceutical agents that is outside of FDA-approved labelling. This information is intended solely for CME and is not intended to promote off-label use of these medications. If you have any questions, contact the medical affairs department of the manufacturer for the most recent pre-scribing information.

TO ENROLL

To enroll in the *Radiologic Clinics of North America* Continuing Medical Education program, call customer service at 1-800-654-2452 or sign up online at http://www.theclinics.com/home/cme. The CME program is available to subscribers for an additional annual fee of USD $327.60.

METHOD OF PARTICIPATION

In order to claim credit, participants must complete the following:

1. Complete enrolment as indicated above.
2. Read the activity.
3. Complete the CME Test and Evaluation. Participants must achieve a score of 70% on the test. All CME Tests and Evaluations must be completed online.

CME INQUIRIES/SPECIAL NEEDS

For all CME inquiries or special needs, please contact elsevierCME@elsevier.com.

RADIOLOGIC CLINICS OF NORTH AMERICA

THE CLINICS ARE AVAILABLE ONLINE!
Access your subscription at:
www.theclinics.com

RADIOLOGIC CLINICS OF NORTH AMERICA

FORTHCOMING ISSUES

July 2018
Dual Energy CT
Savvas Nicolaou and Mohammed F. Mohammed,
Editors

September 2018
Imaging of the Small Bowel and Colorectum
Judy Yee, Editor

November 2018
Imaging of the Pelvis and Lower extremity
Laura Bancroft and Kurt Scherer, Editors

RECENT ISSUES

March 2018
MR Imaging of the Prostate
Aytekin Oto, Editor

January 2018
Oral and Maxillofacial Radiology
Dania Tamimi, Editor

November 2017
Imaging and Cancer Screening
Dushyant V. Sahani, Editor

ISSUE OF RELATED INTEREST

PET Clinics, April 2018 (Vol. 13, No. 2)
Prostate Cancer: Imaging and Therapy
Abass Alavi and Sandip Basu, Editors
Available at: www.pet.theclinics.com

Preface

Imaging of Lung Cancer: Update on Screening, Staging, and Therapy

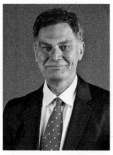
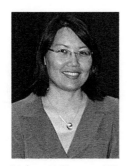

Jeremy J. Erasmus, MD   Mylene T. Truong, MD

Editors

Imaging pertaining to screening, staging, and therapy has been dramatically impacted by new knowledge and understanding of non–small cell lung cancer. Lung cancer screening is now recommended as a result of the finding of a reduction in lung cancer–specific mortality by the National Lung Cancer Screening Trial. With the subsequent approval for reimbursement of low-dose CT screening in the appropriate patient population by the Centers for Medicare and Medicaid Services, screening programs have proliferated. This has necessitated new guidelines to image and manage screen-detected lung nodules. New guidelines have also been issued by the Fleischner Society to address the management of lung nodules, both solid and subsolid, detected incidentally on multidetector CT imaging. To address advances in oncology, molecular biology, pathology, and radiology, the American Thoracic Society/European Respiratory Society/International Association for the Study of Lung Cancer (ATS/ERS/IASLC) revised the pathologic classification of lung adenocarcinoma. This classification provides a standard for pathologic diagnosis not only for patient care but also for clinical trials and TNM classification. The new 8th edition of the TNM staging system has been externally validated and is based on a detailed analysis of a new international database by the Staging and Prognostic Factors Committee of the IASLC. Because of significant differences in survival between patients with different

T and M descriptors, modifications of individual descriptors and overall stage groups have been implemented. Understanding the key revisions in TNM-8 will allow accurate staging of patients with lung cancer and optimize therapy. In terms of imaging to stage and assess treatment response, CT and PET/CT remain the most widely used modalities. However, advances in MR imaging, such as contrast-enhanced MR angiography, short-time inversion recovery turbo spin-echo sequence, diffusion-weighted imaging, whole-body MR imaging, and PET/MR imaging, provide an additional means to assess oncologic patients. Finally, there has been a paradigm shift in lung cancer therapeutic approach. Advances in immunotherapy as well as chemotherapy with targeted agents contribute to the personalization of cancer care. In personalized lung cancer care, the identification of genetic abnormalities and use of biomarkers, such as gene mutations in epidermal growth factor receptor and anaplastic lymphoma kinase, aid in determining treatment options, such as targeted and immunotherapeutic agents. In lung cancer, expression of programmed death ligand-1 (PD-L1, B7-H1) is a method for cancer cells to evade elimination by the immune system. Knowledge of tumor-immune interactions has enabled the development of immune checkpoint inhibitors as new treatment strategies in advanced lung cancer. Advances in radiation therapy include the use of focused beam techniques, such as

Radiol Clin N Am 56 (2018) xv–xvi
https://doi.org/10.1016/j.rcl.2018.03.009
0033-8389/18/© 2018 Published by Elsevier Inc.

3-dimensional conformal radiation therapy, intensity-modulated radiotherapy, stereotactic body radiotherapy, and proton therapy, to precisely deliver high radiation dose and improve local tumor control. The continued development and use of immunotherapeutic strategies incorporating combinations of targeted immunomodulators and immune checkpoint blockade with radiation therapy have increased the relevance of the abscopal effect, the ability of localized radiation to trigger systemic antitumor effects.

The reviews in this issue provide a comprehensive analysis of these challenging and timely topics in the imaging of lung cancer. We would like to thank the authors for their expertise and contributions, Dr Frank H. Miller, Consulting Editor, for the opportunity to provide an update in lung cancer imaging to radiologists in both private and academic practice, and John Vassallo, Associate Publisher, and his team for their support in this endeavor.

Jeremy J. Erasmus, MD
Department of Diagnostic Radiology
The University of Texas
MD Anderson Cancer Center
1515 Holcombe Boulevard, Unit 1478
Houston, TX 77030, USA

Mylene T. Truong, MD
Department of Diagnostic Radiology
The University of Texas
MD Anderson Cancer Center
1515 Holcombe Boulevard, Unit 1478
Houston, TX 77030, USA

E-mail addresses:
jerasmus@mdanderson.org (J.J. Erasmus)
mtruong@mdanderson.org (M.T. Truong)

Management of Incidental Lung Nodules
Current Strategy and Rationale

Jeffrey B. Alpert, MD*, Jane P. Ko, MD

KEYWORDS

- Incidental nodule • Lung nodule • Fleischner Society • Nodule management • Subsolid
- Computed tomography

KEY POINTS

- Incidental lung nodules often require additional evaluation in a manner that balances risk of clinically relevant disease, patient anxiety and inconvenience, and overimaging.
- The Fleischner Society has recently published updated management guidelines for solid and subsolid lung nodules incidentally detected on computed tomography (CT).
- Lung nodule size remains the primary factor that determines the likelihood of malignancy. Nodule attenuation, morphology, and location factor into the determination of malignancy probability.
- Continued technological advancements in CT imaging show promise in differentiating potentially malignant nodules, based on quantitative features such as nodule volume and texture analysis.

INTRODUCTION

Lung nodules incidentally detected on computed tomography (CT) comprise a large and complex group of pathologic entities that often require additional evaluation. Whether discovered on CT of the neck, chest, or abdomen, these lung nodules are identified in conjunction with or in the absence of other diagnostic imaging findings. This is in clear distinction to nodules discovered in the context of lung cancer screening, in which high-risk current and former smokers undergo formal evaluation with the specific goal of identifying early-stage lung cancers. Extensive literature from numerous lung cancer screening programs address lung nodule management in a high-risk screening population. Screening studies include the National Lung Screening Trial, International Early Lung Cancer Action Program, Canadian screening studies Pan-Canadian Early Detection of Lung Cancer Study (PanCan) and British Columbia Cancer Agency, and the European Nederlans-Leuvens Longkanker Screenings Onderzoek (NELSON) screening trial. Although some screening data can be applied to incidentally discovered lung nodules, these incidental nodules must be managed in an appropriate manner that balances risk of clinically relevant disease, undue patient anxiety and inconvenience, and overimaging.

Recently revised management guidelines for incidental lung nodules have been published by the Fleischner Society, an international multidisciplinary group of scientists that includes thoracic radiologists, pulmonologists, surgeons, and pathologists.[1] These guidelines have been recently updated in a continued effort to integrate advancements in knowledge and to appropriately balance the risk of clinically significant disease with the management preferences of clinicians and patients. Recommendations are determined by the risk of malignancy of incidental lung nodules, which can be inferred from data such as

Disclosure Statement: J.P. Ko: Research collaboration, Siemens Healthineers.
Department of Radiology, Thoracic Imaging, NYU Langone Health, 660 First Avenue, 7th Floor, New York, NY 10016, USA
* Corresponding author.
E-mail address: jeffrey.alpert@nyumc.org

radiologic.theclinics.com

nodule size, morphology, and attenuation (ie, solid vs subsolid). Fleischner Society management guidelines typically apply to adult patients older than 35, as younger patients are less likely to develop lung cancer; patients without underlying malignancy, as oncologic patients can have metastases; and immunocompetent individuals, as immunocompromised patients are susceptible to lung infection. The advisory group stresses the importance of using these recommendations in the full clinical context of the patient's potential comorbidities and preferences, while allowing more flexibility in recommendations by radiologists and compliance by clinicians.

The goal of this article is to review important recommendations and changes made by the Fleischner Society to their management guidelines for incidental lung nodules on CT images, as these guidelines create the standard by which incidental nodules are evaluated and managed. Relevant literature pertaining to risk of nodule malignancy is reviewed in the context of a nonscreening population, and future directions are explored.

FLEISCHNER SOCIETY MANAGEMENT GUIDELINES: COMPLIANCE

Awareness of and adherence to Fleischner Society guidelines for management of incidental pulmonary nodules have improved over time. In a survey of members of the Radiological Society of North America, 77.8% of respondents were aware of the recommendations, and nearly 60% of respondents worked in a practice that advocated such guidelines. A significantly higher rate of concordance between radiologist recommendations and Fleischner guidelines was found in academic settings, practices with a written policy available for viewing at work, in groups with at least one dedicated fellowship-trained thoracic radiologist, and among radiologists with fewer than 5 years of practice experience.[2] Other literature has reported low adherence to established guidelines, with one group documenting 34% of recommendations adherent to Fleischner guidelines in a real-world working environment that included both emergency department and outpatient clinics.[3] Noncompliance contributing to overmanagement of small incidental nodules also has been documented.[4,5] Adherence may simply be a matter of mindfulness, with one radiology group's adherence to guidelines as high as nearly 83% after formal discussions and institutional guidelines emphasizing the importance of standardized recommendations.[6] Increased awareness also has strengthened compliance by clinicians and patients. Increased likelihood of

nodule surveillance was associated with direct communication of imaging results to the referring physician or the patient, in addition to the recommendation of a specific CT follow-up time interval by the radiologist.[7] Furthermore, in an age of increasing flexibility and customization of imaging and reporting systems, including the recommendation template with the imaging report may improve compliance with follow-up recommendations by clinicians and their patients. Although only 39% of patients received follow-up imaging as recommended in one reported patient population, those patients were significantly more likely to undergo follow-up when recommendation templates were included in CT reports.[8]

FLEISCHNER SOCIETY MANAGEMENT GUIDELINES: UPDATES

Current Fleischner Society recommendations update guidelines pertaining to both solid and subsolid nodules.[9,10] Rather than specific follow-up imaging intervals, current guidelines now provide a time range, providing greater discretion not only to radiologists who may suggest sooner follow-up for suspicious nodule morphology, for example, but also to clinicians and patients who are more attuned to underlying patient history and preferences. Additional recommendations also are provided for multiple solid and subsolid nodules, as multiplicity may alter the frequency and duration of surveillance. It follows that management for patients with multiple incidental nodules should be guided by the largest or most suspicious-appearing nodule (Fig. 1).

IMAGING CONSIDERATIONS

Appropriate management of incidentally detected lung nodules is based on accurate, high-quality imaging. CT imaging should incorporate thin-section axial images on the order of 1.5 mm or smaller to minimize volume averaging, allow improved nodule detection, and enable accurate characterization of nodule size, morphology, and attenuation[11] (Fig. 2). Thin-section images also facilitate reconstruction of multiplanar coronal and sagittal images, which can be useful in discriminating nodules from oblique areas of linear scarring or atelectasis (Fig. 3). Intravenous contrast is typically not needed for accurate detection and evaluation of lung nodules. In patients who require follow-up imaging, low-dose CT technique is important to reduce cumulative patient radiation dose. The Fleischner guidelines recommend volumetric CT dose index of no more than 3 mGy for a standard-size patient, the

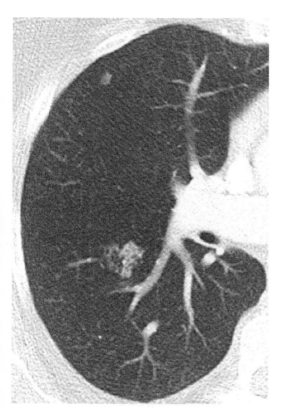

Fig. 1. Two incidentally discovered lung nodules in a 66-year-old woman undergoing CT angiography for thoracic aortic aneurysm. A part-solid 2-cm nodule is in the anterior right lower lobe, and a smaller 0.6-cm solid nodule is adjacent to the right minor fissure. Additional evaluation focused on the suspicious-appearing part-solid nodule, due to size and solid component, later proven to represent lung adenocarcinoma.

same as recommended by the American College of Radiology for lung cancer screening.[12] Automated tube current modulation and iterative reconstruction technique can be used to lower radiation dose.

Assessing Nodule Size

Nodule size should be determined by the average of short-axis and long-axis measurements on the same image in whichever plane yields the largest nodule size, rounded to the nearest millimeter. Average nodule size has achieved better results in malignancy prediction models than a single maximum nodule diameter, as this is thought to correlate better with 3-dimensional volume.[1] There is also recognized variability in the accuracy of manually derived nodule size measurements. In one study examining the intraobserver and interobserver variability in measurement of subsolid lung nodules on initial and follow-up examinations, variability significantly increased when initial and follow-up CT readers were different, and there was a measurement variability of up to approximately 2.2 mm in measurements of both longest and average nodule diameters among CT readers.[13]

Given the variability in manual linear measurements with electronic calipers, there has been growing interest in the role of nodule volume and growth as a predictor of malignancy risk. The Dutch NELSON screening trial used lung nodule volume, volume-doubling time, and volumetry-based nodule diameter to evaluate nearly 10,000 nodules.[14] In this investigation, a nodule volume of 100 mm^3 or smaller, correlating with a maximum

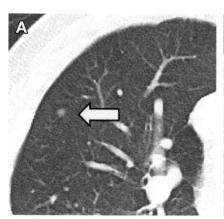
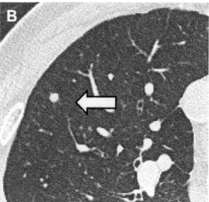

Fig. 2. A 74-year-old man undergoing CT pulmonary angiography for suspected pulmonary embolism. An incidental 5-mm solid nodule in the right upper lobe is initially identified on 5-mm axial lung window image (A, arrow) and appears as a ground-glass nodule; however, on the corresponding 1-mm axial image (B), the nodule (arrow) is solid, and the margin is more distinct.

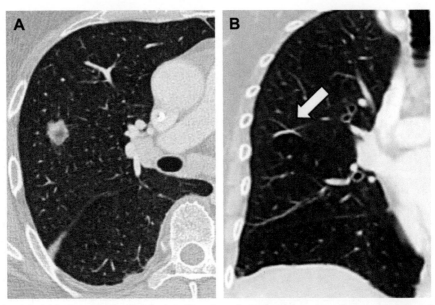

Fig. 3. (*A*) Rounded 1.2-cm nodule with lobulated borders abuts the right minor fissure on 5-mm axial lung window image. Corresponding reformatted coronal image (*B*) demonstrates a flat, discoid appearance (*arrow*) with subtle upward retraction of the fissure; the finding was characterized as a postinflammatory scar.

transverse diameter less than 5 mm, was thought unlikely to reflect malignancy. An intermediate nodule measuring 100 to 300 mm³, correlating with a diameter of approximately 5 to 10 mm, was further assessed by volume-doubling time to predict the likelihood of developing lung cancer within 2 years of the initial CT scan. A high-probability nodule measuring 300 mm³ or more correlated with nodule diameter of 10 mm or larger and was immediately investigated further.[14] Notably, these volumetry-based nodule diameter protocols resulted in equal or higher sensitivity and specificity for malignancy when compared with the widely accepted American College of Chest Physicians nodule management protocol.[14] In a related study, an optimized volume-doubling time cutoff was determined for rapidly growing solid nodules in a lung cancer screening program, resulting in a reduction in false-positive case referrals of up to 33%.[15] Additionally, lung nodule volume was incorporated into a malignancy prediction model for incidental lung nodules detected on CT, resulting in significantly improved performance of the prediction model by approximately 20%.[16] Although several studies show that volumetric measurement provides greater sensitivity of nodule growth, it has yet to become widely used in everyday clinical practice.

Incomplete Initial Imaging of the Chest

If a lung nodule is incidentally detected on CT of the neck, heart, or abdomen, there is often uncertainty regarding the need for and timing of full CT evaluation of the lungs. There is limited literature to guide radiologists and clinicians in this regard. Postinflammatory changes at the lung apices are a common finding that may be encountered on CT of the neck. Nodule calcification can occur at the apices, and multiple pleural-based opacities may be suggestive of a benign etiology, with reconstructed coronal or sagittal views demonstrating an elongated or bandlike shape suggestive of scarring. At the lung bases, among a small number of patients with newly discovered lung nodules reported on abdominal CT, only 7% of patients had malignant nodules, all of which represented metastatic disease; no malignant lung nodules were detected in abdominal CT patients without a history of malignancy, suggesting the likelihood of a new primary lung cancer is low.[17] A similar study found significant differences in patient age, history of malignancy, and incidental nodule size between groups of benign and malignant lung nodules detected on abdominal CT, concluding that lung nodules smaller than 8 mm on abdominal CT in patients younger than 50 years with no history of malignancy were unlikely to be malignant.[18] Updated Fleischner Society management guidelines address potential uncertainty: if an incidental nodule is large or has a suspicious appearance, or the patient has compelling clinical history, full CT imaging of the thorax may be warranted without delay.[1] Intermediate-size nodules should be followed with complete CT chest after the appropriate follow-up time interval determined by size to document stability. No additional follow-up imaging of small nonsuspicious nodules smaller than 6 mm is advised by the Fleischner Society (Fig. 4).

Notably, if CT neck or CT abdomen examinations were performed using thicker axial sections, or if an outside CT chest was performed with thick sections, for instance, future CT imaging of the chest should be performed with thin-section images. The improved spatial resolution and less volume averaging of thin-section image allows optimal evaluation and serves as a baseline for future follow-up studies. In addition, the improved characterization of nodule density with thin-section CT images can influence nodule management.

ASSESSING NODULE RISK

Management of incidentally discovered lung nodules is based on the likelihood of clinically significant malignancy. Several features contribute to the overall suspicion and risk for malignancy of a newly discovered nodule, such as nodule size, attenuation, morphology, and location. Although some of these elements rely on well-established literature, others are still influenced by evolving research.

Nodule Size: Solid Nodules

The primary nodule feature that conveys risk of malignancy is nodule size. The nodule size

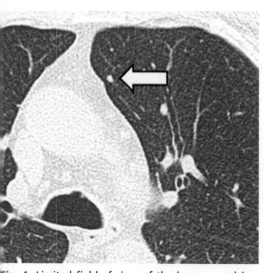

Fig. 4. Limited field-of-view of the lungs on calcium scoring CT in a 69-year-old male nonsmoker. This 1-mm axial image demonstrates a solid 3-mm nodule in the left upper lobe (*arrow*). No surveillance imaging was recommended for this nodule, in accordance with Fleischner guidelines.

threshold for surveillance has increased from earlier recommendations and now parallels several lung cancer screening study results. Specifically, the minimum size threshold for follow-up imaging of an incidental solid nodule is 6 mm per Fleischner Society guidelines, based on an estimated cancer risk of 1% or greater above this threshold.[1] Importantly, nodule size is determined by the average of short-axis and long-axis measurements rather than a single maximum nodule diameter. In cases of both solitary and multiple solid nodules smaller than 6 mm, no routine follow-up is required for low-risk individuals (see **Fig. 4; Fig. 5**), in contrast to prior recommendations based on a nodule size of 4 mm. This change in size threshold is based on extrapolated data from high-risk screening populations in which the average risk of cancer in solid nodules smaller than 6 mm was found to be less than 1%.[14,19] In contrast to high-risk patients in lung cancer screening programs, a solid nodule or multiple solid nodules in low-risk never smokers and younger patients, without history of malignancy, have an even lower risk of malignancy, further supporting this position.[20] In high-risk patients with a solitary solid nodule or multiple solid nodules all smaller than 6 mm, follow-up imaging is not required but could be considered in 12 months, especially in instances whereby lung nodule morphology or upper lobe location may raise the risk of cancer as high as 5%.[1]

For solitary solid nodules 6 to 8 mm in size, a follow-up imaging is now recommended between 6 and 12 months, with the time interval influenced by nodule appearance and patient preference (**Fig. 6**). Notably, updated Fleischner guidelines indicate that strict 2-year follow-up may not be required for all benign-appearing nodules to establish long-term stability, as earlier recommendations were based on older literature that incorporated thick-section CT images, hard-copy images, and radiographs.[14,19,21,22] In a low-risk patient with a well-defined, accurately measured solitary solid nodule with a benign morphology, the Fleischner Society states that 6-month to 12-month follow-up may be adequate for these intermediate-size nodules, and further follow-up 18 to 24 months from the original CT can be considered at the discretion of the radiologist and clinician.[1] However, in a high-risk patient with a solitary solid 6-mm to 8-mm nodule, further follow-up is recommended to 18 to 24 months, as there is an estimated risk of malignancy as high as 2% for these larger nodules, as determined by several screening trials.[14,19] For example, among participants in the NELSON screening trial, a small number of high-risk screening participants were

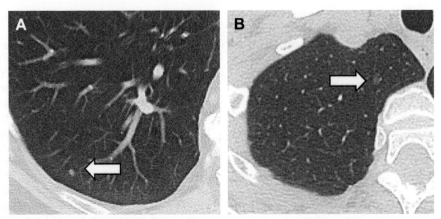

Fig. 5. (*A*) Incidental 3-mm solid right lower lobe nodule (*arrow*) in a 69-year-old nonsmoker with shortness of breath. (*B*) Incidental 5-mm right upper lobe ground-glass nodule (*arrow*) in a 57-year-old nonsmoker. No CT surveillance is required in either of these instances.

diagnosed with lung cancers during a 2-year screening period: 56% in the first year and 44% in the second year.[23] Current guidelines for nodules 8 mm or larger remain the same and are influenced by nodule morphology in addition to nodule size (**Fig. 7**). Options for these larger nodules include 3-month follow-up CT imaging, PET/CT imaging to determine metabolic activity, or tissue sampling. The decision to pursue further investigation is ultimately up to the patient and referring clinician and should take into consideration the risk for malignancy based on imaging.

In instances of multiple solid nodules with 1 or more measuring 6 mm or larger, initial management recommendations are the same for both low-risk and high-risk patients. Follow-up is initially suggested between 3 and 6 months, with

greater concern placed on the possibility of newly discovered metastatic malignancy. Metastases to the lungs often have a lower lung or peripheral lung predominance and typically progress within 3 months. The possibility of an infectious etiology such as bronchiolitis also may be considered and will typically demonstrate change within a 3-month interval. Interestingly, results from the NELSON screening trial indicate an increased risk of primary lung cancer for nodules numbering up to 4, and a decreased risk associated with 5 or more nodules.[1]

Nodule Size: Subsolid Nodules

Similar to solid nodules, management of subsolid lung nodules is determined by size, with less

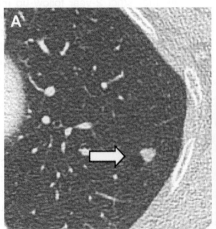
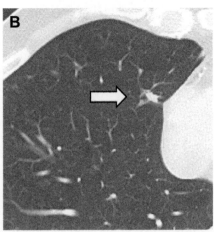

Fig. 6. Incidental solitary 7-mm solid nodules in 2 patients, both imaged for cardiovascular disease. (*A*) Triangular left upper lobe nodule (*arrow*) in a 53-year-old woman; initial 6-month to 12-month follow-up CT was recommended according to Fleischner guidelines. (*B*) Ovoid anterior right middle lobe nodule (*arrow*) with irregular margins in a 49-year-old man; initial follow-up CT imaging was advised in 6 months, given its somewhat suspicious appearance. Note this recommendation is independent of whether the patient is low or high risk.

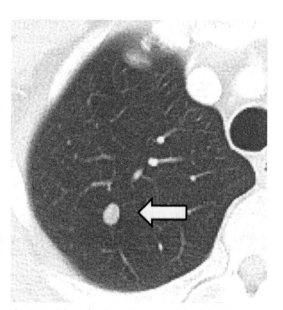

Fig. 7. Incidental solitary 9-mm ovoid solid right upper lobe nodule (*arrow*) in a 66-year-old woman with mitral regurgitation. The referring clinician and the patient opted for initial follow-up CT surveillance in 3 months, rather than PET imaging or tissue sampling, given the well-circumscribed nodule margin favoring a benign etiology and the patient's low risk of malignancy. The nodule was stable at initial follow-up.

emphasis on whether patients are low-risk or high-risk. Again, it is important to note that nodule size is determined by the average of short-axis and long-axis measurements rather than a single maximum nodule diameter. For a single subsolid nodule smaller than 6 mm, no follow-up is required, regardless of whether a nodule is considered pure ground-glass or part-solid density (see **Fig. 5**). In practice, reliable detection of a solid component within a small subsolid nodule smaller than 6 mm is very difficult, and suspected part-solid nodules are therefore managed in the same fashion as their pure ground-glass counterparts. Fleischner Society guidelines suggest an overall likelihood of malignancy of less than 1% among subsolid nodules smaller than 6 mm, although one study in an Asian population reported that approximately 10% of solitary ground-glass nodules 5 mm or smaller did grow over a period of 6 years (**Fig. 8**); nearly 1% of all these small lesions developed into adenocarcinoma with the development of a suspicious solid component with an average time of approximately 3.5 years.[24] Clinical context is paramount in patient management; in an elderly patient, for example, the prolonged time required for a small growing subsolid nodule to develop into a clinically significant malignancy

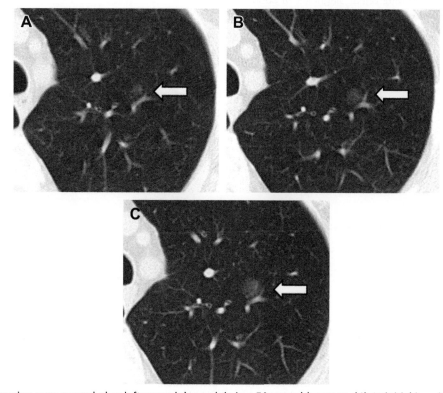

Fig. 8. Growing pure ground-glass left upper lobe nodule in a 54-year-old woman. (*A*) At initial imaging, a 4-mm ground-glass nodule (*arrow*) was detected. (*B*) Three years later, the nodule has grown to 6 mm. (*C*) In 6 years, the nodule has developed a subtle solid density at its lateral margin and has grown to 9 mm, likely an evolving adenocarcinoma lesion.

may not impact the patient's life. For larger nodules measuring an average of 6 mm or larger, the Fleischner Society guidelines have slightly changed. For solitary pure ground-glass nodules 6 mm or larger, follow-up imaging is now recommended between 6 and 12 months rather than the previously advised 3 months, as earlier follow-up is unlikely to influence the outcome of a slowly growing ground-glass focus of neoplasia, even with suspicious imaging features, such as size larger than 10 mm or internal bubbly lucency.[25–28] This change in strategy also aims to reduce the total number of follow-up examinations. Follow-up imaging of these solitary nodules (6 mm or larger) can then be considered every 2 years up to 5 years, as current literature suggests up to 20% to 25% of pure ground-glass nodules grow over time, and an average of up to 4 years is required to reliably determine nodule growth, as these nodules typically grow slowly.[29–31]

In distinction to pure ground-glass lung nodules, solitary part-solid nodules larger than 6 mm are characterized by the size of a solid component (Fig. 9). In nodules with a solid component smaller than 6 mm, malignancy is more likely to reflect preinvasive (in situ) or minimally invasive adenocarcinoma.[28,32] Infection or inflammation also is considered in the differential diagnosis of such a nodule, and therefore, short-term follow-up imaging in 3 to 6 months is advised by the Fleischner Society to document resolution, improvement, or persistence, and to determine the need for additional evaluation.[1,33] A solid component measuring 6 mm or larger is considered more suspicious, as reported by numerous studies, suggesting a much higher likelihood of local tissue invasion.[32,34–39] In nodules that demonstrate lobulated borders or cystic components, an enlarging solid component, or a solid component larger than 8 mm, management recommendations from the Fleischner Society include PET/CT imaging, tissue sampling, or even surgical excision[1] (Fig. 10).

In instances of multiple ground-glass or part-solid nodules, the Fleischner Society suggests follow-up imaging in 3 to 6 months, as an infectious etiology should be considered (Fig. 11). Persistent nodules can then be evaluated appropriately over time, as multiple lesions can represent various entities in the adenocarcinoma spectrum, such as atypical adenomatous hyperplasia or adenocarcinoma in situ. For multiple subsolid nodules smaller than 6 mm, additional CT follow-up can be considered at 2 and 4 years. Notably, in cases of multiple nodules, management should be guided by the most suspicious-appearing nodule (see Fig. 1). Prolonged follow-up imaging to reassess several

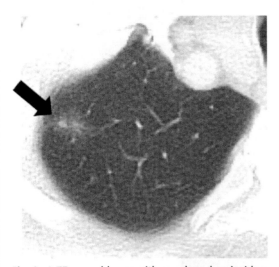

Fig. 9. A 77-year-old man with cough and an incidentally discovered 1.4-cm right upper lobe solitary part-solid nodule with a 4-mm solid component (*arrow*). Initial follow-up CT imaging was advised in 3 months, according to Fleischner guidelines; the nodule was unchanged. Accordingly, annual CT should be performed for 5 years, as recommended by Fleischner guidelines.

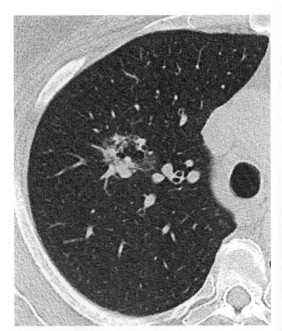

Fig. 10. A 2.4-cm right upper lobe nodule was incidentally discovered on CT in a 66-year-old woman imaged before liver transplantation. This part-solid nodule is suspicious for malignancy and shows ground-glass attenuation, nodular solid components, and internal bubbly lucencies. The patient was referred to cardiothoracic surgery, and adenocarcinoma was later confirmed.

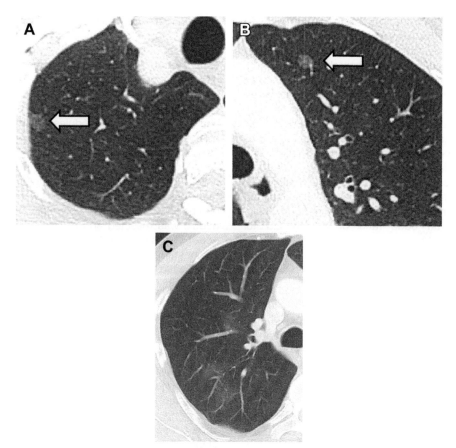

Fig. 11. Two patients with multiple ground-glass nodules 6 mm and larger. (*A, B*) Incidental right and left upper lobe 7-mm ground-glass nodules (*arrows*) in a 48-year-old woman. (*C*) Several poorly marginated ground-glass right lung nodules were discovered in an asymptomatic 41-year-old man before becoming a kidney donor. Initial follow-up CT imaging was recommended in 3 to 6 months for both patients.

slowly growing lesions in the setting of multifocal adenocarcinoma is often required to determine patient management.

Nodule Doubling Time

The frequency of follow-up imaging is based on the expected doubling time of a malignant lung nodule, and doubling time is dependent on nodule attenuation and presumed histology. The volumetric doubling time of a solid nodule is reported between 100 and 400 days, and thus detectable growth should be evident between 1 and 2 years of surveillance.[40] This is in contrast to subsolid lung nodules, specifically part-solid and pure ground-glass nodules on the adenocarcinoma spectrum. These indolent lesions demonstrate longer volumetric doubling times: subsolid nodules typically double within 3 to 5 years (see **Fig. 8**), with a reported range of 300 to 450 days for part-solid nodules and 600 to 900 days for pure ground-glass lung nodules.[29,41] In this regard, among malignant nonsolid (ground-glass)

nodules, Yankelevitz and colleagues[41] reported a median transition time from nonsolid to part-solid density of 25 months, with a successful postsurgical survival rate of 100%, concluding that nonsolid nodules can be safely followed with CT at 12-month intervals. This is supported by a subsequent prospective multicenter study of the natural progression of more than 1200 subsolid lung nodules, which reports a mean time for progression of pure ground-glass to part-solid nodule density of 3.8 ± 2.0 years.[42] This literature justifies both longer imaging surveillance intervals and longer duration of surveillance.

Nodule Attenuation and Morphology

Thin-section CT images viewed in a lung window setting and reconstructed using a sharp kernel are considered the best imaging practice for discriminating ground-glass and solid nodule components. Improved spatial resolution aids the radiologist in accurately evaluating nodule composition and morphology. The presence of fat or calcification within a nodule can frequently determine a benign appearance and should be viewed using mediastinal window setting with images reconstructed using a soft kernel[43–45] (Fig. 12).

Earlier literature has established nodule shape and margination as important features in determining risk of malignancy. Round and ovoid nodules with smooth regular borders are more likely to be benign, whereas lobulated, irregular, or spiculated nodule margins have long been considered suspicious for malignancy[43,45,46] (see Figs. 6 and 7); such conclusions have been reinforced with more recent screening trials, such as the PanCan screening trial that reported nodule spiculation with an odds ratio of 2.2 to 2.5 for malignancy.[19,47]

Nodule Location

Lung nodule location impacts the likelihood of malignancy. Lung cancer is more frequently identified in an upper lobe location, specifically the right upper lobe.[46,48] One recent screening trial described upper lobe location as a risk factor for malignancy, conveying an odds ratio of approximately 2.0.[19]

Perifissural Lung Nodules

In terms of nodule location, incidental lung nodules in a perifissural location are typically benign. Many radiologists assume such nodules are small intrapulmonary lymph nodes, based in part on a prior report of a small number of pathologically proven cases.[49] Updated Fleischner Society guidelines advise no further follow-up of perifissural nodules, even if 6 mm or larger in average size, provided the nodule has an ovoid or triangular configuration on axial images and a discoid or lentiform appearance on reformatted multiplanar images[1] (Fig. 13).

Perifissural nodules with an ovoid or triangular configuration are considered benign, even when growth is documented. As part of the NELSON screening trial, nearly 20% of more than 4000 nodules detected at baseline screening were classified as perifissural nodules (solid nodules attached to a fissure with an ovoid or triangular shape) and had a mean size of 4.4 mm.[50] Despite 15.5% of the nodules increasing in size at 1 year follow-up and 8.3% with a doubling time of fewer than 400 days, none of the nodules were malignant on imaging follow-up. Notably, only 1 perifissural nodule was resected and proven to be a lymph node. This study bolsters the conclusions of an earlier study of another high-risk screening population, which found 28% of more than 800 noncalcified nodules were perifissural, often triangular (44%), oval (42%), below the carina (84%), or with a septal connection (73%) and a mean maximum length of less than 4 mm.[51] After 2 years of follow-up imaging, no registered cancers from this screening population originated from a perifissural nodule, despite nodule growth among some patients. However, follow-up imaging of a perifissural nodule may be warranted in a patient with underlying malignancy, or if a nodule demonstrates a spiculated irregular margin or distortion of the adjacent fissure, as these features would increase the probability of malignancy.[1]

FUTURE DIRECTIONS

Continued technical advancements in imaging have the ability to shape future management of

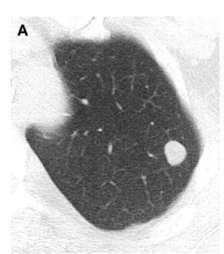
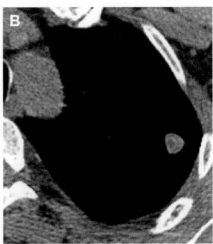

Fig. 12. Incidentally detected 1.4-cm left upper lobe nodule in a 47-year-old man with chest pain, viewed on axial images in lung (A) and mediastinal/soft tissue windows (B). The nodule has fat density on thin mediastinal windows reconstructed with soft tissue kernel and is consistent with a hamartoma.

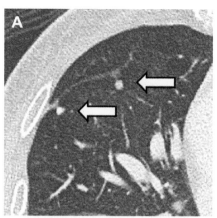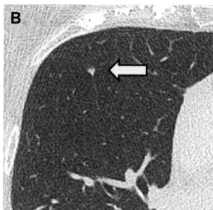

Fig. 13. Examples of round (*A*) and triangular (*B*) perifissural lung nodules (*arrows*), none larger than 4 mm. Because of the typical location, size, and appearance of these perifissural nodules, no further evaluation is required.

incidental lung nodules. Specifically, there has been growing interest in the capabilities of quantitative CT imaging, including volumetric nodule assessment as well as CT histogram and texture analysis, in which nodule CT attenuation values are examined. Nodule volumetry has shown promising results in its ability to evaluate the composition of subsolid lung nodules, potentially differentiating lesions on the lung adenocarcinoma spectrum.[52,53] Studies have also shown the ability of histogram analysis to assist in histologic subtyping of subsolid lung adenocarcinomas, and other work seeks to differentiate specific biomarker lesions, such as epidermal growth factor receptor mutation, using texture analysis.[53–56] Automated computer analysis of lung nodules is also a topic of ongoing research, with efforts to establish computerized deep learning using huge data sets to better predict potentially malignant lung nodules.[57–59]

The use of prediction models also has garnered attention, especially those that incorporate lung nodule features and clinical risk factors to predict the likelihood of nodule malignancy. The Brock model, or the PanCan model, named for its analysis of thousands of nodules from the lung cancer screening trial of the same name, includes both clinical and nodule features, such as nodule density, location, and spiculation, to distinguish between benign and malignant nodules in a screening population. The model shows excellent predictive accuracy and an area under the receiver operating curve of 0.94.[1,19] The clinical utility of this model has yet to be firmly established.

SUMMARY

In distinction to lung nodules discovered in high-risk screening populations, incidentally detected nodules are increasingly common in routine diagnostic CT imaging, with an estimated frequency of detection greater than 30% on CT.[60] Management recommendations for these incidental lung nodules, such as those outlined by the Fleischner Society, reflect the balance of risk of malignancy and the clinical context in which nodules are discovered. Nodule size, attenuation, morphology, and location all influence the likelihood of malignancy and, thus, the necessity and timing of follow-up, according to current Fleischner recommendations. As technological advancements in imaging continue, semiautomated and other advanced computerized analysis of lung nodule features may have an increasing role in determining the risk of malignancy.

REFERENCES

1. MacMahon H, Naidich DP, Goo JM, et al. Guidelines for management of incidental pulmonary nodules detected on CT images: from the Fleischner Society 2017. Radiology 2017;284(1):228–43.
2. Eisenberg RL, Bankier AA, Boiselle PM. Compliance with Fleischner Society guidelines for management of small lung nodules: a survey of 834 radiologists. Radiology 2010;255(1):218–24.
3. Lacson R, Prevedello LM, Andriole KP, et al. Factors associated with radiologists' adherence to Fleischner Society guidelines for management of pulmonary nodules. J Am Coll Radiol 2012;9(7): 468–73.
4. Masciocchi M, Wagner B, Lloyd B. Quality review: Fleischner criteria adherence by radiologists in a large community hospital. J Am Coll Radiol 2012; 9(5):336–9.
5. Esmaili A, Munden RF, Mohammed TL. Small pulmonary nodule management: a survey of the members of the Society of Thoracic Radiology with

comparison to the Fleischner Society guidelines. J Thorac Imaging 2011;26(1):27–31.

6. Eisenberg RL, Fleischner S. Ways to improve radiologists' adherence to Fleischner Society guidelines for management of pulmonary nodules. J Am Coll Radiol 2013;10(6):439–41.

7. Ridge CA, Hobbs BD, Bukoye BA, et al. Incidentally detected lung nodules: clinical predictors of adherence to Fleischner Society surveillance guidelines. J Comput Assist Tomogr 2014;38(1):89–95.

8. McDonald JS, Koo CW, White D, et al. Addition of the Fleischner Society guidelines to chest CT examination interpretive reports improves adherence to recommended follow-up care for incidental pulmonary nodules. Acad Radiol 2017;24(3):337–44.

9. MacMahon H, Austin JH, Gamsu G, et al. Guidelines for management of small pulmonary nodules detected on CT scans: a statement from the Fleischner Society. Radiology 2005;237(2):395–400.

10. Naidich DP, Bankier AA, MacMahon H, et al. Recommendations for the management of subsolid pulmonary nodules detected at CT: a statement from the Fleischner Society. Radiology 2013;266(1):304–17.

11. Godoy MC, Kim TJ, White CS, et al. Benefit of computer-aided detection analysis for the detection of subsolid and solid lung nodules on thin- and thick-section CT. AJR Am J Roentgenol 2013;200(1):74–83.

12. Kazerooni EA, Armstrong MR, Amorosa JK, et al. ACR CT accreditation program and the lung cancer screening program designation. J Am Coll Radiol 2016;13(2 Suppl):R30–4.

13. Kim H, Park CM, Song YS, et al. Measurement variability of persistent pulmonary subsolid nodules on same-day repeat CT: what is the threshold to determine true nodule growth during follow-up? PLoS One 2016;11(2):e0148853.

14. Horeweg N, van Rosmalen J, Heuvelmans MA, et al. Lung cancer probability in patients with CT-detected pulmonary nodules: a prespecified analysis of data from the NELSON trial of low-dose CT screening. Lancet Oncol 2014;15(12):1332–41.

15. Heuvelmans MA, Oudkerk M, de Bock GH, et al. Optimisation of volume-doubling time cutoff for fast-growing lung nodules in CT lung cancer screening reduces false-positive referrals. Eur Radiol 2013;23(7):1836–45.

16. Mehta HJ, Ravenel JG, Shaftman SR, et al. The utility of nodule volume in the context of malignancy prediction for small pulmonary nodules. Chest 2014; 145(3):464–72.

17. Alpert JB, Fantauzzi JP, Melamud K, et al. Clinical significance of lung nodules reported on abdominal CT. AJR Am J Roentgenol 2012;198(4):793–9.

18. Wu CC, Cronin CG, Chu JT, et al. Incidental pulmonary nodules detected on abdominal computed tomography. J Comput Assist Tomogr 2012;36(6): 641–5.

19. McWilliams A, Tammemagi MC, Mayo JR, et al. Probability of cancer in pulmonary nodules detected on first screening CT. N Engl J Med 2013;369(10): 910–9.

20. Samet JM, Avila-Tang E, Boffetta P, et al. Lung cancer in never smokers: clinical epidemiology and environmental risk factors. Clin Cancer Res 2009; 15(18):5626–45.

21. Shin KE, Lee KS, Yi CA, et al. Subcentimeter lung nodules stable for 2 years at LDCT: long-term follow-up using volumetry. Respirology 2014;19(6): 921–8.

22. Zhao B, James LP, Moskowitz CS, et al. Evaluating variability in tumor measurements from same-day repeat CT scans of patients with non-small cell lung cancer. Radiology 2009;252(1):263–72.

23. Horeweg N, Scholten ET, de Jong PA, et al. Detection of lung cancer through low-dose CT screening (NELSON): a prespecified analysis of screening test performance and interval cancers. Lancet Oncol 2014;15(12):1342–50.

24. Kakinuma R, Muramatsu Y, Kusumoto M, et al. Solitary pure ground-glass nodules 5 mm or smaller: frequency of growth. Radiology 2015;276(3):873–82.

25. Lee HY, Choi YL, Lee KS, et al. Pure ground-glass opacity neoplastic lung nodules: histopathology, imaging, and management. AJR Am J Roentgenol 2014;202(3):W224–33.

26. Lee SM, Park CM, Goo JM, et al. Invasive pulmonary adenocarcinomas versus preinvasive lesions appearing as ground-glass nodules: differentiation by using CT features. Radiology 2013;268(1):265–73.

27. Hwang IP, Park CM, Park SJ, et al. Persistent pure ground-glass nodules larger than 5 mm: differentiation of invasive pulmonary adenocarcinomas from preinvasive lesions or minimally invasive adenocarcinomas using texture analysis. Invest Radiol 2015; 50(11):798–804.

28. Lee JH, Park CM, Lee SM, et al. Persistent pulmonary subsolid nodules with solid portions of 5 mm or smaller: their natural course and predictors of interval growth. Eur Radiol 2016;26(6):1529–37.

29. Kobayashi Y, Fukui T, Ito S, et al. How long should small lung lesions of ground-glass opacity be followed? J Thorac Oncol 2013;8(3):309–14.

30. Aoki T. Growth of pure ground-glass lung nodule detected at computed tomography. J Thorac Dis 2015; 7(9):E326–8.

31. Lim HJ, Ahn S, Lee KS, et al. Persistent pure ground-glass opacity lung nodules >/= 10 mm in diameter at CT scan: histopathologic comparisons and prognostic implications. Chest 2013;144(4):1291–9.

32. Cohen JG, Reymond E, Lederlin M, et al. Differentiating pre- and minimally invasive from invasive adenocarcinoma using CT-features in persistent pulmonary part-solid nodules in Caucasian patients. Eur J Radiol 2015;84(4):738–44.

33. Lee SM, Park CM, Goo JM, et al. Transient part-solid nodules detected at screening thin-section CT for lung cancer: comparison with persistent part-solid nodules. Radiology 2010;255(1):242–51.

34. Saito H, Yamada K, Hamanaka N, et al. Initial findings and progression of lung adenocarcinoma on serial computed tomography scans. J Comput Assist Tomogr 2009;33(1):42–8.

35. Matsuguma H, Mori K, Nakahara R, et al. Characteristics of subsolid pulmonary nodules showing growth during follow-up with CT scanning. Chest 2013;143(2):436–43.

36. Lee KH, Goo JM, Park SJ, et al. Correlation between the size of the solid component on thin-section CT and the invasive component on pathology in small lung adenocarcinomas manifesting as ground-glass nodules. J Thorac Oncol 2014;9(1):74–82.

37. Hwang EJ, Park CM, Ryu Y, et al. Pulmonary adeno-carcinomas appearing as part-solid ground-glass nodules: is measuring solid component size a better prognostic indicator? Eur Radiol 2015;25(2):558–67.

38. Liao JH, Amin VB, Kadoch MA, et al. Subsolid pulmonary nodules: CT-pathologic correlation using the 2011 IASLC/ATS/ERS classification. Clin Imaging 2015;39(3):344–51.

39. Saji H, Matsubayashi J, Akata S, et al. Correlation between whole tumor size and solid component size on high-resolution computed tomography in the prediction of the degree of pathologic malignancy and the prognostic outcome in primary lung adenocarcinoma. Acta Radiol 2015;56(10):1187–95.

40. Hasegawa M, Sone S, Takashima S, et al. Growth rate of small lung cancers detected on mass CT screening. Br J Radiol 2000;73(876):1252–9.

41. Yankelevitz DF, Yip R, Smith JP, et al. CT screening for lung cancer: nonsolid nodules in baseline and annual repeat rounds. Radiology 2015;277(2):555–64.

42. Kakinuma R, Noguchi M, Ashizawa K, et al. Natural history of pulmonary subsolid nodules: a prospective multicenter study. J Thorac Oncol 2016;11(7):1012–28.

43. Siegelman SS, Khouri NF, Leo FP, et al. Solitary pulmonary nodules: CT assessment. Radiology 1986;160(2):307–12.

44. Siegelman SS, Khouri NF, Scott WW Jr, et al. Pulmonary hamartoma: CT findings. Radiology 1986;160(2):313–7.

45. Erasmus JJ, Connolly JE, McAdams HP, et al. Solitary pulmonary nodules: part I. Morphologic evaluation for differentiation of benign and malignant lesions. Radiographics 2000;20(1):43–58.

46. Lindell RM, Hartman TE, Swensen SJ, et al. Five-year lung cancer screening experience: CT appearance, growth rate, location, and histologic features of 61 lung cancers. Radiology 2007;242(2):555–62.

47. Xu DM, van Klaveren RJ, de Bock GH, et al. Role of baseline nodule density and changes in density and nodule features in the discrimination between benign and malignant solid indeterminate pulmonary nodules. Eur J Radiol 2009;70(3):492–8.

48. Horeweg N, van der Aalst CM, Thunnissen E, et al. Characteristics of lung cancers detected by computer tomography screening in the randomized NELSON trial. Am J Respir Crit Care Med 2013;187(8):848–54.

49. Bankoff MS, McEniff NJ, Bhadelia RA, et al. Prevalence of pathologically proven intrapulmonary lymph nodes and their appearance on CT. AJR Am J Roentgenol 1996;167(3):629–30.

50. de Hoop B, van Ginneken B, Gietema H, et al. Pulmonary perifissural nodules on CT scans: rapid growth is not a predictor of malignancy. Radiology 2012;265(2):611–6.

51. Ahn MI, Gleeson TG, Chan IH, et al. Perifissural nodules seen at CT screening for lung cancer. Radiology 2010;254(3):949–56.

52. Scholten ET, Jacobs C, van Ginneken B, et al. Detection and quantification of the solid component in pulmonary subsolid nodules by semiautomatic segmentation. Eur Radiol 2015;25(2):488–96.

53. Ko JP, Suh J, Ibidapo O, et al. Lung adenocarcinoma: correlation of quantitative CT findings with pathologic findings. Radiology 2016;280(3):931–9.

54. Li Q, Fan L, Cao ET, et al. Quantitative CT analysis of pulmonary pure ground-glass nodule predicts histological invasiveness. Eur J Radiol 2017;89:67–71.

55. Ozkan E, West A, Dedelow JA, et al. CT gray-level texture analysis as a quantitative imaging biomarker of epidermal growth factor receptor mutation status in adenocarcinoma of the lung. AJR Am J Roentgenol 2015;205(5):1016–25.

56. Sacconi B, Anzidei M, Leonardi A, et al. Analysis of CT features and quantitative texture analysis in patients with lung adenocarcinoma: a correlation with EGFR mutations and survival rates. Clin Radiol 2017;72(6):443–50.

57. He X, Sahiner B, Gallas BD, et al. Computerized characterization of lung nodule subtlety using thoracic CT images. Phys Med Biol 2014;59(4):897–910.

58. Reeves AP, Xie Y, Jirapatnakul A. Automated pulmonary nodule CT image characterization in lung cancer screening. Int J Comput Assist Radiol Surg 2016;11(1):73–88.

59. Nibali A, He Z, Wollersheim D. Pulmonary nodule classification with deep residual networks. Int J Comput Assist Radiol Surg 2017;12(10):1799–808.

60. Gould MK, Tang T, Liu IL, et al. Recent trends in the identification of incidental pulmonary nodules. Am J Respir Crit Care Med 2015;192(10):1208–14.

Pulmonary Nodule Management in Lung Cancer Screening
A Pictorial Review of Lung-RADS Version 1.0

Myrna C.B. Godoy, MD, PhD*, Erika G.L.C. Odisio, MD,
Mylene T. Truong, MD, Patricia M. de Groot, MD,
Girish S. Shroff, MD, Jeremy J. Erasmus, MD

KEYWORDS

- Lung cancer • Lung cancer screening • Pulmonary nodule • Computed tomography
- Low-dose computed tomography • Lung-RADS

KEY POINTS

- The American College of Radiology has established the Lung-RADS classification to standardize the low-dose computed tomography lung cancer screening lexicon, interpretation, reporting, and recommendations for management.
- Lung-RADS assessment categories facilitate communication with clinicians and clarify management of screen-detected nodules.
- Lung-RADS facilitates auditing of lung cancer screening programs and data collection for research and outcome analysis for future refinement of lung cancer screening practices.
- The use of a standardized reporting system is a requirement for lung cancer screening reimbursement by the Centers for Medicare and Medicaid Services.
- Currently, although most radiologists in the United States have adopted the use of Lung-RADS, there are similar management recommendations, including those from the National Comprehensive Cancer Network.

INTRODUCTION

The US Preventive Services Task Force has given a grade B recommendation for lung cancer screening (LCS) with low-dose computed tomography (LDCT) scanning for high-risk current and former smokers.[1] This recommendation is based primarily on the results from the National Lung Screening Trial, a randomized clinical trial of more than 50,000 high-risk smokers, which reported a 20% reduction in lung cancer–specific mortality rate associated with LDCT screening compared with screening with chest radiography.[2,3] In this study, lung cancer was diagnosed in 1.1% of participants undergoing LDCT scanning with a sensitivity and specificity of 93.8% and 73.4, respectively.[3]

Private insurance and Centers for Medicare and Medicaid Services are now reimbursing the cost of LCS in the appropriate population. As a result, the number of detected lung nodules is expected to increase as LDCT screening is implemented nationally. The American College of Radiology (ACR) in association with the Society of Thoracic Radiology (STR) has published standardized guidelines for image acquisition to optimize image quality and patient safety in LCS programs.[4] These guidelines provide recommendations for radiation

Department of Diagnostic Radiology, The University of Texas MD Anderson Cancer Center, 1515 Holcombe Boulevard, Unit 371, Houston, TX 77030, USA
* Corresponding author.
E-mail address: mgodoy@mdanderson.org

Radiol Clin N Am 56 (2018) 353–363
https://doi.org/10.1016/j.rcl.2018.01.003
0033-8389/18/© 2018 Elsevier Inc. All rights reserved.

radiologic.theclinics.com

exposure factors, CT detector configuration, image slice thickness and interval, field of view and matrix size, window and level settings, reconstruction algorithms, reformatted images, and advanced noise reduction techniques.[4]

Standardization of the definition of a positive result in LDCT screening and appropriate management of positive screening results are essential to optimize the cost-effectiveness of LCS.[5] These proposals will decrease inappropriate nodule evaluation, decrease patient radiation dose owing to unnecessary reevaluation with imaging, and decrease invasive diagnostic procedures. In this regard, the ACR has established the Lung-RADS classification[6] to standardize the LDCT screening lexicon, interpretation, reporting, and recommendations for management of identified nodules. The first and current version of this classification was released in April 2014.[6] The use of Lung-RADS assessment categories will facilitate communication with clinicians and standardization of patient management, improving the quality of patient care. It will allow auditing of LCS programs and facilitate data collection for research and outcome analysis for future refinement of LCS practices. The use of a standardized reporting system is a requirement for reimbursement of LCS by the Centers for Medicare and Medicaid Services. Currently, although most radiologists in the United States have adopted the use of Lung-RADS, there are similar management recommendations, including those from the National Comprehensive Cancer Network.

Another important consideration in LCS is appropriate documentation and communication of results. In this regard, the ACR Practice Parameter for Communication of Diagnostic Imaging Findings has defined new practice parameters and technical standards for LDCT in LCS. This educational tool is designed to assist practitioners in providing appropriate radiologic care for patients.[4] Providers can request a database application that facilitates management of patient intake, scheduling, and follow-up.[4]

In this article, we discuss image acquisition and reconstruction, nodule evaluation, and current guidelines for pulmonary nodule management in the LCS setting. Each Lung-RADS category will be reviewed and practical cases encountered in clinical practice will be presented. It is important to emphasize that recommendations of management are flexible, and guidelines should be interpreted using clinical judgment on a case-by-case basis. For challenging cases, a multidisciplinary review can be useful to determine the best management for a particular patient, taking into consideration clinical aspects such as age, comorbidities, life expectancy, and imaging findings.

CONSIDERATIONS ON IMAGE ACQUISITION, RECONSTRUCTION, AND ANALYSIS

The ACR-STR practice parameters recommend LCS be performed with a multidetector helical CT technique in a single breath hold at full inspiration.[4] The CT scan should be performed without intravenous contrast administration and should extend from the lung apices to the costophrenic recesses. The field of view should be optimized for each patient to include the entire transverse and anteroposterior dimensions of the lungs.

Axial image reconstruction with slice thickness of 2.5 mm or less, with reconstruction intervals equal to or less than the slice thickness, is recommended for image review.[4] However, image reconstruction at 1 mm or less minimizes volume-averaging effects and, therefore, should be available to optimize characterization of small lung nodules, particularly in the assessment of nodule size and morphology pertaining to solid and subsolid components.[4] Multiplanar reconstruction can be useful to improve the characterization of nodule location and shape (Fig. 1), particularly nodules located along the pleural surface, because these perifissural nodules have a low potential for malignancy.[4,7] Maximum intensity projection images increase nodule detection.[8,9] Computer-aided detection systems can be used as a second reader to increase detection and nodule characterization.[10–12] Although semiautomated volumetric assessment of nodule size and growth by computer analysis has some technical limitations, it is more accurate and reproducible than 2-dimensional measurements.[4,13,14]

In terms of patient safety, the radiation dose should be as low as reasonably achievable without compromising image quality. For LCS, the CT technique should be set to yield a CTDIvol of less or equal 3 mGy for a standard-sized patient (height, 5 feet 7 inches [170 cm]; weight, 155 pounds [69.75 kg]) and should be decrease for smaller sized patients and increased for larger sized patients.[4]

Nodules are defined according to Fleischner Society's glossary of terms as a rounded opacity, well or poorly defined, and less than 3 cm in diameter.[15] Nodule size should be measured on lung window (high spatial frequency algorithm) images. Size of a screen-detected nodule is defined as the average of the longest diameter and the perpendicular diameter on a single axial CT image, rounded to the nearest whole number. Comparison with prior examinations should be performed whenever available to assess changes over time.

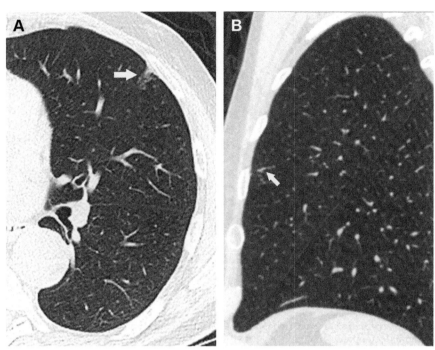

Fig. 1. Usefulness of multiplanar reconstruction for the characterization of lung lesions. (*A*) Axial low-dose computed tomography (LDCT) image shows a left upper lobe ground glass nodular opacity (*arrow*). (*B*) Sagittal LDCT image reconstruction demonstrates a linear configuration of the left upper lobe lesion, characterizing focal scarring rather than a true ground glass nodule (*arrow*).

A diameter difference of at least 1.5 mm is used to determine nodule growth. When multiple nodules are identified, a single final Lung-RADS category should be given to the LCS examination, based on the most worrisome nodule. Depending on the presence of prior history of lung cancer or CT findings of clinically significant or potentially clinically disease not related to lung cancer, a modifier C or S, respectively, is added to the assessment category of 0 to 4.

AMERICAN COLLEGE OF RADIOLOGY LUNG-RADS ASSESSMENT CATEGORIES
Lung-RADS Category 0: Incomplete

Category descriptor: Incomplete.

This category includes LCS examinations that are considered incomplete for 1 of 2 reasons: (1) There is incomplete image visualization of the lung parenchyma, or (2) comparison with a prior image is required before a final assessment category can be given.

Estimated population prevalence: 1%.

Management: Additional LCS CT images or comparison to prior chest CT examinations is needed. After additional image acquisition or image comparison is performed, a final assessment should be given.

Lung-RADS Category 1: Negative

Category descriptor: No nodules and definitely benign nodules.

Includes LDCT with no nodules or with nodule(s) that have benign characteristics, such as nodule(s) with specific calcifications: complete, central, popcorn, concentric rings; and fat containing nodules (−40 to −120 Hounsfield units in attenuation; **Fig. 2**).

Estimated population prevalence: 90% (combined category 1 and 2).

Probability of malignancy: Less than 1%.

Management: Continue annual screening with LDCT in 12 months.

Lung-RADS Category 2: Benign Appearance or Behavior

Category descriptor: Nodules with a very low likelihood of becoming a clinically active cancer owing to size or lack of growth.

Includes the following findings on baseline screening:

- Solid nodule less than 6 mm (**Fig. 3**);
- Part-solid nodule less than 6 mm in total diameter; and
- Nonsolid nodule less than 20 mm (**Fig. 4**).

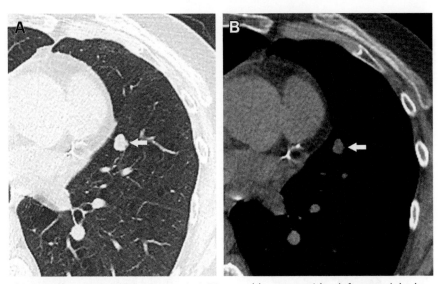

Fig. 2. Negative screening: Lung-RADS category 1. A 74-year-old woman with a left upper lobe hamartoma. (*A*) Axial LDCT image with lung window settings shows a 10 × 8-mm lobulated nodule in the lingual (*arrow*). (*B*) Mediastinal window settings allows characterization of focal areas of low attenuation (−60 Hounsfield units) within the nodule (*arrow*), consistent with a hamartoma. Management recommendation for Lung-RADS category 1 lesions is to continue annual screening.

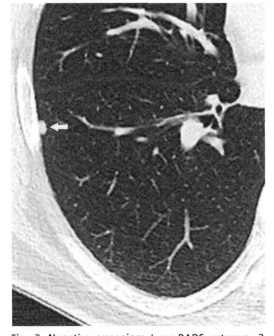

Fig. 3. Negative screening: Lung-RADS category 2. Axial LDCT image shows a noncalcified 6 × 4 mm (5 mm mean diameter) right lower lung nodule (*arrow*). The nodule size threshold for a positive screening in Lung-RADS is 6 mm or greater mean diameter (not 6 mm maximum diameter). Management recommendation for Lung-RADS category 2 lesions is to continue annual screening.

Includes the following findings on subsequent screenings:

- New solid nodule less than 4 mm;
- Nonsolid nodule 20 mm or greater and unchanged or slowly growing;
- Category 3 or 4 nodules unchanged for 3 months or longer.

Estimated population prevalence: 90% (combined category 1 and 2)

Probability of malignancy: Less than 1%.

Additional comments: The solid nodule size threshold for a positive baseline CT screening (6 mm mean diameter) has been modified in Lung-RADS compared with the one initially used in at the National Lung Screening Trial (4 mm maximum diameter). The new threshold resulted from studies that evaluated alternative nodule size thresholds in participants undergoing LCS in the International Early Lung Cancer Action Program (I-ELCAP) and the National Lung Screening Trial.[16–18] In a study by Yip and colleagues,[16] a comparison using alternative nodule size thresholds of 6.0, 7.0, 8.0, and 9.0 mm showed frequencies of positive LCS results of 10.5% (2700 of 25,813), 7.2% (1847 of 25,813), 5.3% (1362 of 25,813), and 4.1% (1007 of 25,813), respectively. The corresponding proportional reduction in additional CT scans was 33.8% (1380 of 4080), 54.7% (2233 of 4080), 66.6% (2718 of 4080), and 73.8% (3013 of 4080), respectively. However, the proportion of lung cancer diagnoses determined within

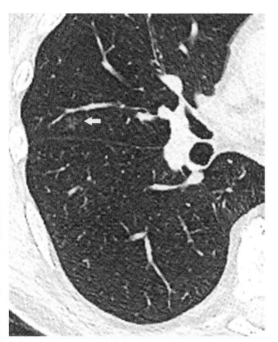

Fig. 4. Negative screening: Lung-RADS category 2. Axial LDCT image shows a nonsolid 8 × 6 right middle lung nodule (*arrow*). Nonsolid nodules less than 20 mm are considered lesions of benign appearance or behavior given their usually indolent behavior, even though persistent nonsolid nodules have a relatively high likelihood of representing lung adenocarcinoma with a lepidic growth pattern on pathology. Management recommendation for Lung-RADS category 2 lesions is to continue annual screening. This approach reduces overdiagnosis in lung cancer screening. A significant growth or interval development of a solid component within a nonsolid nodule, however, should raise concern for an actively growing cancer and a more aggressive management should be considered.

the first 12 months that would have been delayed up to 9 months was 0.9% (2 of 232), 2.6% (6 of 232), 6.0% (14 of 232), and 9.9% (23 of 232) of the patients, respectively. Based on these data and similar results from the I-ELCAP study,[16–18] a higher threshold of nodule size (6 mm mean diameter) was adopted by Lung-RADS with the intent of increasing the positive predictive value of LCS without causing a significant delay in the diagnosis of lung cancer.

Management: Continue annual screening with LDCT in 12 months.

Lung-RADS Category 3: Probably Benign

Category descriptor: Nodules with a low likelihood of becoming a clinically active cancer.

Includes the following findings on baseline screening:

- Solid nodule 6 mm or greater to less than 8 mm (Fig. 5);
- Part solid nodule 6 mm or greater in total diameter with solid component less than 6 mm; and
- Nonsolid nodule 20 mm or greater (Fig. 6).

Includes the following findings on subsequent screenings:

- New solid nodule 4 mm to less than 6 mm;
- New part solid nodule less than 6 mm in total diameter; and
- New nonsolid nodule.

Estimated population prevalence: 5%.
Probability of malignancy: 1% to 2%.
Additional comments: Despite the low malignancy risk, nodules in this group require workup to confirm benign etiology. For this reason, a lung-RADS category 3 represents a positive LCS.

Management: Perform LDCT follow-up in 6 months.

Lung-RADS Category 4A: Suspicious

Category descriptor: Findings for which additional diagnostic testing and/or tissue sampling is recommended.

Includes the following findings on baseline screening:

- Solid nodule 8 mm or greater to less than 15 mm;
- Part solid nodule 6 mm or greater in total diameter with solid component 6 mm or greater to less than 8 mm; and
- Endobronchial nodule (Fig. 7).

Includes the following findings on subsequent screenings:

- New solid nodule 6 mm to less than 8 mm;
- Growing solid nodule less than 8 mm (Fig. 8); and
- Part-solid nodule with a new or growing solid component less than 4 mm.

Estimated population prevalence: 2%.
Probability of malignancy: 5% to 15%.
Management: Perform LDCT follow-up scan in 3 months; PET/CT scanning may be used when there is a solid component that is 8 mm or greater.

Lung-RADS Category 4B: Suspicious

Category descriptor: Findings for which additional diagnostic testing and/or tissue sampling is recommended.

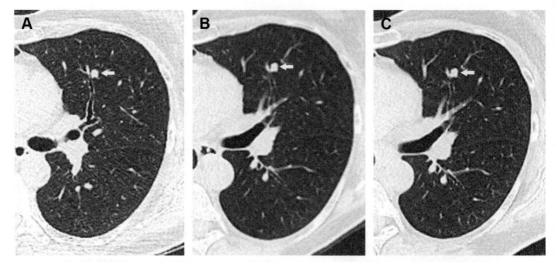

Fig. 5. Positive screening. Lung-RADS category 3. Probably benign left upper lobe nodule in a 71-year-old woman. (*A*) Axial LDCT image shows a noncalcified solid 7-mm mean diameter left upper lobe nodule (*arrow*), consistent with a Lung-RADS category 3 lesion. Management recommendation for these lesions is LDCT follow-up scanning in 6 months. (*B*) The lesions remained stable at 6 months follow-up (*arrow*). Category 3 or 4 nodules unchanged for 3 months or longer are reclassified as Lung-RADS category 2 lesions and management recommendation is to return to annual screening (12 months from the baseline LDCT scanning). (*C*) On subsequent annual screening, the lesion remained stable (lung-RADS 2 category; *arrow*).

Includes the following findings on baseline screening:

- Solid nodule 15 mm or greater; and
- Part solid nodule with solid component 8 mm or greater (**Fig. 9**).

Includes the following findings on subsequent screenings:

- New or growing solid nodule 8 mm or greater (**Fig. 10**); and
- Part solid nodule with a new or growing solid component 4 mm or greater.

Estimated population prevalence: 2% (combined category 4A and 4X).
Probability of malignancy: Greater than 15%.

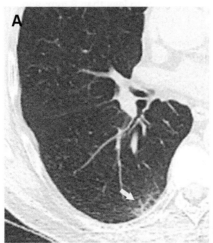
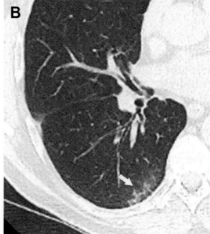

Fig. 6. Positive screening. Lung-RADS category 3. Probably benign right lower lung nonsolid nodule in a 60-year-old man. (*A*) Axial LDCT image shows a greater than 20 mm nonsolid right lower lung nodule (*arrow*), consistent with Lung-RADS category 3 lesion. Management recommendation for these lesions is low-dose computed tomography follow-up scanning in 6 months. (*B*) The lesion remained stable at 6 months follow-up (*arrow*) and was reclassified as a Lung-RADS category 2. It remained stable on subsequent annual screening (not shown).

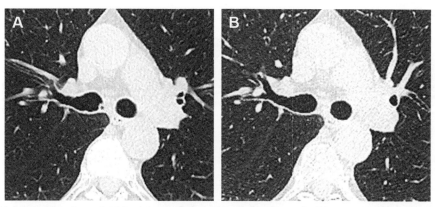

Fig. 7. Positive screening. Lung-RADS category 4A (suspicious). Endobronchial lesion in a 68-year-old woman. (*A*) Axial LDCT image shows a small endobronchial filling defect in the right main bronchus (*asterisk*), consistent with a Lung-RADS category 4A lesion. The differential diagnosis includes retained secretions or a primary or secondary neoplasm of the airways. Lung-RADS management recommendation for these lesions is LDCT follow-up scanning in 3 months. The National Comprehensive Cancer Network management recommendation for endobronchial lesions is follow-up in 1 month, which may give radiologists more flexibility for lesions of greater concern. In this particular case, images were reviewed immediately after acquisition and repeat images were acquired at the level of the carina after coughing maneuver (*B*), showing resolution of the finding. Therefore, the LDCT scanning was classified as Lung-RADS category 1 (negative).

Management: Chest CT scan with or without contrast, PET/CT scan, and/or tissue sampling depending on the probability of malignancy and comorbidities. PET/CT scan may be used when there is a solid component that is 8 mm or greater.

Lung-RADS Category 4X: Suspicious

Category descriptor: Findings for which additional diagnostic testing and/or tissue sampling is recommended.

Includes category 3 or 4 nodules with additional features or imaging findings that increases the suspicion of malignancy, including spiculation, a nonsolid nodule that doubles in size in 1 year, enlarged lymph nodes etc (**Figs. 11** and **12**).

Additional comments: Bubbly or internal lucencies within a lesion may also raise concern for lung cancer, because this finding has an association with lung adenocarcinoma. Additionally, for nodules adjacent to a cystic airspace, imaging manifestations that are concerning for lung

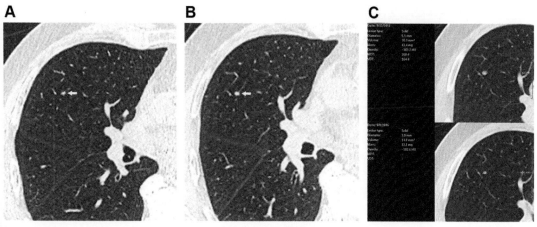

Fig. 8. Positive screening. Lung-RADS category 4A (suspicious). Growing solid nodule less than 8 mm in a 64-year-old man. (*A*) Axial LDCT image shows a solid 3 mm mean diameter right upper lung nodule (*arrow*), consistent with a Lung-RADS category 2 lesion. (*B*) On subsequent annual screening, the lesion shows interval growth, measuring 5.1 mm mean diameter (*arrow*), and was reclassified as a Lung-RADS category 4A lesion, requiring a LDCT follow-up scan to be performed in 3 months. (*C*) Volumetric analysis increases confidence in characterization of lung nodules for interval growth. In this case, a volume doubling time of 164 days was demonstrated.

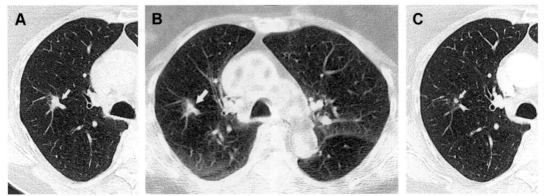

Fig. 9. Positive screening. Lung-RADS category 4B (suspicious). Part solid nodule 6 mm or greater in total diameter with a solid component 8 mm or greater in a 70-year-old woman. (*A*) Axial LDCT image shows a 20 × 14-mm (17 mm mean diameter) part solid right upper lung nodule with a 12 × 8 (10 mm mean diameter) solid component (*arrow*), consistent with a Lung-RADS category 4B lesion. Management recommendation for these lesions includes repeat chest CT scanning with or without contrast, PET/CT scanning, and/or tissue sampling. (*B*) Fused axial PET/CT image shows low fluorodeoxyglucose uptake (*arrow*). A decision was made to follow the lesion in 3 months, which showed marked decrease in size of the solid component (*C*), measuring 6 × 5 mm (*arrow*). Therefore, the LDCT follow-up scan was reclassified as Lung-RADS 2 (negative).

adenocarcinoma include an increase in wall thickness or the development of a new peripheral solid component. These features can result in the designation of nodule as Lung-RADS 4X category.[19] The inclusion of the category 4X in the Lung-RADS classification increases malignancy yield among experienced radiologists. In a study by Chung and colleagues,[20] the malignancy rate for 4X subsolid nodules varied from 46% to 57% and was substantially higher than the malignancy

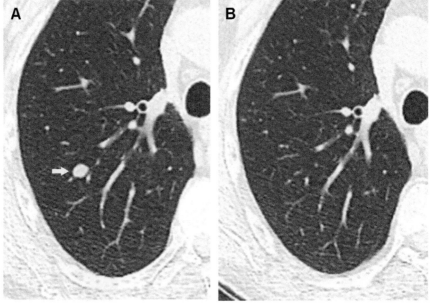

Fig. 10. Positive screening. Lung-RADS category 4B (suspicious). New or growing solid nodule 8 mm or larger. (*A*) Axial LDCT image shows a 10 mm × 8 mm (9 mm mean diameter) solid right upper lung nodule (*arrow*) in a 67-year-old man, which was not present on prior annual LDCT screening (*B*), consistent with a Lung-RADS category 4B lesion. The management recommendation for these lesions includes repeat chest CT scan with or without contrast, PET/CT scan, and/or tissue sampling. A multidisciplinary review reached a shared decision to perform a lung biopsy.

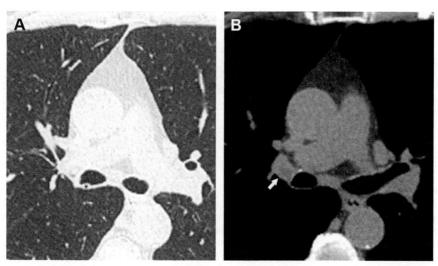

Fig. 11. Positive screening. Lung-RADS category 4X. Suspicious findings in a 74-year-old man. (*A*) Axial LDCT image shows a subtle endobronchial filling defect in the right main bronchus (*asterisk*). (*B*) LDCT image with mediastinal window settings shows associated right hilar lymphadenopathy measuring 13 mm in short axis (*arrow*), with a central area of lower attenuation suggesting necrosis. Given the associated lymphadenopathy, these findings are consistent with Lung-RADS category 4X. Endobronchial biopsy showed squamous cell carcinoma.

rates of categories 3, 4A, and 4B subsolid nodules without observer intervention (9%, 19%, and 23%, respectively).[20] Most false positives in this study represented transient lesions, emphasizing the need for short-term follow-up before performing an interventional procedure.[20]

Estimated population prevalence: 2% (combined category 4A and 4X).

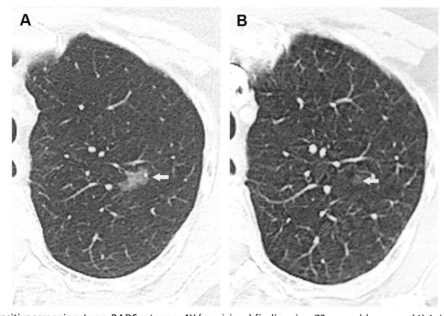

Fig. 12. Positive screening. Lung-RADS category 4X (suspicious) findings in a 72-year-old woman. (*A*) Axial LDCT image shows 20 × 8 mm nonsolid left upper lobe nodule (*arrow*). This lesion would have been characterized as a Lung-RADS category 2 lesion; however, comparison with available prior diagnostic CT image (*B*) acquired 5 years earlier for another reason shows a significant increase in size of the nodule (*arrow*), concerning for an active lung cancer. A multidisciplinary review reached a shared decision to perform a lung biopsy, which demonstrated well to moderately differentiated adenocarcinoma. Left upper lobectomy was performed with a final diagnosis of moderately differentiated invasive adenocarcinoma, predominately acinar and lepidic.

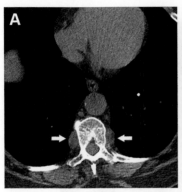 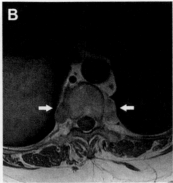 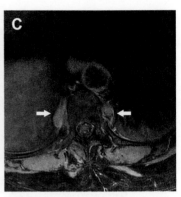

Fig. 13. Modifier S: Clinically significant or potentially significant non-lung cancer finding. Extramedullary hematopoiesis in a 62-year-old woman. (A) A low-dose computed tomography image on mediastinal window settings shows bilateral paraspinal masses at the level of T10 vertebral body (*arrows*). MR T1-weighted precontrast (B) and T1-weighted postcontrast (C) images show postcontrast enhancement of the paraspinal masses (*arrows*) consistent with vascularity. Lesions did not invade the adjacent bony structures but were contiguous with T10 vertebral body. Biopsy showed extramedullary hematopoiesis.

Probability of malignancy: Greater than 15%.

Management: Chest CT scan with or without contrast, PET/CT scan, and/or tissue sampling depending on the probability of malignancy and comorbidities. PET/CT scanning may be used when there is a solid component that is 8 mm or larger.

MODIFIER S

A modifier "S" may be added on to category 0 to 4 coding (eg, "Lung-RADS 2S") if there is a clinically significant or potentially significant non–lung cancer finding (**Figs. 13** and **14**).[21] Findings should be reported in accordance with currently available guidelines for management of incidental findings.

MODIFIER C

A modifier "C" should be added on to category 0 to 4 coding (eg, "Lung-RADS 1C") in patients with a prior diagnosis of lung cancer who are eligible for LCS.

SUMMARY

The ACR Lung-RADS is a classification dedicated to risk stratification of findings and standardization of management decisions in low dose CT screening for lung cancer. The system is similar to the National Comprehensive Cancer Network guidelines and most recently published Fleischner Society guidelines, but is designed for the subset of patients intended for low-dose screening studies.

Fig. 14. Modifier S: Clinically significant or potentially significant non-lung cancer finding. Severe coronary artery calcification. A low-dose computed tomography image on mediastinal window settings shows heavy left anterior descending coronary artery calcification (*arrow*). Vascular abnormalities including moderate and heavy coronary artery and aortic wall calcification, as well as aortic dilatation, are among the most common causes of potentially significant non-lung cancer finding in lung cancer screening.

REFERENCES

1. Moyer VA. Screening for lung cancer: U.S. Preventive Services Task Force recommendation statement. Ann Intern Med 2014;160(5):330–8.
2. Aberle DR, Adams AM, Berg CD, et al. Reduced lung-cancer mortality with low-dose computed tomographic screening. N Engl J Med 2011; 365(5):395–409.

3. National Lung Screening Trial Research Team, Church TR, Black WC, Aberle DR, et al. Results of initial low-dose computed tomographic screening for lung cancer. N Engl J Med 2013; 368(21):1980–91.

4. Kazerooni EA, Austin JH, Black WC, et al. ACR-STR practice parameter for the performance and reporting of lung cancer screening thoracic computed tomography (CT): 2014 (Resolution 4). J Thorac Imaging 2014;29(5):310–6.

5. Black WC. Computed tomography screening for lung cancer in the National Lung Screening Trial: a cost-effectiveness analysis. J Thorac Imaging 2015;30(2):79–87.

6. American College of Radiology (ACR). Lung CT screening reporting and data system (lung-RADS). 2014. Available at: https://www.acr.org/Quality-Safety/Resources/LungRADS. Accessed September 12, 2017.

7. Ahn MI, Gleeson TG, Chan IH, et al. Perifissural nodules seen at CT screening for lung cancer. Radiology 2010;254(3):949–56.

8. Jankowski A, Martinelli T, Timsit JF, et al. Pulmonary nodule detection on MDCT images: evaluation of diagnostic performance using thin axial images, maximum intensity projections, and computer-assisted detection. Eur Radiol 2007;17(12):3148–56.

9. Bastarrika Aleman G, Dominguez Echavarri PD, Noguera Tajadura JJ, et al. Usefulness of maximum intensity projections in low-radiation multislice CT lung cancer screening. Radiologia 2008;50(3):231–7 [in Spanish].

10. Huang P, Park S, Yan R, et al. Added value of computer-aided CT image features for early lung cancer diagnosis with small pulmonary nodules: a matched case-control study. Radiology 2018; 286(1):286–95.

11. Jacobs C, van Rikxoort EM, Scholten ET, et al. Solid, part-solid, or non-solid?: classification of pulmonary nodules in low-dose chest computed tomography by a computer-aided diagnosis system. Invest Radiol 2015;50(3):168–73.

12. Christe A, Leidolt L, Huber A, et al. Lung cancer screening with CT: evaluation of radiologists and different computer assisted detection software (CAD) as first and second readers for lung nodule detection at different dose levels. Eur J Radiol 2013;82(12):e873–8.

13. Horeweg N, van Rosmalen J, Heuvelmans MA, et al. Lung cancer probability in patients with CT-detected pulmonary nodules: a prespecified analysis of data from the NELSON trial of low-dose CT screening. Lancet Oncol 2014;15(12):1332–41.

14. Gietema HA, Wang Y, Xu D, et al. Pulmonary nodules detected at lung cancer screening: interobserver variability of semiautomated volume measurements. Radiology 2006;241(1):251–7.

15. Hansell DM, Bankier AA, MacMahon H, et al. Fleischner Society: glossary of terms for thoracic imaging. Radiology 2008;246(3):697–722.

16. Yip R, Henschke CI, Yankelevitz DF, et al. CT screening for lung cancer: alternative definitions of positive test result based on the national lung screening trial and international early lung cancer action program databases. Radiology 2014;273(2): 591–6.

17. Henschke CI, Yip R, Yankelevitz DF, et al. Definition of a positive test result in computed tomography screening for lung cancer: a cohort study. Ann Intern Med 2013;158(4):246–52.

18. Henschke CI, Yankelevitz DF, Naidich DP, et al. CT screening for lung cancer: suspiciousness of nodules according to size on baseline scans. Radiology 2004;231(1):164–8.

19. Farooqi AO, Cham M, Zhang L, et al. Lung cancer associated with cystic airspaces. AJR Am J Roentgenol 2012;199(4):781–6.

20. Chung K, Jacobs C, Scholten ET, et al. Lung-RADS category 4X: does it improve prediction of malignancy in subsolid nodules? Radiology 2017;284(1): 264–71.

21. Godoy MCB, Pereira HAC, Carter BW, et al. Incidental findings in lung cancer screening: which ones are relevant? Semin Roentgenol 2017;52(3): 156–60.

Missed Lung Cancer

Rydhwana Hossain, MD[a], Carol C. Wu, MD[b], Patricia M. de Groot, MD[b],
Brett W. Carter, MD[b], Matthew D. Gilman, MD[a], Gerald F. Abbott, MD[a],*

KEYWORDS

• Lung cancer • Lung nodule • Chest radiography • Computed tomography • Observer performance

KEY POINTS

- Early detection of lung cancer can change therapeutic and surgical management options for patients.
- Familiarity with frequently encountered blind spots, lesion characteristics (such as size, location, and density), observer errors, and imaging quality issues that may contribute to missed lung cancer can help radiologists improve detection of suspicious lesions.
- Recognizing normal anatomy, developing a thorough search pattern, and scrutinizing for causes of unexplained findings (such as lymphadenopathy or pleural effusion) can help radiologists avoid missed lung cancer.

INTRODUCTION

In the United States, lung cancer is the leading cause of cancer-related deaths; early detection can significantly change both therapeutic options and the long-term prognosis for patients. Early diagnosis and complete surgical resection remain the key to improved survival, but more than two-thirds of patients are diagnosed at an advanced stage. Radiologists play an important role in lung cancer detection, particularly in incidental cancers found on imaging performed for unrelated reasons, as up to 39% of patients with lung cancer are asymptomatic at the time of diagnosis. Chest radiographs (CXRs) are the most frequently ordered imaging study for numerous clinical indications. The increased clinical demand on radiologists has resulted in less time for interpretation of studies, with a potential risk for more errors to occur. Missed lung cancer is one of the leading causes of medical malpractice among radiologists. About 90% of the missed cancers involved CXR, whereas computed tomography (CT) and other imaging studies account for the remaining 10%.[1]

FACTORS LEADING TO MISSED LUNG CANCER

Three types of observer errors have been described by Kundel and colleagues[2]: (1) scanning, (2) recognition, and (3) decision-making. Failure to fixate on the lesion region of interest causes scanning error and requires the observer to focus on the lesion of interest for at least 360 milliseconds on the fovea of the retina. If a nodule is adequately scanned but not detected, this is considered a recognition error. In a study by Kundel and colleagues,[2] both scanning and recognition errors each accounted for 30% of observer errors. The most common observer error in the study was due to a decision-making error (45%), which is the result of adequate detection of the abnormality but misinterpretation of a malignant lesion as a benign or a normal finding.

Other confounding factors that may cause failure to detect a lesion include reader fatigue, satisfaction of search, and intentional underreading. With increasing emphasis on turnaround time, radiologists are forced to interpret a larger volume of images in a shorter period of time, resulting in

a Thoracic Imaging and Interventions, Massachusetts General Hospital, 55 Fruit Street FND 202, Boston, MA 02114, USA; b Thoracic Imaging, University of Texas MD Anderson Cancer Center, 1515 Holcombe Boulevard, Houston, TX 77030, USA
* Corresponding author.
E-mail address: gabbott@mgh.harvard.edu

Radiol Clin N Am 56 (2018) 365–375
https://doi.org/10.1016/j.rcl.2018.01.004
0033-8389/18/© 2018 Elsevier Inc. All rights reserved.

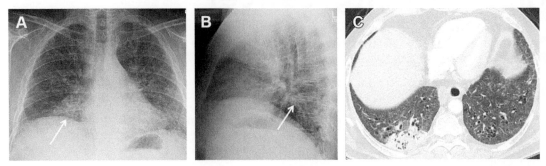

Fig. 1. (*A*) PA chest demonstrates bilateral diffuse hazy opacities and low lung volume thought to be related to patient's known non-specific interstitial pneumonia (NSIP). Focal opacity in the right lower lobe (*arrow*) was not recognized. (*B*) Lateral chest radiograph shows positive spine sign (*arrow*), absence of normal progressive lucency over the lower thoracic vertebral bodies, which was not recognized. (*C*) Chest CT performed months later demonstrates bilateral groundglass opacities and traction bronchiectasis consistent with NSIP and a right lower lobe consolidation, eventually proven to represent adenocarcinoma. The lung cancer was missed on chest radiograph due to satisfaction of search and failure to recognize the "spine sign" on the lateral chest radiograph.

both visual fatigue and central nervous system fatigue. Satisfaction of search is another potential observer error that occurs when a second but more visually alarming or obvious finding results in loss of attention to more subtle abnormalities (**Fig. 1**). As more imaging studies are ordered and performed, there is increasing detection of incidentalomas. Perceived pressure from referring colleagues to decrease the number of reported incidentalomas and recommended additional workup can result in intentional underreading by radiologists.

MISSED LUNG CANCER ON CHEST RADIOGRAPH

In general, poor image quality and poor viewing conditions can play a role in observer error. In addition, some of the most common reasons for missed lung cancer on CXR are largely poor nodule conspicuity due to small size, ill-defined margins, ground-glass density, and overlying structures.

Locations of Most Common Missed Cancers

In the hallmark retrospective study performed by Austin and colleagues[3] in 1992, twenty-seven cases of missed lung cancers were reviewed. The investigators concluded that up to 81% of missed lung cancers are located in the upper lobes, favoring the right upper lobe particularly (56%). This predominance could be explained by the higher frequency of lung cancer occurrence in the upper lobes[4] and the presence of overlapping clavicle and ribs (**Fig. 2**). The perihilar region is the second most common location for missed lung cancers. Lin and colleagues[5] described 17 out of 37 missed lung cancers that were hilar in location. Centrally

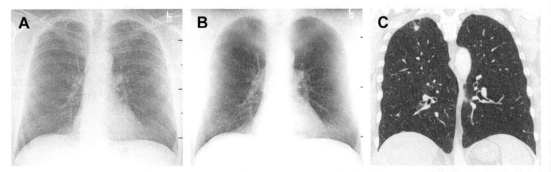

Fig. 2. (*A*) PA chest radiograph shows a subtle right upper lobe nodule which is obscured due to overlying bone. (*B*) Dual energy chest radiograph with bone subtraction significantly improves the conspicuity of the right upper lobe nodule. (*C*) Coronal chest CT shows the spiculated right upper lobe nodule. This nodule was missed on the initial chest radiograph due to overlying osseous structures.

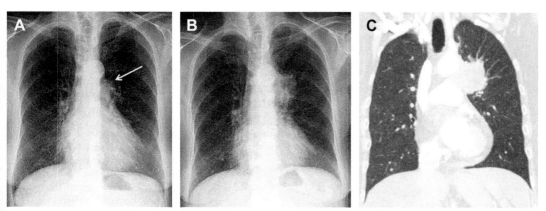

Fig. 3. (*A*) PA chest radiograph demonstrates subtle abnormal convex margin (*arrow*) instead of normal concave margin at the AP window which was missed. (*B*) PA chest radiograph 6 months later shows enlarging soft tissue mass in the AP window. (*C*) Coronal chest CT confirms the presence of the mass which was proven to be a poorly differentiated carcinoma.

located missed tumors are usually larger in size in comparison with a peripheral lesion, implying that these lesions are overlooked because of superimposed structures. Other overlying structures that can obscure lesions include ribs, vessels, diaphragm, mediastinum (**Fig. 3**), and the heart (**Fig. 4**). Airway lesions are often subtle on CXR; but careful examination of the tracheal and proximal bronchial air columns, particularly in patients presenting with stridor, wheezing, or hemoptysis, can help detection of these lesions (**Fig. 5**). Familiarity with the normal

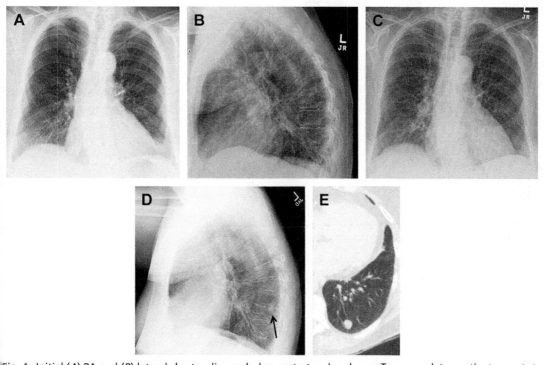

Fig. 4. Initial (*A*) PA and (*B*) lateral chest radiograph demonstrates clear lungs. Two years later, patient reports to the ER with chest pain and cough. (*C*) PA and (*D*) lateral chest radiograph showing a new 1cm nodular opacity which is obscured by the heart on the frontal radiograph and better appreciated on the lateral view (*arrow*). (*E*) A chest CT shows the 10mm nodule in the left lower lobe. This nodule was missed on the chest radiograph due to failure to compare prior lateral radiographs.

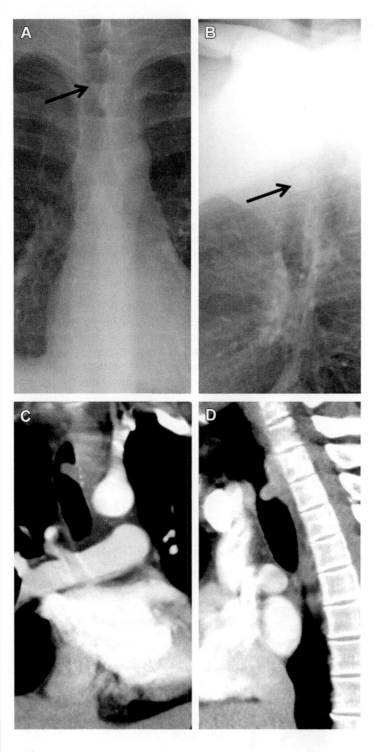

Fig. 5. (A) PA and (B) Lateral chest radiograph shows a subtle upper tracheal nodule (arrows) in a patient presenting with hoarseness and cough. (C) Coronal and (D) Sagittal chest CT reformation images demonstrate an endobronchial nodule, a biopsy proven adenoid cystic carcinoma, arising from the left posterolateral wall of the trachea with at least 50% narrowing of the trachea at this level. Careful examination of the central airways should be an integral part of the routine search pattern for chest radiograph.

radiographic anatomy, including the mediastinal lines and stripes, and knowledge of the most common locations for missed lung cancer (Fig. 6) can help radiologists decrease observer error.

Lesion Characteristics

Size does matter

The mean diameter of missed lung cancers varies from 1.3 to 1.6 cm. The smallest detectable lesion

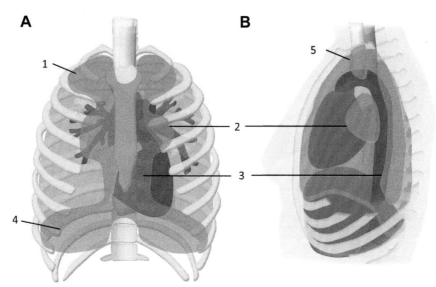

Fig. 6. Diagram of a PA (*A*) and lateral (*B*) chest radiograph of the most common areas of missed lung cancers: 1 upper lobes right greater than left, 2 perihilar region, 3 paramediastinal area, 4 inferior lower lobes and 5 endo-bronchial location.

on a CXR is 4 mm. However, the detection rate varies even for larger lesions, implying that other factors besides size influence the rate of detection.[1]

Conspicuity

Shape, density, and margins of a lesion constitute the conspicuity of a nodule. Ground-glass or part-solid nodules on a CT can be difficult to discern on CXR or may even be imperceptible. The sharper the margins of the lesion, the more readily the lesion is detected.

Image Quality

Technical factors, such as patient positioning, field of view, projections, and imaging quality, also play an important role in the failure of detection of lung cancers. Every CXR should be first assessed for adequate patient positioning to include the entire thorax, including costophrenic angles, lateral edges of the ribs, and lung apices. Patient motion may result in blurred margins and poor definition of the lesion.

Standard CXRs should include 2 projections: posteroanterior (PA) and lateral views with patients upright and with full suspended inspiration. Some studies have reported that 2% to 4% of lung cancers are only seen on the lateral view[3] (see **Fig. 4**). In patients with PA and lateral CXRs, Tala[6] reported that the lateral projection allowed for confident interpretation in 20% of patients. Anteroposterior (AP) views performed at

the bedside have lower image quality in comparison with the PA view.

In terms of image quality, exposure is another important factor; moderately high peak kilovoltage (140 kVp) is generally used to allow for appropriate penetration of the lung and surrounding structures, and adequate penetration includes visibility of the vertebrae posterior to the heart and diaphragmatic contours. Digital correction can compensate for an improperly exposed image. Some artifacts are unavoidable on CXRs, such as medical devices, which can obscure anatomic structures. Other less common radiographic artifacts include jewelry and clothing that have not been removed. However, technical factors are of less consequence than observer performance and lesion characteristics in missed lung cancers.[1]

MISSED LUNG CANCER ON COMPUTED TOMOGRAPHY

In comparison with standard CXR, CT is much more sensitive for the detection of lesions. Similar to CXR, perihilar (**Fig. 7**) and paramediastinal (**Fig. 8**) regions can be difficult to evaluate, particularly in the absence of intravenous contrast.[7] Pulmonary nodules with low attenuation and small size (**Figs. 9** and **10**) or lesions within atelectatic lung can also result in missed lung cancers. White and colleagues[1] reported that most missed parenchymal lesions were in the lower lobes. Possible explanations include partial obscuration of early lung cancer by atelectasis or fibrosis

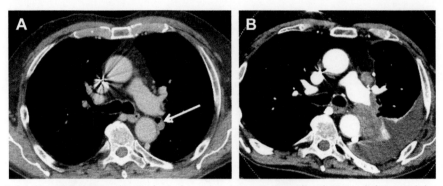

Fig. 7. (A) Axial chest CT using mediastinal windows demonstrates a small enhancing left lower lobe nodule (*arrow*) adjacent to the descending aorta. (B) Follow-up CT 10 months later shows rapid progression of left lower lobe mass which is now non-resectable. There is encasement of the left pulmonary artery, new AP window lymph node, as well a moderate sized malignant pleural effusion. This nodule was missed due to its central location and small size.

more commonly seen in the lower lobes and relative reader fatigue or satisfaction of search, as many radiologists take a cranial to caudal approach during interpretation of chest CTs. In a recent study analyzing negative lung cancer screening CTs, 44 of 1060 (4.2%) participants subsequently developed lung cancer within a year of a negative CT screen. Analysis showed that most of these cancers arose in nodules that had been overlooked, peripheral or endobronchial (**Figs. 11** and **12**). A similar study from the Dutch-Belgium lung cancer screening program, reviewing cases of lung cancer that developed after a negative screening study, found detection error of nodules, bulla wall thickening or nodularity (**Fig. 13**), or endobronchial location to be the major causes of missed cancer.[8] Recent studies by Fintelmann and colleagues,[9] Mascalchi and colleagues,[10] and Farooqi and colleagues[11] have all described associations of lung cancer and cystic airspaces. Careful inspection of the walls of cystic lesions using axial as well as coronal or sagittal

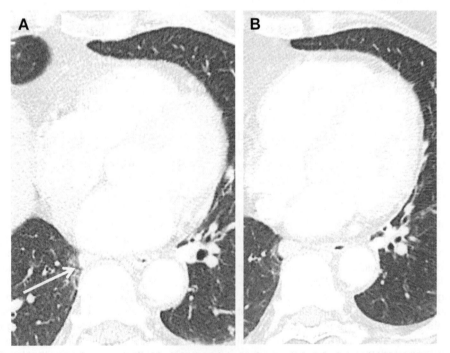

Fig. 8. (A) Axial chest CT shows a small subpleural nodule in the medial right lower lobe, posterior to the left atrium and anterior to the spine (*arrow*). (B) One year later, this nodule has increased in size. This nodule was missed on the first CT due to its paramediastinal location.

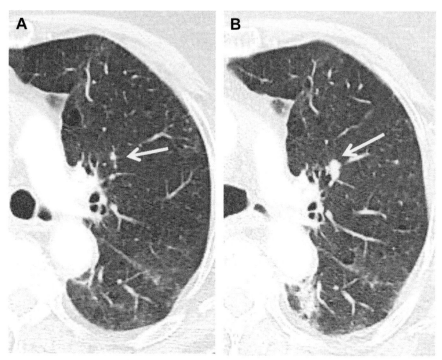

Fig. 9. (A) Axial chest CT shows a small 3 mm nodule (*arrow*) in the left upper lobe in the perihilar region. (B) Axial chest CT 2 years later demonstrates an interval increase in size of central left upper lobe nodule now measuring 9 mm. This nodule was missed due to its small size as well as misinterpreting it for a normal vascular structure.

reformation images can help detect these lesions (Fig. 14).

Maximum intensity projections (MIPs) can aid the radiologists in detection of small nodules[12] on CT, particularly in the central lung, by elongating vascular structures and, hence, increasing the conspicuity of small nodules (Fig. 15). Furthermore, use of modern technologies, such as computer-aided

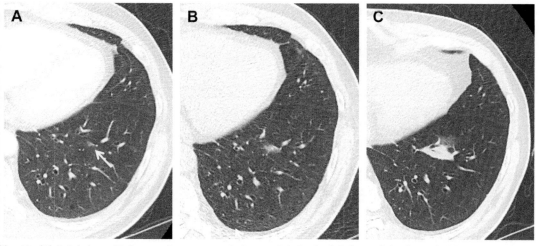

Fig. 10. (A) Axial chest CT shows a 3 mm ground glass nodule in the left lower lobe (*arrow*). (B) One year follow up CT shows increase in size and density of the left lower lobe nodule. (C) Two years following the initial CT, there has been a significant increase in size and density of left lower lobe mass. This nodule was missed on the first two scans, largely due to the poor conspicuity of the nodule.

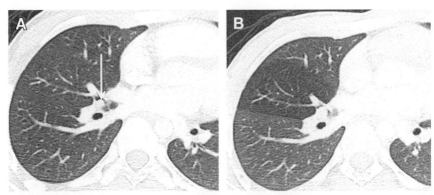

Fig. 11. (A) Axial chest CT shows a small right middle lobe endobronchial nodule (arrow) which was missed. (B) Chest CT 8 months later shows increase in size of the endobronchial nodule, later proven to be a carcinoid tumor, with development of associated air trapping of the right middle lobe.

detection (CAD), can improve the detection of smaller nodules.

METHODS AND HELPFUL TOOLS TO REDUCE INCIDENCES OF MISSED LUNG CANCER ON CHEST RADIOGRAPH AND COMPUTED TOMOGRAPHY
Reading Condition/Technical Factors

Optimal viewing conditions, such as correct lighting, quiet surrounding environment, and appropriate viewing distance, are basic strategies to reduce observer error.

Experience and Knowledge

Familiarity with normal lines, stripes, and spaces can aid in the detection of subtle abnormalities. With experience, the reader will gain confidence in interpretation if conscious efforts are made to

correlate CT to radiographic findings to improve sensitivity and knowledge.[13,14]

Comparison

Comparison with prior imaging can improve the detection of changes and lead to a prompt workup and correct diagnosis in many patients. Comparisons should be made with the most recent study as well as with more remote studies. Up to 16% of successful malpractice actions for delay of lung cancer diagnosis were due to failure of comparison with a prior study.[1] Change in contours of the hila or ancillary signs, such as volume loss or air trapping from an endobronchial lesion, are important features that can be more easily detected when compared with prior imaging. In cases of suspected infection, follow-up imaging to ensure complete resolution is important in the detection of a possible underlying lesion.[15] Incomplete resolution of pulmonary opacities

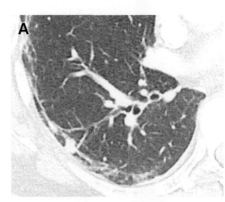
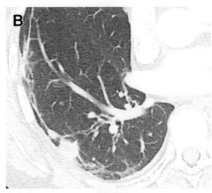

Fig. 12. (A) Baseline axial chest CT shows right lower lobe subpleural reticular opacities related to scarring and fibrosis and two small subpleural nodules that were missed. (B) One year later, chest CT shows interval increase in size of one of the right lower lobe nodules later proven to represent an adenocarcinoma. Presence of parenchymal abnormalities can obscure small nodules or distract readers and result in missed lung cancer.

7/2014　　　　5/2016　　　　11/2016

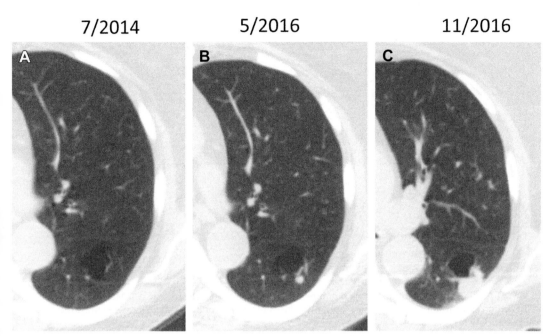

Fig. 13. (*A*) Initial axial chest CT demonstrates a thin walled cyst in the left lower lobe. (*B*) Follow-up CT shows a new nodule in the posterior wall of the cyst measuring 7 mm. (*C*) Chest CT 6 months later shows significant increase in size of the nodule. Careful evaluation of cyst wall for nodularity and thickening is key to avoid missing early lung cancer.

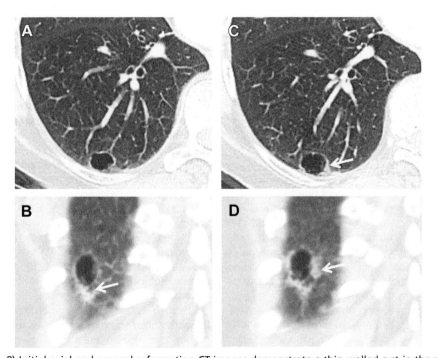

Fig. 14. (*A, B*) Initial axial and coronal reformation CT images demonstrate a thin walled cyst in the right lower lobe. Coronal image shows the small nodule along the inferior cyst wall (*arrow*) to better advantage. (*C, D*) Follow-up CT 6 months later shows increased thickness and nodularity of the medial cyst wall. The inferior wall nodule also grew (not shown). Coronal and sagittal reformation CT images improve evaluation of cyst wall nodularity and thickness.

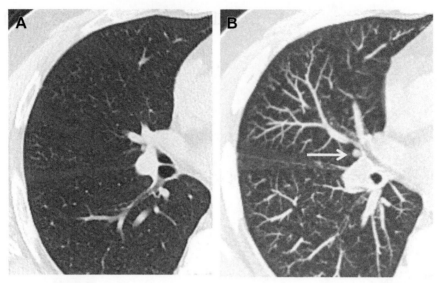

Fig. 15. (*A*) Axial CT image demonstrate a 4 mm peri-hilar right middle lobe nodule. (*B*) Maximum intensity projection (MIP) reformation CT image, by elongating the central pulmonary vessels, increases the conspicuity of small pulmonary nodule (*arrow*).

despite adequate antibiotic treatments should prompt further investigation.

Search Pattern/Blind Spots

A meticulous systematic approach to the interpretation of CXRs and CTs that evaluates blind spots and common locations for lung cancer can minimize observer error.[13,14] Knowledge of normal PA and lateral CXR anatomy will also improve the detection of lung cancer. Likewise, an understanding of the normal central pulmonary arterial and venous anatomy is useful in detecting hilar or perihilar abnormalities. The systematic approach can also reduce detection error due to satisfaction of search.

New Technology and Techniques

To address missed lung cancers due to overlying anatomic structures, such as ribs and clavicles, bone suppression techniques using an algorithm-based software subtract the bones from the standard radiograph, producing a soft tissue–only image. Many of these software techniques can be applied to already existing picture archiving and communication systems, without purchasing new equipment or increasing the radiation dose to patients. The use of bone suppression software results in increased detection of lung cancer. Similarly, dual-energy CXRs also improve the detection of lung cancers. Dual-energy radiographs that are acquired at 2 different peak kilovoltages emphasize the differences in attenuation of soft tissue and bones structures. After the acquisition of

2 separate radiographs with different peak kilovoltages, overlying osseous structures can be removed to improve conspicuity of pulmonary nodules (see **Fig. 2**). A study published by Li and colleagues[16] compared the two techniques and concluded that dual-energy imaging had higher rates of detecting small lung cancers in comparison with bone suppression software. However, some of the disadvantages of dual-energy imaging include a slightly higher radiation dose due to acquisition of 2 images and the need to purchase new equipment.

CAD systems, developed to serve as a secondary reader, can improve the detection of pulmonary nodules for both CXR and CT.[17] Several studies showed improved detection of missed lung cancer using CAD, particularly among less experienced readers. A study by Armato and colleagues[18] reported an 84% detection of missed cancers using CAD. However, the usage of CAD does result in false positives, particularly due to vascular structures.[18] A more recent study published in 2017 evaluated the utility of CAD with radiomics in a large chest CT database of 1004 cases and demonstrated 88.9% sensitivity for the detection of lung nodules.[19]

Effective and efficient communication of the detected imaging abnormalities to referring clinicians and appropriate follow-up recommendations by radiologists are also important factors in reduction of missed lung cancer. Automated result notification software[20,21] and decision support tools for radiologists are increasingly available to improve the workflow.[22,23]

SUMMARY

Radiologists have an important role in the diagnosis of lung cancer. Failure to detect lung cancer is one of the leading causes of medical malpractice for radiologists in the United States. Knowledge of the normal anatomy and most common locations of missed lung cancers on both CXR and CT together with a comprehensive search pattern reduce the incidence of missed lesions. Meticulous attention to technical factors, optimal reading conditions, comparison with prior studies, and awareness of the spectrum of interpretation pitfalls all contribute to a reduction in missed lung cancers.

REFERENCES

1. White CS, Salis AI, Meyer CA. Missed lung cancer on chest radiography and computed tomography: imaging and medicolegal issues. J Thorac Imaging 1999;14(1):63–8.
2. Kundel HL, Nodine CF, Carmody D. Visual scanning, pattern recognition and decision-making in pulmonary nodule detection. Invest Radiol 1978;13(3): 175–81.
3. Austin JH, Romney BM, Goldsmith LS. Missed bronchogenic carcinoma: radiographic findings in 27 patients with a potentially resectable lesion evident in retrospect. Radiology 1992;182(1):115–22.
4. Byers TE, Vena JE, Rzepka TF. Predilection of lung cancer for the upper lobes: an epidemiologic inquiry. J Natl Cancer Inst 1984;72(6):1271–5.
5. Lin G, Ko SF, Cheung YC, et al. Chest radiographic findings of missed lung cancers. Chin J Radiol 2004; 29:315–21.
6. Tala E. Carcinoma of the lung. A retrospective study with special reference to pre-diagnosis period and roentgenographic signs. Acta Radiol Diagn (Stockh) 1967;(Suppl 268):1–127.
7. Gierada DS, Pinsky PF, Duan F, et al. Interval lung cancer after a negative CT screening examination: CT findings and outcomes in National Lung Screening Trial participants. Eur Radiol 2017;27:3249.
8. Scholten ET, Horeweg N, de Koning HJ, et al. Computed tomographic characteristics of interval and post screen carcinomas in lung cancer screening. Eur Radiol 2015;25:81.
9. Fintelmann FJ, Brinkmann JK, Jeck WR, et al. Lung cancers associated with cystic airspaces: natural history, pathologic correlation, and mutational analysis. J Thorac Imaging 2017;32(3):176–88.
10. Mascalchi M, Attinà D, Bertelli E, et al. Lung cancer associated with cystic airspaces. J Comput Assist Tomogr 2015;39(1):102–8.
11. Farooqi AO, Cham M, Zhang L, et al, International Early Lung Cancer Action Program Investigators. Lung cancer associated with cystic airspaces. AJR Am J Roentgenol 2012;199(4):781–6.
12. Gruden JF, Ouanounou S, Tigges S, et al. Incremental benefit of maximum-intensity-projection images on observer detection of small pulmonary nodules revealed by multidetector CT. AJR Am J Roentgenol 2002;179(1):149–57.
13. Wu MH, Gotway MB, Lee TJ, et al. Features of non-small cell lung carcinomas overlooked at digital chest radiography. Clin Radiol 2008;63:518–28.
14. de Groot PM, Carter BW, Abbott GF, et al. Pitfalls in chest radiographic interpretation: blind spots. Semin Roentgenol 2015;50(3):197–209.
15. Little BP, Gilman MD, Humphrey KL, et al. Outcome of recommendations for radiographic follow-up of pneumonia on outpatient chest radiography. AJR Am J Roentgenol 2014;202(1):54–9.
16. Li F, Engelmann R, Pesce LL, et al. Small lung cancers: improved detection by use of bone suppression imaging – comparison with dual-energy subtraction chest radiography. Radiology 2011; 261(3):937–49.
17. Li Q, Li F, Suzuki K, et al. Computer-aided diagnosis in thoracic CT. Semin Ultrasound CT MR 2005;26(5): 357–63.
18. Armato SG III, Li F, Giger ML, et al. Lung cancer: performance of automated lung nodule detection applied to cancers missed in a CT screening program. Radiology 2002;225:685–92.
19. Ma J, Zhou Z, Ren Y, et al. Computerized detection of lung nodules through radiomics. Med Phys 2017; 44(8):4148–58.
20. O'Connor SD, Dalal AK, Sahni VA, et al. Does integrating nonurgent, clinically significant radiology alerts within the electronic health record impact closed-loop communication and follow-up? J Am Med Inform Assoc 2016;23(2):333–8.
21. Gale BD, Bissett-Siegel DP, Davidson SJ, et al. Failure to notify reportable test results: significance in medical malpractice. J Am Coll Radiol 2011;8(11):776–9.
22. Lu MT, Rosman DA, Wu CC, et al. Radiologist point-of-care clinical decision support and adherence to guidelines for incidental lung nodules. J Am Coll Radiol 2016;13(2):156–62.
23. Alkasab TK, Bizzo BC, Berland LL, et al. Creation of an open framework for point-of-care computer-assisted reporting and decision support tools for radiologists. J Am Coll Radiol 2017;14(9):1184–9.

Lung Cancer Biopsies

Amita Sharma, MD*, Jo-Anne O. Shepard, MD

KEYWORDS

- Image-guided percutaneous transthoracic needle biopsy • Lung cancer diagnosis • Biomarkers
- Preoperative localization • Pneumothorax • Pulmonary hemorrhage • Hemothorax • Air embolus

KEY POINTS

- Image-guided percutaneous thoracic needle biopsy (PTNB) is a safe and effective method of obtaining a diagnosis in suspected malignancy, focal benign lesions, or infection.
- Planning for PTNB involves careful discussion with the clinical team, review of all available imaging, and optimization of the patient's medical condition.
- Conscious sedation, a stable patient position, and low-level patient respirations create a controlled environment for PTNB.
- A saline column in the coaxial needle protects from air embolus during needle exchanges.
- Complications of PTNB include pneumothorax, hemothorax, pulmonary hemorrhage, nondiagnostic sample, air embolism, and seeding of the biopsy tract. Major complications are rare.

INTRODUCTION

Image-guided percutaneous thoracic needle biopsy (PTNB) is a safe and effective method of obtaining a diagnosis in suspected malignancy, focal benign lesions, or infection.[1–5] It is the preferred technique for diagnosis of new or growing pulmonary nodules, or when bronchoscopy is negative for a persistent airspace opacity or hilar mass.[6,7] PTNB has a sensitivity and specificity of 93% to 98% and 98% to 100%, respectively, for the diagnosis of malignancy. Sensitivity for the evaluation of benign lesions is significantly lower than for malignant lesions and varies from 17% to 91%.[8,9]

Methods of image guidance include fluoroscopy, ultrasonography, computed tomography (CT), and magnetic resonance imaging. Most procedures are performed with CT guidance but ultrasonography is often preferred for subpleural lung masses or those that extend across the chest wall.[9–11]

INDICATIONS FOR COMPUTED TOMOGRAPHY–GUIDED PERCUTANEOUS THORACIC NEEDLE BIOPSY

PTNB forms part of the armamentarium for the diagnosis of pulmonary malignancy, infection, and benign disease. Options for diagnostic intervention are bronchoscopy, including navigational bronchoscopy, PTNB, and surgical excision. PTNB is preferable for evaluation of peripheral lesions, or if a bronchoscopy is negative for evaluation of air space opacity, central nodules, and hilar masses.[7] Open surgical wedge resection or video-assisted thoracoscopic surgery (VATS) biopsy is indicated for diffuse lung disease, for suspicious nodules undergoing definitive resection, or previously nondiagnostic needle biopsy.[12] Surgical candidates can be referred for PTNB to provide preoperative confirmation of malignancy before definitive resection. This confirmation allows a more streamlined approach to planning and consenting for surgery and also avoids

Disclosures: The authors have no relevant financial disclosures.
Division of Thoracic Imaging and Intervention, Department of Radiology, Massachusetts General Hospital, 55 Fruit Street, Founders 202, Boston, MA 02114, USA
* Corresponding author.
E-mail address: asharma2@mgh.harvard.edu

Radiol Clin N Am 56 (2018) 377–390
https://doi.org/10.1016/j.rcl.2018.01.001

radiologic.theclinics.com

surgical resection of benign lesions, infection, and lymphoma.[13–16] Nonsurgical candidates with lung cancer or metastases may be referred for PTNB to confirm malignancy before radiotherapy, ablation, or chemotherapy. In patients with known lung cancer, PTNB provides adequate tissue for molecular analysis to identify biomarkers and mutations amenable to treatment with targeted agents and enrollment into clinical trials.[17–21]

PATIENT SELECTION

Potential patients for PTNB should be approved by clinicians who perform PTNB and have an understanding of the indications, contraindications, and alternatives to PTNB. Before approval, assessment of all available imaging can identify an extrathoracic target, such as a liver or adrenal lesion that would appropriately upstage the tumor. Multidisciplinary evaluation and adequate surgical support are inherent to safe practice, particularly with high-risk patients.

PTNB is a safe procedure provided that patients are selected carefully, and the benefit of the procedure outweighs the risks. A patient should be able to lie flat and still for at least 1 hour, breathing gently without coughing or talking. Factors that reduce a patient's suitability for PTNB include underlying acute and chronic medical conditions that impair compliance and the ability to tolerate complications.

Acute reversible conditions should be treated before biopsy, such as cardiac arrhythmias or ischemia, pulmonary edema, metabolic dysfunction, neurologic injury, and pulmonary infection. Chronic conditions can also reduce a patient's tolerance to complications. Severe chronic obstructive pulmonary disease or emphysema resulting in forced expiratory volume in 1 second (FEV_1) of less than 1 L/s or FEV_1 less than 35% predicted are relative contraindications to PTNB. Bronchoscopy, including navigational bronchoscopy, is preferable to PTNB in such scenarios, because of the significantly lower risk of pneumothorax. Development of a pneumothorax during PTNB can halt the procedure before any diagnostic tissue can be obtained and can precipitate respiratory arrest. A pneumonectomy is considered a relative contraindication to PTNB, but a peripheral nodule in the remaining lung may be biopsied with adequate surgical support.[22] PTNB can precipitate respiratory failure in patients with pulmonary fibrosis. Pulmonary artery hypertension greater than 50 mm Hg can increase the risk of pulmonary

hemorrhage, although mild pulmonary hypertension has not been associated with increased complications.[23] Chronic renal or hepatic insufficiency can also increase the risk of significant pulmonary hemorrhage as well as adversely affect metabolism of drugs used for conscious sedation or general anesthesia.[10] A patient categorized as American Society of Anesthesiologists (ASA) Physical Status Classification IV or who has a compromised airway cannot receive conscious sedation and may require general anesthesia or monitored anesthesia care (MAC).

NODULE SELECTION

It is important to confirm that a nodule or opacity persists on short-term follow-up imaging (4–6 weeks), because infection or inflammatory change can mimic malignancy, particularly in the presence of underlying chronic lung disease such as emphysema or fibrosis. Nodule features that affect the likelihood of successful biopsy include size, location, and attenuation.

Size

Nodules that are typically amenable to PTNB are 8 mm or larger, although nodules as small as 5 mm can be successfully biopsied. Diagnostic accuracy rates of 82% to 95% are reported for subcentimeter nodules.[24,25]

Location

The feasibility of biopsy depends largely on the location of the nodule, particularly when it is less than 2 cm. Ideally, a nodule should be motionless during PTNB. In this regard, respiratory motion has less effect on nodules in the apical segment of the upper lobes and superior segment of the lower lobes. However, respiratory motion near the diaphragm can be significant even with the use of conscious sedation. CT fluoroscopy is helpful in assisting biopsy of small mobile nodules. Crossing a fissure during a biopsy contributes to the risk of pneumothorax, because the incidence is directly related to the number of pleural surfaces crossed. The posterior segments of the upper lobes and the middle lobe are challenging locations because the fissures are often along the path of the biopsy needle. Biopsy of a lesion in a subpleural location or within atelectatic lung is associated with fewer complications than when aerated lung is traversed.[26] However, if a nodule is small and in the subpleural region, there is a risk that the coaxial needle in the shortest direct path will move in and out of the lung during respiration. This risk can be avoided by an oblique approach through adjacent lung, creating a longer path in the lung.

Attenuation

PTNB has value in the evaluation of both ground-glass and part-solid nodules. Although early studies reported a low sensitivity and diagnostic accuracy, more recent publications have shown sensitivity and specificity rates for PTNB of sub-solid nodules between 92% to 97% and 90% to 100%, respectively.[27] Diagnostic accuracy is reported to be 91%. Greater sensitivity is found with core biopsies than with fine-needle aspiration (FNA) alone. Biopsy of cavitary nodules can be optimized using FNA of the intracavitary contents or wall and core biopsy of the wall.

TECHNIQUE

Most radiologists use a coaxial technique using 18-G or 19-G coaxial needles. Once the tip of the coaxial needle is within the nodule, a 22-G FNA needle or a 20-G core biopsy needle can be exchanged for the central stylet (Fig. 1). The following step-by-step description explains the principles of a coaxial technique but is also applicable to a single-needle technique (Fig. 2, Table 1).

Patient Preparation

Patients should be able to give consent and to tolerate the procedure. In addition, certain medications that increase the risk of pulmonary hemorrhage or hemothorax should be withheld to restore normal coagulation. Coumadin, full-dose aspirin,

and nonsteroidal antiinflammatory drugs should be discontinued 5 days before biopsy. Heparin and Lovenox are discontinued 6 and 12 hours before biopsy, respectively, with confirmation of normalization of blood coagulation factors. The platelet count should be greater than 50,000/μL but preferably more than 100,000/μL and International Normalized Ratio and a prothrombin time ratio greater than 1.4. If a patient uses continuous positive airway pressure or bilevel positive airway pressure ventilation, this should be stopped for at least 24 hours following PTNB to prevent a delayed pneumothorax. Patients who live alone or have severe comorbidities may require overnight admission. Patients receiving conscious sedation or general anesthesia need to refrain from solids for 8 hours and fluids for 2 hours or as per institutional policy.

Sedation

PTNB can be performed with local anesthesia, conscious sedation, monitored anesthesia care, or general anesthesia. Institutional preferences often depend on resources and work-flow management. If local anesthesia only is used, the patient should practice breath holding with the radiologist before the procedure. Whether performed at midinspiration or end expiration, the phase of breath holding should be consistent during imaging, all needle maneuvers, and during procurement of the biopsy. It is helpful for the radiologist to breath hold at the same time as the patient because this reminds the radiologist to instruct the patient to restart breathing. The authors perform PTNB with intravenous

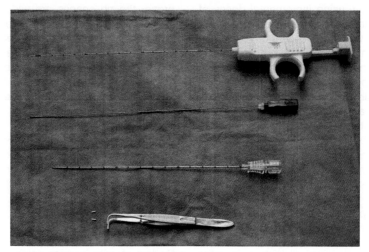

Fig. 1. The biopsy needles that are commonly used for PTNB. From the top: 20-gauge core biopsy needle; 22-gauge FNA needle; 19-gauge coaxial needle through which pass core biopsy and FNA needles during the biopsy; metal tweezers adjacent to 2 3 mm × 0.8 mm gold fiducial markers. The fiducial markers are placed through the coaxial needle to aid nodule localization during minimally invasive surgical resection or radiation planning.

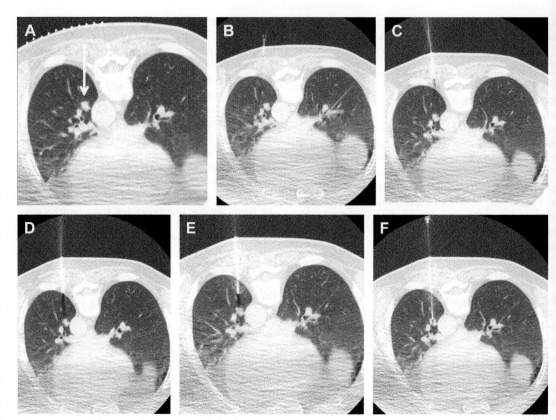

Fig. 2. A 74-year-old man with 1.2-cm adenocarcinoma in the left lower lobe. Selected axial lung window CT images from a PTNB show the step-by-step technique. (*A*) The patient is in the prone position, with a grid placed on the patient's back. Limited 5-mm axial sections locate the lesion and 2.5-mm axial sections determine the optimal table position and entry point for biopsy of the lung nodule (*arrow*). (*B*) A 25-gauge local anesthetic needle confirms the entry point. (*C*) A 19-gauge coaxial needle is advanced incrementally through the subcutaneous tissues to the extrapleural space. (*D*) Local anesthetic is injected before pleural puncture. (*E*) The coaxial needle is advanced with a sharp, firm jab through the pleural space and the tip rests within the lung parenchyma. (*F*) The needle tip is advanced into the nodule in preparation for biopsy.

conscious sedation, using incremental doses of an anxiolytic (midazolam) and a narcotic for analgesia (fentanyl). Conscious sedation produces restful, low-volume, reproducible respiratory excursions without need for breath holding. Needle maneuvers are performed during a plateau in respiration, usually at end expiration. Oversedation can cause paradoxic hyperactivity, particularly in elderly patients. General anesthesia may be necessary if conscious sedation is contraindicated or for urgent biopsies in noncooperative patients. A double-lumen endotracheal tube can be useful in high-risk patients at risk for pulmonary hemorrhage. Low-volume ventilation is preferable because positive pressure can cause a small pneumothorax to rapidly enlarge.

Patient Positioning

Patient stability during the procedure is best achieved in the supine or prone position. When prone, the rib spaces are wide and the patient cannot see the needle. Recovery in the dependent, supine position is often easier for patients to tolerate. The subclavian vessels, prominent costochondral cartilages, and breast tissue can hinder the anterior approach in the upper zones. The lateral approach renders the patient less stable; the ribs are closer together, reducing access; and there is a higher incidence of pneumothorax compared with the supine or prone approach.[28] Some centers report preference for a decubitus position with the biopsy side down following the procedure, because dependent atelectasis can be protective for pneumothorax.[29]

Localizing the Nodule

Review of prior imaging confirms the position of the nodule. A radio-opaque grid is placed on the patient's skin at the level of the suspected nodule. After sedation has been initiated, localized 5-mm

Table 1
Percutaneous transthoracic needle biopsy technique, step by step

Action	Steps
Sedation	None/conscious sedation/general anesthesia with cardiorespiratory monitoring
Patient position	Supine/prone if possible. Stabilize with straps
Needle	Coaxial 18-G/19-G needle at least 3–4 cm longer than distance from skin to nodule
Find the nodule	Review imaging, place radio-opaque skin grid, scout views, limited 5-mm axial sections
Find the window	2.5 mm axial ± gantry angulation. Mark skin entry site
Insert needle	Sterilize field/local anesthetic infiltration, image 25-G needle to confirm window, measure skin to pleura distance, advance coaxial needle to pleural surface
Pierce nodule	Confirm correct trajectory toward nodule. Local anesthetic injected into the extrapleural space/intravenous fentanyl dose before pleural puncture. Cross pleura, advance into nodule
Biopsy	Inject saline into coaxial needle, rapid exchange of stylet with FNA or core biopsy needle, FNA/core biopsy, refill saline during each exchange
Specimen	FNA smear onto slides (on-site cytology), or into saline (flow cytometry and cell block)/transport medium; cores in formalin; microbiology aspirate in saline
Needle removal	Remove all monitoring leads/blood pressure cuff first. Remove needle, rapid rollover
Recovery	Recover in dependent position for 3 h, chest radiograph at 1 and 3 h
Discharge	Home with overnight support. Postbiopsy/sedation instructions

sections are obtained during gentle respiration to localize the nodule. Then 2.5-mm sections are obtained, centered on the nodule, to find a window for biopsy. Dose reduction is achieved by minimizing the milliamperage and kilovoltage. CT fluoroscopy can assess respiratory motion effects on the position of the nodule.

Finding the Window

An appropriate path from the skin to the nodule should be visible on at least 3 axial 2.5-mm sections. This window should avoid ribs, vessels, and fissures. Underlying lung disease, including emphysema, should be avoided if possible and can require a different path into the nodule. Determination of an adequate window can necessitate angulation of the gantry. During evaluation of the preliminary CT images, the appropriate window can be above or below the axial image that shows the nodule. In this case the gantry should be angled superiorly or inferiorly, such that the access route and the nodule are present on the same slice. Increments of 2° to 4° superiorly or inferiorly can be required. Once the required table position has been defined, a line is drawn from the nodule upward to the skin to mimic the trajectory of the biopsy needle. The corresponding line on the grid is determined and the table is moved to the required table position. Using the scanner's laser light, a cross is marked on the patient's skin that intersects the table position with the line on the grid.

Preparation of the Biopsy Site

The marked skin is sterilized with iodine or chlorhexidine following removal of the grid. Sterile towels cover the remainder of the patient's chest. Any movement, coughing, or talking by the patient is discouraged. Lidocaine 1% is injected through a 25-G needle into the subcutaneous tissues at the level of the marked cross. The syringe is detached from the local anesthetic needle that is left in the subcutaneous tissues. A repeat limited axial scan is performed to confirm that the local anesthetic needle is correctly positioned.

Choosing the Coaxial Needle

The distance between the skin and pleura along the needle trajectory is measured. The distance between the skin and nodule is also measured in order to enable the correct length choice of the 19-G coaxial needle. The 19-G coaxial needles are available in a range of lengths, usually 10 cm, 15 cm, and 20 cm. The choice of needle length should be adequate to compensate for an oblique path through the chest, gantry angulation, and nodule movement; 3 to 4 cm of extra needle length allow manipulation of the needle. The core biopsy and aspiration needle (22-G FNA) should be longer than the coaxial needle, and these are available in 5-cm increments from 10 cm to 25 cm.

Advancing the Coaxial Needle into the Nodule

A 4-mm incision is made in the sterilized skin with a scalpel blade and the coaxial needle is advanced into the subcutaneous tissues at the confirmed skin entry site. The angle of entry mimics the gantry angulation and the medial or lateral angulation mimics the chosen trajectory during the planning scans. The coaxial needle may need to be supported by gauze swabs if the subcutaneous tissue is limited. A repeat stack of axial images with the same gantry angulation is performed to confirm the correct position of the coaxial needle. It is important to evaluate the relative position of the tip of the coaxial needle to the nodule. A line is drawn on the workstation along the length of the needle and extending into the nodule. This line is fixed and reviewed along the stack of images. Review may show that the needle tip is heading up or down in relation to the nodule or that the tip is too medial or lateral to the nodule. Any alterations in needle angulation should be performed while the needle is in the chest wall and during the plateau phases of respiration, typically at end expiration. The needle is then advanced through the muscles and up to the pleural surface with the aim that the full length of the needle will be aligned with the nodule on a single 2.5-mm axial image, before pleural puncture. Only minor changes in angulation are feasible once the coaxial needle has traversed the pleura.

Before pleural puncture, 1 to 2 mL of local anesthetic injected through the center of the coaxial needle and an additional dose of fentanyl may ensure patient comfort and immobility during pleural puncture, which can be painful.

Without changing the angulation of the coaxial needle, the pleura is punctured as respiration plateaus, usually during the plateau of end expiration. Pleural puncture usually requires a short, sharp movement of the coaxial needle. The tip should be advanced at least 1 cm beyond the pleura to prevent the needle moving in and out of the pleura during respiration. Following confirmation of the needle trajectory remaining on course toward the lung nodule, the needle is advanced incrementally until the tip lies within the nodule. This technique prevents the needle bouncing off the nodule during biopsy and decreases pulmonary hemorrhage in the adjacent lung.

Obtaining Biopsy Material

The central stylet is exchanged for the 22-G FNA needle over a saline seal to prevent air embolism (Fig. 3). In order to achieve this, a 2-mL syringe with a blunt-ended needle is filled with injectable saline and is used to drip saline into the central core of the coaxial needle as the inner stylet is slowly removed. The coaxial needle should be completely filled with saline before a rapid exchange of the inner stylet with the FNA needle. The FNA needle is allowed to fall to the level of the nodule and advanced rapidly in and out of the coaxial needle by a few millimeters while aspirating with a syringe placed on the end of the needle. Short, sharp jabbing movements cut into the

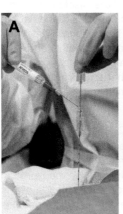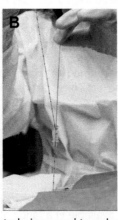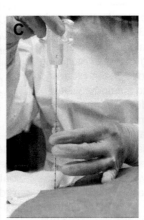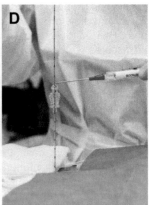

Fig. 3. The saline injection technique used to reduce risk of air embolism during needle exchanges. (A) Once the coaxial needle is positioned within the nodule, the central trocar is exchanged with the aspiration needle or core biopsy needle. Before the central stylet of the coaxial needle is removed, a 2-mL syringe with a blunt-tipped needle is used to drip sterile saline into the hollow bore of the coaxial needle until saline is visible at the top of the trocar. (B) A rapid exchange of the central stylet with the biopsy needle is performed through the saline seal. (C) The biopsy is performed. (D) Before removal of the biopsy needle, the saline is dripped again into the bore of the coaxial needle. A rapid exchange of the biopsy needle with the central stylet is performed through the saline seal.

nodule and negative pressure on the syringe aspirates cells into the needle. Saline is again dripped into the trocar of the coaxial needle and the FNA needle is rapidly exchanged with the central stylet. Once the central stylet is replaced, the sample can be smeared onto a glass slide or into cytology transfer media. Slides are analyzed on site by a cytologist for adequacy and preliminary diagnosis. On-site cytology has been shown to improve diagnostic accuracy without affecting complication rates.[30]

A repeat limited CT scan confirms that the position of the coaxial needle remains within the nodule and that no complications have occurred during aspiration. If lymphoma is suspected, 2 further aspirations are injected into a sterile tube with saline and can be spun down to create a cell block or submitted for flow cytometry while the cytologist is reviewing the slides. If there is a suspicion of infection, a dedicated FNA is performed for microbiological evaluation.

Once the cytotechnologist has confirmed that there are diagnostic cells present, a core biopsy specimen can be performed in this area. If no cells are seen for diagnosis, repositioning of the coaxial needle may be necessary for further aspirates.

A core biopsy is obtained in a similar fashion with exchange of the central stylet for the biopsy needle over a column of saline within the coaxial needle. The cores are placed in a sterile container of saline and then transferred into formalin for histopathology assessment. Multiple core biopsies and FNAs can be performed through the center of the coaxial needle for cytology, pathology, biomarkers, and clinical trial enrollment. A core is preferable for biomarkers but a cell block can also be used for molecular analysis.

Safe Removal of the Biopsy Needle and Recovery

Once adequate samples have been obtained, a final limited scan with the needle in the nodule may be performed to exclude complications. The authors do not routinely image after the needle has been removed. Once all the specimens have been obtained, the patient's skin is cleaned and monitoring equipment, sterile towels, and drapes are removed. The needle remains in the nodule until the end of the procedure. Once the patient's stretcher is positioned next to the CT table, the radiologist swiftly removes the needle, applies a dressing over the skin incision, and the patient is rolled over onto the stretcher to lie on the puncture site. Recovery in this position creates atelectasis in the dependent lung adjacent to the pleural puncture, reducing airflow and the potential need for

chest tube. The patient is transferred to the recovery area and is observed for 3 hours with continuous monitoring and oxygen per nasal cannula. During this recovery time the patient is not allowed to move, eat, drink, or talk. A portable chest radiograph is performed 1 hour after the needle is removed and an anteroposterior erect radiograph is performed 3 hours after the needle is removed. Patients are discharged home but, if they live alone or have severe comorbidities, they can be admitted for overnight observation.

LOCALIZATION OF SMALL NODULES FOR TREATMENT: FIDUCIAL MARKER PLACEMENT

A similar technique can be used for preoperative localization of small lung nodules.[31,32] Localization is useful for minimally invasive surgical resection of peripheral nodules that are too small or of too low density to be palpated by the surgeon during VATS. Using the same approach as PTNB, gold fiducial markers can be placed through the bore of a coaxial needle within or adjacent to a lung nodule (Fig. 4). The procedure is well tolerated and patients are asymptomatic after insertion. It can be performed on an outpatient basis, allowing flexibility in scheduling surgical resection on another day. The fiducial markers are visible by on-table fluoroscopy in the operating room and indicate the position of nonpalpable, nonvisible nodules. They are inert and do not induce a reaction around them that could potentially affect histologic assessment of the lesion.

Several other techniques have been described for preoperative nodule localization. Hook-wires and microcoils extend from the pleural surface or chest wall to the nodule and the surgeon uses the wire as a pathway to resect the nodule.[33–35] Image-guided or bronchoscopic injection of radioopaque contrast or dye can indicate the approximate location of the nodule or the closest pleural surface.[36–38] Radioisotopes can also be injected into the nodule immediately before surgery.[39–41] Radioactivity is detected by a Geiger counter passed along the lung surface at thoracoscopy, to locate the nodule. Percutaneous image-guided insertion of fiducial markers can also be performed as an aid to radiation planning and can be combined with a biopsy for confirmation of malignancy.[42,43]

COMPLICATIONS

Minor complications are frequent but major complications of PTNB are rare. Complications include pneumothorax, hemothorax, pulmonary hemorrhage, nondiagnostic sample, air embolism, and seeding of the biopsy tract.

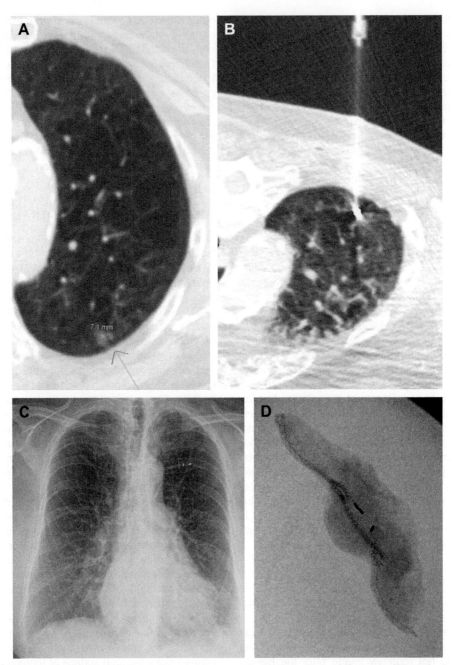

Fig. 4. A 68-year-old woman with 2 prior lung cancers and enlarging 7-mm left upper lobe adenocarcinoma referred for preoperative localization with fiducial markers. (*A*) Axial lung window CT image shows a posterior left upper lobe nodule (*arrow*) surrounded by emphysema. (*B*) Prone image shows 2 gold fiducial markers placed via a coaxial needle medial to the nodule. Direct discussion with the surgeon is important to confirm the exact position of the markers relative to the nodule. (*C*) Chest radiograph 3 hours after procedure shows 2 fiducial markers in the left upper lobe. (*D*) Fluoroscopy image of wedge resection specimen confirms that 2 markers have been excised. Frozen section confirmed complete excision of adenocarcinoma and adequate surgical margins.

A recent meta-analysis reported that the most common risk factors for complications after FNA included smaller lesion size, increased needle gauge, and length of lung parenchyma traversed by the needle.[44]

Pneumothorax

Pneumothorax is the most common complication of PTNB (Fig. 5). The incidence depends on the method of detection (chest radiograph or CT)

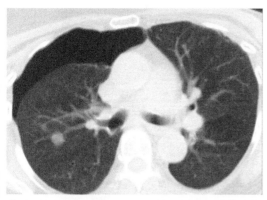

Fig. 5. A 54-year-old woman with 1.8-cm middle lobe adenocarcinoma. Axial lung window CT image obtained following development of chest pain 1 hour after PTNB shows a moderate anterior right pneumothorax that required drainage with an 8-French pigtail pleural catheter.

and is reported to be between 10% and 60%.[26,45–49] Most pneumothoraces are asymptomatic, necessitating conservative management only. The incidence of chest tube insertion for a large or symptomatic pneumothorax varies between 2% and 20%. Risk factors for pneumothorax are large needle size; emphysema, particularly in the region of the needle tract; a noncooperative patient; a lateral approach; multiple pleural punctures; crossing a fissure; and biopsy of deep or cavitary lesions.[26,45–50] The specific methods that the authors use to reduce the risk of a significant pneumothorax include use of conscious sedation and discouraging talking or coughing, because this reduces patient movement and respiratory excursions. The anterior or posterior approach is used whenever possible because there is a higher incidence of pneumothorax with a lateral approach.[28] A coaxial technique allows for multiple biopsies from a single pleural puncture. At the end of the procedure the authors perform a rapid roll-over technique whereby the pleural puncture site is immediately made dependent as the needle is removed.[51] This technique reduces movement of the pleura and maximizes adjacent dependent atelectasis, both protective factors that aid in sealing the pleural puncture site.

In high-risk patients, sealants such as blood (blood patch), fibrin glue, and slurry may be injected through the coaxial needle as it is pulled out of the lung.[52–54] Alternatively, if the patient develops a small pneumothorax during the biopsy, a length of tubing can be attached to the coaxial needle and, using a 20-mL syringe and 3-way stopcock, the pneumothorax can be aspirated as the coaxial needle is removed.[55] A

pneumothorax in the presence of emphysema is more likely to cause a large air leak that requires treatment with a wide-bore surgical chest tube.[13,56]

Once a pneumothorax develops, the risk associated with flying in a pressurized aircraft is often a cause for concern. Although there are limited data, most guidelines recommend a delay of 1 to 2 weeks after radiographic resolution of the pneumothorax.[57–59]

Pulmonary Hemorrhage

The reported incidence of pulmonary hemorrhage is approximately 5% but most of the cases are self-limiting and asymptomatic.[60,61] Risk factors for pulmonary hemorrhage include underlying coagulopathy and vascular lesions of neoplastic, inflammatory, or infective causes. Mild or moderate pulmonary artery hypertension is not associated with increased risk of hemorrhage.[23,62] It is common to detect pulmonary hemorrhage manifesting as ground-glass opacity surrounding the nodule or in the tract during the biopsy; a greater extent of hemorrhage can be segmental or lobar (Figs. 6 and 7).

Methods of reducing hemorrhage include avoidance of large vessels in the trajectory of the needle. The tip of the needle should lie within the nodule before an aspiration or core biopsy, so that any bleeding occurs within the nodule rather than in the surrounding lung. Biopsy of areas of consolidation should be limited to the periphery of the consolidation, avoiding large vessels.

PTNB should be temporarily halted if pulmonary hemorrhage occurs and a repeat CT performed after a short interval to assess progression of hemorrhage. If there is significant hemoptysis the procedure should be stopped, the mouth suctioned, and supportive care administered. The needle should be removed and the patient placed with the biopsy site dependent in an attempt to limit aspirated blood to the biopsied lung only. Once the needle has been removed, coughing should be encouraged and airway suction performed because hemoptysis can result in airway irritation and potentially induce respiratory arrest. Nebulized epinephrine can treat persistent hemoptysis by inducing vasoconstriction. Uncontrollable hemorrhage may necessitate urgent bronchoscopy and isolation of the affected side with bronchial blockers. Persistent hemoptysis may require embolization.

Hemothorax

Injury to intercostal and internal mammary vessels is rare but has been described with a

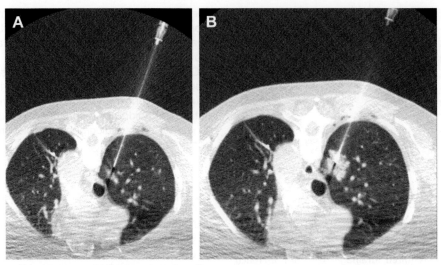

Fig. 6. A 70-year-old man with right upper lobe adenocarcinoma. (*A*) Axial prone lung window CT image obtained during PTNB shows the coaxial needle proximal to the 1.4-cm nodule. (*B*) Following FNA, a repeat image shows development of minor pulmonary hemorrhage that obscures the nodule. This hemorrhage may have been caused by the needle tip lying in lung rather than within the lesion at the time of biopsy. The patient was asymptomatic.

posterior paravertebral or anterior parasternal approach (**Fig. 8**). Careful evaluation of visible vessels in the chest wall during the planning stage is required to avoid these complications.[63]

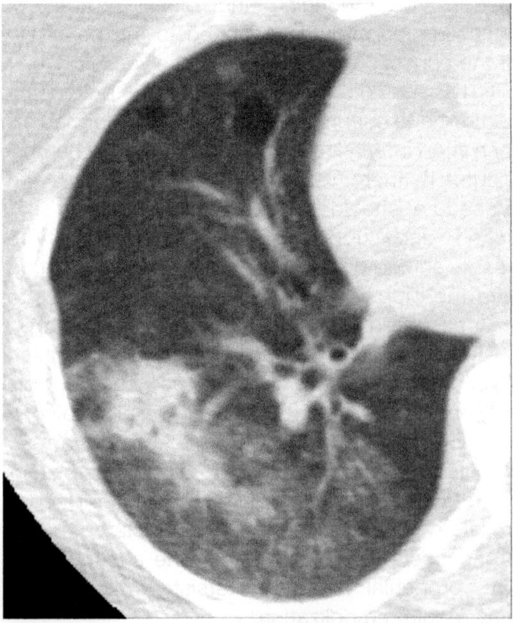

Fig. 7. A 66-year-old woman with history of Sjögren syndrome and 2-cm right lower lobe nodule caused by lymphoma. Axial lung window CT image following PTNB shows moderate hemorrhage that resulted in an episode of self-limiting hemoptysis after PTNB.

Significant hemothorax should be managed in conjunction with thoracic surgery (see **Fig 7**).

Nondiagnostic Sample

A nonspecific, nonmalignant diagnosis following PTNB can be caused by a nondiagnostic specimen as a result of sampling error. The nondiagnostic rate of CT-guided PTNB is up to 15%.[64,65] False-negative results are reported in 7% to 29% of malignant lesions following an initial benign nonspecific biopsy.[66,67]

If a PTNB is negative, a follow-up chest CT scan should be performed to confirm resolution or stability of the lesion. If there is a strong suspicion of malignancy or follow-up CT shows growth of the nodule, repeat PTNB or surgical excision should be considered.

Seeding of the Needle Tract

Seeding of the needle tract is rare and the rate has been reported to be 0.016% to 0.018%.[61,68] The use of a coaxial technique reduces the risk of seeding because aspirated cells are retained within the lumen of the coaxial needle.

Air Embolism

Air embolism is an extremely rare, but often fatal, complication of PTNB (**Fig. 9**).[69] It can occur if room air passes through the coaxial needle into a pulmonary vein and into the left atrium, left ventricle, and to the systemic

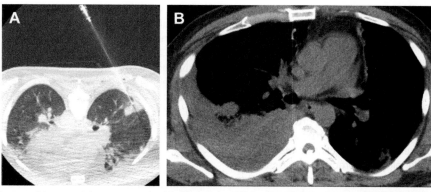

Fig. 8. A 49-year-old man with acute myeloid leukemia and fungal pneumonia. (*A*) Prone axial lung window CT image during PTNB shows the tip of the coaxial needle in the nodule. (*B*) Immediately following removal of the coaxial needle the patient developed pleuritic chest pain. Chest CT showed high-density fluid in the right pleural space secondary to hemothorax requiring emergent drainage.

circulation. Also, the coaxial needle may create a fistula between an airway and a pulmonary artery or vein. The risk of air embolism can be exacerbated with coughing or rapid respiratory excursion.

The authors have encountered only 1 case of air embolism in our facility over 30 years. Our techniques for minimizing the risk of air embolism include strict immobilization of the patient during the procedure. The patient is discouraged from talking, coughing, or breathing deeply during the biopsy. Conscious sedation is extremely helpful in this situation. Careful planning of the passage of the coaxial needle through the lung and confirmation that the needle tip lies within the nodule before biopsy reduces the risk of a fistula between the vessel and airway within the lung or air entering into a vein through the coaxial needle. During the biopsy, we create a fluid seal by injecting a few drops of saline into the coaxial needle as the inner stylet is removed and rapidly exchange the inner stylet for the FNA needle or core biopsy needle to minimize exposure of the center of the coaxial needle to room air.

If air is detected in the pulmonary veins or heart during a biopsy, the procedure should be immediately stopped. The patient should be moved into the supine or Trendelenburg position without turning right side down. One-hundred percent oxygen should be administered via facemask and emergent referral to an intensive care unit or activation of the rapid response team is required. Hyperbaric oxygen therapy reduces morbidity and mortality in patients with air embolism.[70,71]

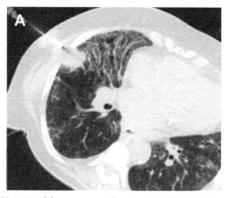
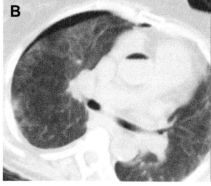

Fig. 9. A 60-year-old woman with air embolism and cardiac arrest after PTNB performed at another hospital. (*A*) Axial lung window CT image shows coaxial needle in the chest wall and a 2.5-cm middle lobe nodule. (*B*) Repeat CT after the patient's condition deteriorated shows a small right pneumothorax and air in the ascending aorta secondary to an air embolus.

SUMMARY

PTNB is a safe, effective method of obtaining tissue in pulmonary nodules. Major complications are rare. Factors that increase the likelihood of success include close communication with the clinical team, optimization of patient factors, use of conscious sedation, adherence to careful technique, and on-site cytology. PTNB provides invaluable information for biomarker-based targeted therapy and enrollment into clinical trials. It can aid radiation planning and preoperative localization of nodules with image-guided percutaneous fiducial marker placement. Such advances have expanded the role of the interventional thoracic radiologist in managing patients with lung cancer.

REFERENCES

1. National Lung Screening Trial Research Team, Aberle DR, Berg CD, Black WC, et al. The National Lung Screening Trial: overview and study design. Radiology 2011;258(1):243–53.

2. MacMahon H, Austin JH, Gamsu G, et al. Guidelines for management of small pulmonary nodules detected on CT scans: a statement from the Fleischner Society. Radiology 2005;237(2):395–400.

3. Rosenkrantz AB, Matza BW, Foran MP, et al. Recommendations for additional imaging on emergency department CT examinations: comparison of emergency- and organ-based subspecialty radiologists. Emerg Radiol 2013;20(2):149–53.

4. Westcott JL. Direct percutaneous needle aspiration of localized pulmonary lesions: result in 422 patients. Radiology 1980;137(1 Pt 1):31–5.

5. Henschke CI, Yankelevitz D, Westcott J, et al. Workup of the solitary pulmonary nodule. American College of Radiology. ACR appropriateness criteria. Radiology 2000;215(Suppl):607–9.

6. Carrafiello G, Lagana D, Nosari AM, et al. Utility of computed tomography (CT) and of fine needle aspiration biopsy (FNAB) in early diagnosis of fungal pulmonary infections. Study of infections from filamentous fungi in haematologically immunodeficient patients. Radiol Med 2006;111(1):33–41.

7. Ferretti GR, Jankowski A, Rodiere M, et al. CT-guided biopsy of nonresolving focal air space consolidation. J Thorac Imaging 2008;23(1):7–12.

8. Greif J, Marmor S, Schwarz Y, et al. Percutaneous core needle biopsy vs. fine needle aspiration in diagnosing benign lung lesions. Acta Cytol 1999; 43(5):756–60.

9. Klein JS, Zarka MA. Transthoracic needle biopsy: an overview. J Thorac Imaging 1997;12(4):232–49.

10. Moore EH. Technical aspects of needle aspiration lung biopsy: a personal perspective. Radiology 1998;208(2):303–18.

11. Liao WY, Chen MZ, Chang YL, et al. US-guided transthoracic cutting biopsy for peripheral thoracic lesions less than 3 cm in diameter. Radiology 2000;217(3):685–91.

12. Lettieri CJ, Veerappan GR, Helman DL, et al. Outcomes and safety of surgical lung biopsy for interstitial lung disease. Chest 2005;127(5):1600–5.

13. Poe RH, Tobin RE. Sensitivity and specificity of needle biopsy in lung malignancy. Am Rev Respir Dis 1980;122(5):725–9.

14. Welker JA, Alattar M, Gautam S. Repeat needle biopsies combined with clinical observation are safe and accurate in the management of a solitary pulmonary nodule. Cancer 2005;103(3):599–607.

15. Watanabe N, Fujioka I, Aota Y, et al. Primary pulmonary Hodgkin lymphoma diagnosed by CT-guided percutaneous biopsy. Rinsho Ketsueki 2015;56(1):41–3.

16. Gupta S, Sultenfuss M, Romaguera JE, et al. CT-guided percutaneous lung biopsies in patients with haematologic malignancies and undiagnosed pulmonary lesions. Hematol Oncol 2010;28(2):75–81.

17. Solomon SB, Zakowski MF, Pao W, et al. Core needle lung biopsy specimens: adequacy for EGFR and KRAS mutational analysis. AJR Am J Roentgenol 2010;194(1):266–9.

18. Yoon HJ, Lee HY, Lee KS, et al. Repeat biopsy for mutational analysis of non-small cell lung cancers resistant to previous chemotherapy: adequacy and complications. Radiology 2012;265(3):939–48.

19. Liao BC, Bai YY, Lee JH, et al. Outcomes of research biopsies in clinical trials of EGFR mutation-positive non-small cell lung cancer patients pretreated with EGFR-tyrosine kinase inhibitors. J Formos Med Assoc 2017. [Epub ahead of print].

20. Tam AL, Kim ES, Lee JJ, et al. Feasibility of image-guided transthoracic core-needle biopsy in the BATTLE lung trial. J Thorac Oncol 2013;8(4):436–42.

21. Stevenson M, Christensen J, Shoemaker D, et al. Tumor acquisition for biomarker research in lung cancer. Cancer Invest 2014;32(6):291–8.

22. Cronin CG, Sharma A, Digumarthy SR, et al. Percutaneous lung biopsy after pneumonectomy: factors for improving success in the care of patients at high risk. AJR Am J Roentgenol 2011;196(4):929–34.

23. Digumarthy SR, Kovacina B, Otrakji A, et al. Percutaneous CT guided lung biopsy in patients with pulmonary hypertension: assessment of complications. Eur J Radiol 2016;85(2):466–71.

24. Wallace MJ, Krishnamurthy S, Broemeling LD, et al. CT-guided percutaneous fine-needle aspiration biopsy of small (< or =1-cm) pulmonary lesions. Radiology 2002;225(3):823–8.

25. Choi SH, Chae EJ, Kim JE, et al. Percutaneous CT-guided aspiration and core biopsy of pulmonary nodules smaller than 1 cm: analysis of outcomes of 305 procedures from a tertiary referral center. AJR Am J Roentgenol 2013;201(5):964–70.

26. Haramati LB, Austin JH. Complications after CT-guided needle biopsy through aerated versus nonaerated lung. Radiology 1991;181(3):778.

27. Kim TJ, Lee JH, Lee CT, et al. Diagnostic accuracy of CT-guided core biopsy of ground-glass opacity pulmonary lesions. AJR Am J Roentgenol 2008; 190(1):234–9.

28. Ko JP, Shepard JO, Drucker EA, et al. Factors influencing pneumothorax rate at lung biopsy: are dwell time and angle of pleural puncture contributing factors? Radiology 2001;218(2):491–6.

29. Rozenblit AM, Tuvia J, Rozenblit GN, et al. CT-guided transthoracic needle biopsy using an ipsilateral dependent position. AJR Am J Roentgenol 2000;174(6):1759–64.

30. Austin JH, Cohen MB. Value of having a cytopathologist present during percutaneous fine-needle aspiration biopsy of lung: report of 55 cancer patients and metaanalysis of the literature. AJR Am J Roentgenol 1993;160(1):175–7.

31. Sancheti MS, Lee R, Ahmed SU, et al. Percutaneous fiducial localization for thoracoscopic wedge resection of small pulmonary nodules. Ann Thorac Surg 2014;97(6):1914–8 [discussion: 1919].

32. Sharma A, McDermott S, Mathisen DJ, et al. Preoperative localization of lung nodules with fiducial markers: feasibility and technical considerations. Ann Thorac Surg 2017;103(4):1114–20.

33. Finley RJ, Mayo JR, Grant K, et al. Preoperative computed tomography-guided microcoil localization of small peripheral pulmonary nodules: a prospective randomized controlled trial. J Thorac Cardiovasc Surg 2015;149(1):26–31.

34. Dendo S, Kanazawa S, Ando A, et al. Preoperative localization of small pulmonary lesions with a short hook wire and suture system: experience with 168 procedures. Radiology 2002;225(2):511–8.

35. Thaete FL, Peterson MS, Plunkett MB, et al. Computed tomography-guided wire localization of pulmonary lesions before thoracoscopic resection: results in 101 cases. J Thorac Imaging 1999;14(2): 90–8.

36. Lenglinger FX, Schwarz CD, Artmann W. Localization of pulmonary nodules before thoracoscopic surgery: value of percutaneous staining with methylene blue. AJR Am J Roentgenol 1994;163(2):297–300.

37. Choi BG, Kim HH, Kim BS, et al. Pulmonary nodules: CT-guided contrast material localization for thoracoscopic resection. Radiology 1998;208(2): 399–401.

38. Endo M, Kotani Y, Satouchi M, et al. CT fluoroscopy-guided bronchoscopic dye marking for resection of small peripheral pulmonary nodules. Chest 2004; 125(5):1747–52.

39. Galetta D, Bellomi M, Grana C, et al. Radio-guided localization and resection of small or ill-defined pulmonary lesions. Ann Thorac Surg 2015;100(4): 1175–80.

40. Grogan EL, Jones DR, Kozower BD, et al. Identification of small lung nodules: technique of radiotracer-guided thoracoscopic biopsy. Ann Thorac Surg 2008;85(2):S772–7.

41. Stiles BM, Altes TA, Jones DR, et al. Clinical experience with radiotracer-guided thoracoscopic biopsy of small, indeterminate lung nodules. Ann Thorac Surg 2006;82(4):1191–6 [discussion: 1196–7].

42. Kothary N, Heit JJ, Louie JD, et al. Safety and efficacy of percutaneous fiducial marker implantation for image-guided radiation therapy. J Vasc Interv Radiol 2009;20(2):235–9.

43. Yousefi S, Collins BT, Reichner CA, et al. Complications of thoracic computed tomography-guided fiducial placement for the purpose of stereotactic body radiation therapy. Clin Lung Cancer 2007;8(4): 252–6.

44. Heerink WJ, de Bock GH, de Jonge GJ, et al. Complication rates of CT-guided transthoracic lung biopsy: meta-analysis. Eur Radiol 2017;27(1): 138–48.

45. Guimaraes MD, Andrade MQ, Fonte AC, et al. Predictive complication factors for CT-guided fine needle aspiration biopsy of pulmonary lesions. Clinics (Sao Paulo) 2010;65(9):847–50.

46. Hiraki T, Mimura H, Gobara H, et al. Incidence of and risk factors for pneumothorax and chest tube placement after CT fluoroscopy-guided percutaneous lung biopsy: retrospective analysis of the procedures conducted over a 9-year period. AJR Am J Roentgenol 2010;194(3):809–14.

47. Kuban JD, Tam AL, Huang SY, et al. The effect of needle gauge on the risk of pneumothorax and chest tube placement after percutaneous computed tomographic (CT)-guided lung biopsy. Cardiovasc Intervent Radiol 2015;38(6):1595–602.

48. Laspas F, Roussakis A, Efthimiadou R, et al. Percutaneous CT-guided fine-needle aspiration of pulmonary lesions: results and complications in 409 patients. J Med Imaging Radiat Oncol 2008;52(5): 458–62.

49. Nour-Eldin NA, Alsubhi M, Emam A, et al. Pneumothorax complicating coaxial and non-coaxial CT-guided lung biopsy: comparative analysis of determining risk factors and management of pneumothorax in a retrospective review of 650 patients. Cardiovasc Intervent Radiol 2016;39(2): 261–70.

50. Anzidei M, Sacconi B, Fraioli F, et al. Development of a prediction model and risk score for procedure-related complications in patients undergoing

percutaneous computed tomography-guided lung biopsy. Eur J Cardiothorac Surg 2015;48(1):e1–6.

51. O'Neill AC, McCarthy C, Ridge CA, et al. Rapid needle-out patient-rollover time after percutaneous CT-guided transthoracic biopsy of lung nodules: effect on pneumothorax rate. Radiology 2012;262(1):314–9.

52. Tran AA, Brown SB, Rosenberg J, et al. Tract embolization with gelatin sponge slurry for prevention of pneumothorax after percutaneous computed tomography-guided lung biopsy. Cardiovasc Intervent Radiol 2014;37(6):1546–53.

53. Wagner JM, Hinshaw JL, Lubner MG, et al. CT-guided lung biopsies: pleural blood patching reduces the rate of chest tube placement for post-biopsy pneumothorax. AJR Am J Roentgenol 2011;197(4):783–8.

54. Petsas T, Vassilakos PJ, Dougenis D, et al. Fibrin glue for sealing the needle track after percutaneous lung biopsy: part I–experimental study. Cardiovasc Intervent Radiol 1995;18(6):373–7.

55. Yamagami T, Terayama K, Yoshimatsu R, et al. Role of manual aspiration in treating pneumothorax after computed tomography-guided lung biopsy. Acta Radiol 2009;50(10):1126–33.

56. Anderson CL, Crespo JC, Lie TH. Risk of pneumothorax not increased by obstructive lung disease in percutaneous needle biopsy. Chest 1994;105(6):1705–8.

57. Hu X, Cowl CT, Baqir M, et al. Air travel and pneumothorax. Chest 2014;145(4):688–94.

58. Tam A, Singh P, Ensor JE, et al. Air travel after biopsy-related pneumothorax: is it safe to fly? J Vasc Interv Radiol 2011;22(5):595–602.e1.

59. Bunch A, Duchateau FX, Verner L, et al. Commercial air travel after pneumothorax: a review of the literature. Air Med J 2013;32(5):268–74.

60. Yeow KM, See LC, Lui KW, et al. Risk factors for pneumothorax and bleeding after CT-guided percutaneous coaxial cutting needle biopsy of lung lesions. J Vasc Interv Radiol 2001;12(11):1305–12.

61. Richardson CM, Pointon KS, Manhire AR, et al. Percutaneous lung biopsies: a survey of UK practice based on 5444 biopsies. Br J Radiol 2002;75(897):731–5.

62. Tai R, Dunne RM, Trotman-Dickenson B, et al. Frequency and severity of pulmonary hemorrhage in patients undergoing percutaneous CT-guided transthoracic lung biopsy: single-institution experience of 1175 Cases. Radiology 2016;279(1):287–96.

63. Glassberg RM, Sussman SK, Glickstein MF. CT anatomy of the internal mammary vessels: importance in planning percutaneous transthoracic procedures. AJR Am J Roentgenol 1990;155(2):397–400.

64. Minot DM, Gilman EA, Aubry MC, et al. An investigation into false-negative transthoracic fine needle aspiration and core biopsy specimens. Diagn Cytopathol 2014;42(12):1063–8.

65. Fontaine-Delaruelle C, Souquet PJ, Gamondes D, et al. Negative predictive value of transthoracic core-needle biopsy: a multicenter study. Chest 2015;148(2):472–80.

66. Savage C, Walser EM, Schnadig V, et al. Transthoracic image-guided biopsy of lung nodules: when is benign really benign? J Vasc Interv Radiol 2004;15(2 Pt 1):161–4.

67. Calhoun P, Feldman PS, Armstrong P, et al. The clinical outcome of needle aspirations of the lung when cancer is not diagnosed. Ann Thorac Surg 1986;41(6):592–6.

68. Tomiyama N, Yasuhara Y, Nakajima Y, et al. CT-guided needle biopsy of lung lesions: a survey of severe complication based on 9783 biopsies in Japan. Eur J Radiol 2006;59(1):60–4.

69. Cheng HM, Chiang KH, Chang PY, et al. Coronary artery air embolism: a potentially fatal complication of CT-guided percutaneous lung biopsy. Br J Radiol 2010;83(988):e83–5.

70. Hiraki T, Fujiwara H, Sakurai J, et al. Nonfatal systemic air embolism complicating percutaneous CT-guided transthoracic needle biopsy: four cases from a single institution. Chest 2007;132(2):684–90.

71. Hirasawa S, Hirasawa H, Taketomi-Takahashi A, et al. Air embolism detected during computed tomography fluoroscopically guided transthoracic needle biopsy. Cardiovasc Intervent Radiol 2008;31(1):219–21.

Tumor Staging of Lung Cancer
Essential Concepts for the Radiologist

Constantine A. Raptis, MD[a],*, Caroline L. Robb, BS[b],
Sanjeev Bhalla, MD[a]

KEYWORDS

• Lung cancer • Staging • Lung adenocarcinoma • Subsolid • Computed tomography

KEY POINTS

- The recommendations for the eighth edition of the tumor, node, and metastasis staging system for lung cancer improve the prognostic discrimination of the various tumor (T) descriptors.
- New size cutoffs have been determined, demarcated by 1-cm increments and descriptors pertaining to local invasion and associated bronchial involvement have been reclassified.
- There are new T descriptors for adenocarcinoma in situ, minimally invasive adenocarcinoma, and part-solid adenocarcinomas.
- Recommendations for multifocal adenocarcinoma include the classification of the lesion with the highest level T descriptor and indication of the number of (#) or multiple (m) lesions.

INTRODUCTION

The staging of lung cancer substantially evolved with the publication of the seventh edition of the tumor (T), node (N), and metastasis (M) classification of lung cancer in 2009.[1–4] Despite many important advancements, characteristics of tumors important in prognostic determination, such as size and various forms of local invasion, were not addressed.[5] The International Association for the Study of Lung Cancer (IASLC) lung cancer staging project was tasked with addressing these issues with the eighth edition of the TNM classification of lung cancer. The eighth edition is based on a database prospectively acquired from 1999 to 2010 and proposes significant changes to the T and M descriptors. This article focuses on the T descriptor, which is based on the size of the primary tumor, the extent of invasion of local structures, and the presence and location of additional ipsilateral tumor nodules. Along with

changes to the staging system itself, the staging project also made important recommendations on the categorization of subsolid nodules and the classification of multiple primary tumor sites. These recommendations are also integral to understanding the T descriptor and are discussed in detail.

TUMOR DESCRIPTOR

The T descriptor in the staging of lung cancer depends on the size of the primary tumor, the extent of invasion of local structures, and the presence and location of additional ipsilateral tumor nodules. For lung cancers, the clinical T (cT) descriptor is typically assessed with a combination of physical examination, imaging, and biopsy. The final cT descriptor of a lung cancer is determined by the descriptor that confers the most advanced stage. It is important to understand that the cT of lung cancers is inexact. For example, abutment

[a] Mallinckrodt Institute of Radiology, 510 South Kingshighway, St Louis, MO 63110, USA; [b] Washington University School of Medicine, 510 South Kingshighway, St Louis, MO 63110, USA
* Corresponding author.
E-mail address: raptisc@wustl.edu

of the pleura does not definitely mean there is pleural invasion. Likewise, the presence of pulmonary nodules does not automatically confirm intrapulmonary metastatic disease. However, it is desirable to have a means of determining the T descriptor of a lung cancer before pursuing definitive therapy. Understanding the cT descriptor can help determine whether surgery will provide benefit and whether other therapies, such as radiation and chemotherapy, should be used as an alternative or used in an adjuvant or neoadjuvant capacity.

Tumor Size

In the seventh edition of the lung cancer staging system, size cutoffs of 2 cm, 3 cm, 5 cm, and 7 cm were used to separate T1a, T1b, T2a, T2b, and T3 lesions, respectively.[4] In the analysis of the eighth edition prospective database, a progressive degradation of survival was observed with 1-cm increments of tumor size for tumors 1 to 5 cm. The subclassification of T1 to incorporate a separate descriptor for lesions of 1 cm or less (T1a) is important given the increased detection of small and earlier stage lung cancers on both routine chest CT and dedicated lung cancer screening CT examinations.[6–9] Furthermore, tumors between 5 cm and 7 cm had a prognosis similar to T3 tumors, whereas tumors greater than 7 cm had a prognosis similar to T4 tumors.[6] These findings led to revised T descriptors for tumor sizes, which are summarized in **Table 1**.

Given the prognostic and potential therapeutic implications of tumor size, accurate measurement of the primary tumor size on imaging is important. Tumor size is determined by measuring the greatest long axis measurement of the primary tumor and typically requires performing multiplanar reconstructions of the primary lesion because the long axis rarely lies in the axial imaging plane.[6] Measurement of the primary tumor can often be difficult due to adjacent atelectasis. The use of intravenous contrast for CT examinations is often helpful for determining the demarcation between the tumor and the adjacent atelectatic lung. The superior contrast resolution of MR imaging can also be helpful for this assessment.

Local Extent

The prospective database used in the eighth edition T descriptor recommendations is based on cases reporting the extent of local invasion. Specific T descriptors were identified for reclassification based on differences in survival when compared with other descriptors in the same or adjacent category. One important change to the

Table 1
Tumor descriptors in the eighth edition of the staging system for lung cancer

T Descriptor	Criterion	Stage
Size	≤1 cm	T1a
	>1 cm, ≤2 cm	T1b (T1a)
	>2 cm, ≤3 cm	T1c (T1b)
	>3 cm, ≤4 cm	T2a
	>4 cm, ≤5 cm	T2b (T2a)
	>5 cm, ≤7 cm	T3 (T2b)
	>7 cm	T4 (T3)
Local invasion	Visceral pleura	T2
	Parietal pleura	T3
	Parietal pericardium	T3
	Chest wall	T3
	Superior sulcus	T3
	Rib	T3
	Phrenic nerve	T3
	Diaphragm	T4 (T3)
	Mediastinum	T4
	Heart or great vessels	T4
	Trachea	T4
	Esophagus	T4
	Vertebral body	T4
	Recurrent laryngeal nerve	T4
Airway and atelectasis	Mainstem bronchus <2 cm from carina	T2 (T3)
	Mainstem bronchus >2 cm from carina	T2
	Carina	T4
	Atelectasis of whole lung	T2 (T3)
	Atelectasis of part less than whole lung	T2
Nodules	Same lobe as primary tumor	T3
	Ipsilateral lung, different lobe	T4

Changes from the seventh edition staging system are in parentheses. Of note, mediastinal pleural invasion was removed from the local invasion criteria in the eighth edition staging system.

local invasion criteria relates to the distance of primary tumors involving the mainstem bronchus from the carina. In the previous staging system, tumors involving the mainstem bronchus but less than 2 cm from the carina were T3, whereas those greater than 2 cm from the carina were T2. In the eighth edition staging system, the 2-cm cutoff in distance from the carina as a contributor to T descriptor has been eliminated. Tumors involving the mainstem bronchus, regardless of distance from the carina, are T2, whereas invasion of the carina remains a T4 descriptor.[4,6] However, reporting the location of the primary tumor along the mainstem bronchus should still be performed for the purposes of surgical planning.

In the seventh edition staging system, postobstructive atelectasis or pneumonitis was T2 (partial atelectasis of a lung) and T3 (complete atelectasis of a lung). In the eighth edition, partial and complete atelectasis are both given a T2 descriptor.[4,6] Because postobstructive atelectasis or pneumonitis may not be detectable after resection, reporting of this finding on imaging is important. As such, atelectasis or pneumonitis detected on imaging alone can still be used in determining the pathologic T (pT) descriptor.

Visceral pleural involvement, defined as invasion beyond the elastic layer of the pleural connective tissue, retains the T2 descriptor in the eighth edition staging system.[6,10] Visceral pleural invasion is defined via pathologic analysis of a resected specimen and cannot be determined on imaging studies. Extension from 1 lobe to another through the visceral pleura or an incomplete fissure is also a T2 descriptor. Parietal pleural invasion remains a T3 descriptor. Of note, mediastinal pleural invasion has been removed as a discrete descriptor because invasion of the mediastinal pleura without deeper invasion into the mediastinum is rare. Thus, the T descriptor for mediastinal pleural invasion is the same as invasion of the pleura elsewhere.[6]

Evaluation of pleural invasion is not reliable on computed tomography (CT). Extended contact with the pleura (>3 cm) is a sensitive but not specific finding of pleural involvement.[11] Conversely, extension into the subpleural fat is specific but not sensitive. The authors' practice is to report the length of contact of the tumor with the pleura, but not to use this finding to definitively indicate pleural invasion. It is also relevant to note when lesions tether the pleura or are connected to it by soft tissue bands, as tumor can grow through adhesions and invade the subjacent pleura (**Fig. 1**). Newer imaging techniques that are not widely used, including directed ultrasonography and dynamic cine MR imaging, have been used to evaluate for focal pleural adherence. If the lesion and the pleura slide against each other, pleural adherence is not present.[12–14]

Invasion of the chest wall, superior sulcus, phrenic nerve, and parietal pericardium remain as T3 descriptors.[6] Frank chest wall involvement can be identified on CT as extension of a soft tissue mass into the chest wall fat, musculature, or bones. MR imaging, by virtue of its superior contrast resolution, can also be helpful for

determining chest wall invasion. However, it is important to note that lung cancer invasion into the chest wall can be seen pathologically in the absence of invasion on imaging.

Mediastinal, heart, great vessel, trachea, esophagus, vertebral body, and recurrent laryngeal nerve involvement remain as T4 descriptors. Diaphragm invasion, previously a T3 descriptor, is a T4 descriptor in the eighth edition staging system because its prognosis is similar to other T4 descriptors.[6] A summary of the invasion criteria used for the T descriptor in the eighth TNM staging system for lung cancer is provided in **Table 1**.

Additional Ipsilateral Tumor Nodules

T descriptors for tumor nodules in the ipsilateral and contralateral lung are unchanged in the eighth edition staging system. Nodules in the same lobe of the primary tumor are T3, whereas nodules in a lobe in the ipsilateral lung different from the primary tumor are T4.[4] Nodules discovered on imaging studies have a differential diagnosis of metastatic disease, synchronous primary tumor, or benign lesion.[7,15–17] It is important to note the location of nodules so they can be sampled either preoperatively or at the time of surgery if possible and deemed necessary. Evaluation of indeterminate lung nodules may also involve PET-CT or a follow-up CT. In noting the location of indeterminate nodules, radiologists should indicate the specific location of the most distant or concerning nodules, as these will be the determinant of the patient's T (or M) stage.

NEW UNDERSTANDING OF LUNG ADENOCARCINOMA

In 2011, adenocarcinoma in situ (AIS), minimally invasive adenocarcinoma (MIA), and lepidic predominant adenocarcinoma (LPA) were defined by the IASLC/American Thoracic Society/European Radiology Society and later adopted into the 2015 World Health Organization Classification of lung tumors.[18,19] The IASLC lung cancer staging project incorporated these new entities into the TNM staging system. The T descriptor of Tis(AIS) for AIS and T1(mi) for MIA are used. Adenocarcinomas comprise mucinous and nonmucinous tumors. Mucinous AIS, MIA, and LPA typically manifest on CT as solid nodules or foci of airspace opacification with air bronchograms, whereas nonmucinous tumors manifest as solid or subsolid lesions, either nonsolid (pure ground-glass) or part-solid (ground-glass and solid components).[20] In part-solid nodules along the nonmucinous adenocarcinoma spectrum, the ground-glass component on CT typically corresponds to lepidic growth,

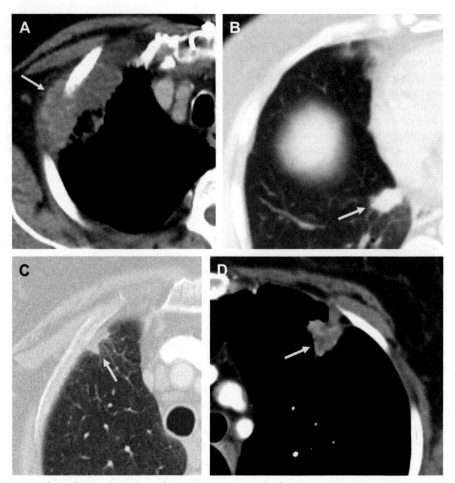

Fig. 1. (*A*) A CT with mediastinal windows shows direct extension of a right upper lobe adenocarcinoma into the chest wall (*arrow*). Visualization of tumor extension into the chest wall is a specific sign of invasion through the pleura. (*B*) A CT with lung widows from a different patient shows a right lower lobe adenocarcinoma (*arrow*) that abuts the mediastinal pleura over a short length (less than 1 cm). On resection, there was invasion of the visceral pleura through adhesions. (*C*) A CT with lung windows shows a right upper lobe squamous cell cancer (*arrow*) in contact with the pleura greater than 1.4 cm. No gross invasion was seen into the subpleural fat or ribs. Despite the proximity of the malignancy with the adjacent pleura, there was no pleural invasion on resection. (*D*) A CT with mediastinal windows, shows a left upper lobe adenocarcinoma (*arrow*) connected to the pleura via soft tissue bands. Despite these soft tissue bands, there was no pleural invasion on resection. Gross extension into the subpleural fat or chest wall is the only definitive sign on CT of pleural invasion, although abutment of the pleura 3 cm or greater is suspicious for pleural involvement and should be described in radiology reports.

whereas the solid component corresponds to the invasive component. In LPA manifesting as a part-solid nodule, the size of the solid component representing the invasive component should be used to determine the T descriptor.[20] Nonmucinous AIS most commonly manifests on CT as a pure ground-glass nodule, although a small solid component can be present owing to collapse of alveolar walls or a benign scar.[21–26] Nonmucinous MIA most often manifests on CT as a part-solid nodule with a total size of 3 cm or less and a solid component of 1 cm or less but also can manifest as a pure ground-glass or, rarely, a solid nodule.[22,27,28] Nonmucinous LPA manifests on CT as a part-solid nodule; a solid nodule; or, rarely, a pure ground-glass nodule.[20] Distinguishing between these entities can be difficult but increasing overall size, increasing size of the solid component, increasing attenuation of the ground-glass component, air bronchograms, distortion of adjacent vasculature, and pleural indentation should suggest nonmucinous MIA or LPA instead of AIS.[20,22,27,28] As a general guideline, on CT, nonmucinous AIS should not have a solid component greater than 0.5 cm and nonmucinous MIA should not have a solid component greater than 1.0 cm.

For any part-solid nodule with a solid component greater than 0.5 cm, invasive adenocarcinoma should also be in the differential diagnosis, and invasive adenocarcinoma should be favored when the solid component is greater than 2 cm[20] (Box 1 and Fig. 2).

The invasive component can be overestimated on CT due to concomitant scarring, whereas small invasive components may not be detectable on CT.[18,20,29] However, CT is used to determine the cT descriptor of the tumor before definitive pathologic confirmation following resection. For lesions with a solid component greater than 0.5 cm, the differential diagnosis should include nonmucinous LPA and invasive adenocarcinoma, both lesions which should be given T descriptors correlating with the size of the solid component of the lesion.

The IASLC lung cancer staging project recommends that part-solid nodules be assessed on thin section (1 mm preferred) CT images. Currently, lung windows are recommended when measuring the size of the invasive component because mediastinal window measurements may underestimate invasion in comparison with pathologic measurements. The solid component should be measured in its largest dimension, which may require multiplanar reconstructions.[20] When the solid component is less than 1 cm, MIA can be included in the differential diagnosis along with LPA and invasive adenocarcinoma. For example, a part-solid tumor with total nodule size of

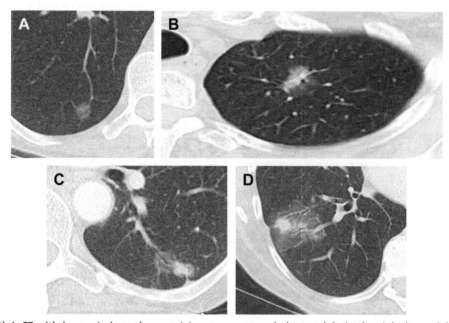

Fig. 2. (A) A CT with lung windows shows a 1.1-cm pure ground-glass nodule in the right lower lobe. The cT descriptor for this nodule is cTis. Following resection, pathologic evaluation confirmed AIS and the pT descriptor is pTis(AIS). Although the most common imaging appearance of AIS is a pure ground-glass nodule, it can have a solid component less than 5 mm due to collapse of alveolar walls or scarring. (B) A CT with lung windows shows a left upper lobe part-solid nodule with a solid component measuring 3 mm. The cT descriptor for this nodule is cT1 minimally invasive (cT1mi), and could represent AIS, MIA, or LPA pathologically. Following resection, pathologic evaluation showed MIA and the pT descriptor is pT1mi. (C) A CT with lung windows shows a left lower lobe part-solid lesion with a 7-mm solid component. The differential diagnosis includes MIA, T1a(mi); LPA, T1a; and invasive adenocarcinoma, T1a. Following resection, pathologic evaluation showed LPA. (D) CT with lung windows shows a right lower lobe part-solid nodule with a 1.1-cm solid component. The differential diagnosis includes LPA T1b and invasive adenocarcinoma T1b. Following resection, pathologic evaluation showed invasive adenocarcinoma. The presence of larger soft tissue components of part-solid nodules should increase the suspicion for invasive adenocarcinoma. ([A] *Courtesy of* Kristopher Cummings, MD, Mayo Clinic, Scottsdale, AZ.)

2.0 cm and a 0.7-cm solid component has the T descriptor of cT1a and the differential pathologic diagnosis includes MIA, LPA, and invasive adenocarcinoma. Total lesion size (ground-glass plus solid component) should also be measured and reported because lesions with a ground-glass component greater than 3 cm without a solid component or with a solid component of less than or equal to 0.5 cm have a cT1a descriptor.

Part-solid nodules can have multiple solid components. There is no consensus about how to estimate the invasive component of these nodules on CT. Pathologically, the sum of the invasive components can be expressed as a percentage of the entire lesion; however, the current recommendation from the IASLC for cT descriptor determination is to measure the long axis of the largest solid component as a means of estimating the invasive component.[20]

MULTIPLE LUNG NODULES

Multiple pulmonary sites of lung cancer can be attributed to (1) a solid primary lung cancer with 1 or more separate solid tumor nodules of the same histologic type (intrapulmonary metastasis), (2) 2 separate primary lung cancers, (3) multiple lung cancer nodules with prominent ground-glass or lepidic features, and (4) pneumonic-type lung cancer manifesting as diffuse or multinodular areas of consolidation. The IASLC lung cancer staging project for the eighth edition of the TNM staging system had subcommittees formulate instructions on how to apply the TNM classification to these 4 manifestations of multifocal lung cancer (see later discussion).

Patients with a solid primary lung cancer are classified as having separate tumor nodules when there is a dominant lung nodule or mass and one (or more) solid separate lung nodules, either presumed or proved to have the same histologic features. A primary lung cancer with one or more separate solid tumor nodules of the same histologic type (intrapulmonary metastasis) has a T3 descriptor if the additional tumor nodules are in the same lobe and T4 if the additional tumor nodules are in an ipsilateral lobe different from the primary tumor. If there are additional tumor nodules in the contralateral lung, the disease is classified as M1a and the T descriptor should be determined by the other characteristics of the primary lesion.[30]

The criterion used to determine whether two tumors are synchronous or separate primary tumors relies on histologic assessment; for example, squamous or adenocarcinoma. Factors suggestive of separate primary tumors include different radiologic appearance or metabolic uptake, different rates of growth, absence of nodal or systemic metastases, and different biomarker patterns. The decision to classify two lesions as synchronous primary cancers is ideally determined by a multidisciplinary team, taking into account clinical, imaging, and histologic factors. The proposed TNM classification for synchronous primary lung cancers is that each cancer is classified separately with its own T, N, and M descriptor.

Primary lung cancers manifesting as multiple subsolid nodules (either pure ground-glass or part-solid) often exhibit a more indolent behavior with a decreased propensity for nodal or systemic spread and an increased propensity to the development of additional subsolid cancers. In patients with an adenocarcinoma manifesting as a subsolid nodule, which could represent AIS, MIA, or LPA, additional nodules with ground-glass features should be considered multiple sites of disease, regardless of whether they have been biopsied or if these additional nodules are proven to be AIS, MIA, or LPA.[30,31] Lesions which are purely ground-glass and less than 5 mm in size should not be counted as additional sites of disease because they may represent a benign or preneoplastic condition such as adenomatous alveolar hyperplasia.[30]

Multifocal adenocarcinoma is classified by the T descriptor of the lesion with the highest T along with the number (#) of lesions or multiple (m) indicated in parentheses, and an N and M category that applies to all of the multiple tumor foci collectively. The T(#/m) multifocal classification should be applied equally whether the lesions are in the same lobe or in different ipsilateral or contralateral lobes. For example, if a patient with an MIA demonstrating a 5 mm solid component also has 5 other subsolid lesions suspicious for additional foci of disease that have solid components less than 5 mm, the T descriptor T1a(mi) (6) would be used. It should be noted that in contrast to patients with intrapulmonary metastases, in patients with multifocal adenocarcinoma with ground-glass or lepidic features, the lobes involved do not affect the T or M staging.[20,30]

Diffuse pneumonic-type adenocarcinomas, typically of mucinous histology, are associated with a worse prognosis but also with a decreased propensity for nodal and distant metastases. Pneumonic-type adenocarcinomas often have poorly demarcated borders and are difficult to measure. Per the IASLC lung cancer staging project, if there is one site of pulmonary involvement in a single lobe, the standard T staging criteria should be used with size measurements as would be given for a solid mass. If the disease is difficult to measure but confined to a single lobe, the T3 descriptor should be used. In cases of pneumonic-type adenocarcinoma that involve multiple lobes, T4 should be used to describe tumors with sites of disease in multiple lobes of the same lung, whereas M1a should be used to describe tumors with sites of disease in both lungs.[30]

EFFECT ON STAGE GROUPINGS

After the T, N, and M descriptors are determined, an overall stage grouping is assigned to describe the burden of disease. Stage groupings are a prognostic factor that help guide, but do not necessarily dictate, treatment recommendations. The IASLC issued a full report on recommendations for changes to the stage groupings for lung cancer in the new eighth edition staging system. These recommendations were based on analysis of the new prospective database used for the eighth edition revisions of the TNM staging system.[32] In light of the many changes to the TNM staging system, modifying the stage groupings is complex as the stage groupings needed to be adjusted to incorporate the changes to the TNM staging system itself. Consequently, given the increased number of T descriptors, particularly related to the new 1-cm cutoff points for size, a more complex set of stage groupings was recommended. In addition, the committee reviewed survival using the new database and modified the stages accordingly.

Overall, for non-small cell lung cancer, stage-for-stage survival increased across all stages, likely a reflection of improved diagnosis and treatment of lung cancer. There was, however, a relative worsening of survival for more advanced stages, particularly IIIB. These survival analyses led to reclassification of some disease distributions into other stages, as well as the creation of new stage groupings; for example, the new IIIC stage for patients with a distribution of disease between the IIB and IVA groups.[32] Ultimately, a detailed understanding of the stage groupings is not generally required for imaging interpretation. What is necessary is an appreciation that the imaging characteristics that lead to T, N, and M descriptor assignments are ultimately used to determine an overall stage group to define patient prognosis and management.

SUMMARY

The recommendations for the eighth edition TNM staging system for lung cancer are an important step forward in mitigating the arbitrary nature with which the T descriptor had been assigned to the primary tumor and improving the prognostic discrimination of the various T descriptors. New size cutoffs have been determined, demarcated by 1-cm increments, and descriptors pertaining to local invasion and associated bronchial involvement have been reclassified. In response to improved understanding of adenocarcinoma, the IASLC has also provided new T descriptors for AIS, MIA, and part-solid adenocarcinomas. Recommendations for multifocal adenocarcinoma include the classification of the lesion with the highest level T descriptor and indication of the number of lesions by (#) or (m). In conclusion, the eighth edition of the TNM staging system improves staging and provides guidelines to stratify patients with lung cancer to better determine appropriate management and prognosis.

REFERENCES

1. Raptis CA, Bhalla S. The 7th edition of the TNM staging system for lung cancer. Radiol Clin North Am 2012;50(5):915–33.
2. Sobin L, Gospodarowicz M, Wittekind C. TNM classification of malignant tumors. 7th edition. Hoboken (NJ): Wiley Blackwell; 2009.
3. Groome PA, Bolejack V, Crowley JJ, et al. The IASLC lung cancer staging project: validation of the proposals for revision of the T, N, and M descriptors and consequent stage groupings in the forthcoming (seventh) edition of the TNM classification of malignant tumours. J Thorac Oncol 2007;2(8):694–705.
4. Rami-Porta R, Ball D, Crowley J, et al. The IASLC lung cancer staging project: proposals for the revision of the T descriptors in the forthcoming (seventh) edition of the TNM classification for lung cancer. J Thorac Oncol 2007;2(7):593–602.
5. Rami-Porta R, Bolejack V, Giroux DJ, et al. The IASLC lung cancer staging project: the new database to inform the eighth edition of the TNM classification of lung cancer. J Thorac Oncol 2014;9(11): 1618–24.
6. Rami-Porta R, Bolejack V, Crowley J, et al. The IASLC lung cancer staging project: proposals for the revisions of the T descriptors in the forthcoming eighth edition of the TNM classification for lung cancer. J Thorac Oncol 2015;10(7):990–1003.
7. Henschke CI, McCauley DI, Yankelevitz DF, et al. Early lung cancer action project: overall design and findings from baseline screening. Lancet 1999;354(9173):99–105.
8. Horeweg N, van der Aalst CM, Thunnissen E, et al. Characteristics of lung cancers detected by computer tomography screening in the randomized NELSON trial. Am J Respir Crit Care Med 2013; 187(8):848–54.

9. National Lung Screening Trial Research Team, Aberle DR, Adams AM, Berg CD, et al. Reduced lung-cancer mortality with low-dose computed tomographic screening. N Engl J Med 2011; 365(5):395–409.

10. Travis WD, Brambilla E, Rami-Porta R, et al. Visceral pleural invasion: pathologic criteria and use of elastic stains: proposal for the 7th edition of the TNM classification for lung cancer. J Thorac Oncol 2008;3(12):1384–90.

11. Glazer HS, Duncan-Meyer J, Aronberg DJ, et al. Pleural and chest wall invasion in bronchogenic carcinoma: CT evaluation. Radiology 1985;157(1): 191–4.

12. Bandi V, Lunn W, Ernst A, et al. Ultrasound vs CT in detecting chest wall invasion by tumor. Chest 2008; 133(4):881–6.

13. Kajiwara N, Akata S, Uchida O, et al. Cine MRI enables better therapeutic planning than CT in cases of possible lung cancer chest wall invasion. Lung Cancer 2010;69(2):203–8.

14. Akata S, Kajiwara N, Park J, et al. Evaluation of chest wall invasion by lung cancer using respiratory dynamic MRI. J Med Imaging Radiat Oncol 2008; 52(1):36–9.

15. Kunitoh H, Eguchi K, Yamada K, et al. Intrapulmonary sublesions detected before surgery in patients with lung cancer. Cancer 1992;70(7):1876–9.

16. Keogan MT, Tung KT, Kaplan DK, et al. The significance of pulmonary nodules detected on CT staging for lung cancer. Clin Radiol 1993;48(2):94–6.

17. Swensen SJ, Jett JR, Hartman TE, et al. CT screening for lung cancer: five-year prospective experience. Radiology 2005;235(1):259–65.

18. Travis WD, Brambilla E, Noguchi M, et al. International Association for the Study of Lung Cancer/ American Thoracic Society/European Respiratory Society international multidisciplinary classification of lung adenocarcinoma. J Thorac Oncol 2011; 6(2):244–85.

19. Travis WD, Brambilla E, Burke A, et al. WHO classification of tumours of the lung, pleura, thymus, and heart. 4th edition. Lyon (France): IARC Press; 2015.

20. Travis WD, Asamura H, Bankier AA, et al. The IASLC lung cancer staging project: proposals for coding T categories for subsolid nodules and assessment of tumor size in part-solid tumors in the forthcoming eighth edition of the TNM classification of lung cancer. J Thorac Oncol 2016;11(8):1204–23.

21. Cohen JG, Reymond E, Lederlin M, et al. Differentiating pre- and minimally invasive from invasive adenocarcinoma using CT-features in persistent pulmonary part-solid nodules in Caucasian patients. Eur J Radiol 2015;84(4):738–44.

22. Zhang Y, Qiang JW, Ye JD, et al. High resolution CT in differentiating minimally invasive component in early lung adenocarcinoma. Lung Cancer 2014; 84(3):236–41.

23. Zhang H, Duan J, Li Z-J, et al. Analysis on minimally invasive diagnosis and treatment of 49 cases with solitary nodular ground-glass opacity. J Thorac Dis 2014;6(10):1452–7.

24. Lee HY, Choi Y-L, Lee KS, et al. Pure ground-glass opacity neoplastic lung nodules: histopathology, imaging, and management. AJR Am J Roentgenol 2014;202(3):W224–33.

25. Lee HY, Lee KS. Ground-glass opacity nodules: histopathology, imaging evaluation, and clinical implications. J Thorac Imaging 2011;26(2):106–18.

26. Isaka T, Yokose T, Ito H, et al. Comparison between CT tumor size and pathological tumor size in frozen section examinations of lung adenocarcinoma. Lung Cancer 2014;85(1):40–6.

27. Lee KH, Goo JM, Park SJ, et al. Correlation between the size of the solid component on thin-section CT and the invasive component on pathology in small lung adenocarcinomas manifesting as ground-glass nodules. J Thorac Oncol 2014;9(1):74–82.

28. Lee SM, Goo JM, Lee KH, et al. CT findings of minimally invasive adenocarcinoma (MIA) of the lung and comparison of solid portion measurement methods at CT in 52 patients. Eur Radiol 2015; 25(8):2318–25.

29. Yamada N, Kusumoto M, Maeshima A, et al. Correlation of the solid part on high-resolution computed tomography with pathological scar in small lung adenocarcinomas. Jpn J Clin Oncol 2007;37(12): 913–7.

30. Detterbeck FC, Nicholson AG, Franklin WA, et al. The IASLC lung cancer staging project: summary of proposals for revisions of the classification of lung cancers with multiple pulmonary sites of involvement in the forthcoming eighth edition of the TNM classification. J Thorac Oncol 2016;11(5): 639–50.

31. Detterbeck FC, Marom EM, Arenberg DA, et al. The IASLC lung cancer staging project: background data and proposals for the application of TNM staging rules to lung cancer presenting as multiple nodules with ground glass or lepidic features or a pneumonic type of involvement in the forthcoming eighth edition of the TNM classification. J Thorac Oncol 2016;11(5):666–80.

32. Goldstraw P, Chansky K, Crowley J, et al. The IASLC lung cancer staging project: proposals for revision of the TNM stage groupings in the forthcoming (eighth) edition of the TNM classification for lung cancer. J Thorac Oncol 2016;11(1):39–51.

Staging Lung Cancer
Regional Lymph Node Classification

Ahmed H. El-Sherief, MD[a,b,]*, Charles T. Lau, MD, MBA[c], Brett W. Carter, MD[d],
Carol C. Wu, MD[d]

KEYWORDS

- Lung cancer • Staging • Lymph node • Lymph node map
- International association for the study of lung cancer (IASLC)

KEY POINTS

- N descriptor refers to absence or presence of regional nodal metastatic disease.
- Regional lymph node maps have been created to standardize the assessment of the N descriptor for lung cancer.
- According to the eighth edition of the tumor-node-metastasis staging system for lung cancer, the International Association for the Study of Lung Cancer lymph node map is to be used for the standardization of N descriptor assessment.

INTRODUCTION

In the tumor-node-metastasis (TNM) staging system for lung cancer, the N descriptor refers to the absence or location of cancer spread to a regional lymph node.[1] Lung cancer spread to a nonregional lymph node is considered a distant metastasis (M descriptor in the TNM staging system).[1]

In the eighth edition of the TNM staging system, the N descriptors used in the seventh edition are unchanged because they adequately predict prognosis. The principle has been maintained that the nodal descriptors be based on the anatomic location of the metastatic lymph node in the thorax and not on the number of metastatic lymph nodes (nN). Even though the number of involved nodal stations has prognostic impact on pathologic lymph node(pN)

staging, this has not been validated for clinical lymph node staging (cN) and, hence, is not a recommendation in the eighth edition. It is recommended, however, that the nN (or stations) be recorded.

The clinical determination of the N descriptor requires a multimodality approach. Computed tomography (CT), positron emission tomography/computed tomography (PET/CT) with fluorodeoxyglucose (FDG), esophageal ultrasound (EUS) and/or endobronchial ultrasonography (EBUS), and mediastinoscopy are the common modalities used to clinically determine the N descriptor. This review discusses the N descriptors in the eighth edition of the TNM staging system for lung cancer, the anatomic definitions for describing regional lymph nodes, and the various imaging and invasive techniques for tissue sampling.

[a] Section of Thoracic Imaging, Department of Diagnostic Radiology, Veterans Affairs Greater Los Angeles Healthcare System, 11301 Wilshire Boulevard, Building 500, Los Angeles, CA 90073, USA; [b] David Geffen School of Medicine, University of California, Los Angeles, 10833 Le Conte Avenue, Los Angeles, CA 90095, USA; [c] Section of Cardiothoracic Imaging, Radiology Service, Veterans Affairs Palo Alto Healthcare System, 3801 Miranda Avenue, Palo Alto, CA 94304, USA; [d] Department of Diagnostic Radiology, University of Texas MD Anderson Cancer Center, 1515 Holcombe Boulevard, Unit 1478, Houston, TX 77030, USA
* Corresponding author. Section of Thoracic Imaging, Department of Diagnostic Radiology, Greater Los Angeles Veterans Administration Healthcare System, 11301 Wilshire Boulevard, Building 500, Los Angeles, CA 90073.
E-mail address: ahelsherief@gmail.com

Radiol Clin N Am 56 (2018) 399–409
https://doi.org/10.1016/j.rcl.2018.01.008
0033-8389/18/Published by Elsevier Inc.

INTERNATIONAL ASSOCIATION FOR THE STUDY OF LUNG CANCER LYMPH NODE MAP DEFINITIONS SETS

The location of regional nodal metastasis is important when determining treatment and prognosis.[1] Accordingly, regional lymph node maps have been created to standardize the assessment of the N descriptor. In these maps, lymph nodes are labeled using a system of numerical levels and assigned names based their anatomical location. The first lung cancer lymph node map was created by Naruke and colleagues.[2,3] Subsequently the American Thoracic Society, and the Mountain-Dresler modification of the American Thoracic Society lymph node map were also used to describe nodal metastases.[4–6] Because the discrepancy between the maps resulted in an overall discordance of 31.5% in the assessment of the N descriptor, the International Association for the Study of Lung Cancer (IASLC) proposed a new lymph node map to reconcile the differences among the maps.[7] The IASLC lymph node map is used in the eighth edition of the TNM staging system and defines 14 regional lymph node stations (**Figs. 1–7**).[6]

REGIONAL LYMPH NODE (N) CLASSIFICATION

In lung cancer, the N descriptor in the TNM staging system is classified as N0, N1, N2, N3, or NX. N0 refers to the absence of lung cancer spread to a regional lymph node. N1 refers to lung cancer spread to 1 or more ipsilateral hilar, interlobar,

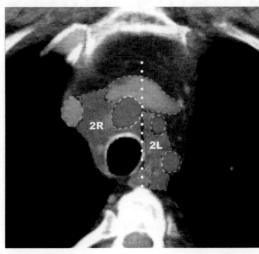

Fig. 2. Stations 2R and 2L. Axial CT image below the level of the apex of the lungs, and above the level where the caudal margin of the left innominate vein intersects with the trachea. The left lateral wall of the trachea (*dotted white line*) separates station 2R (*yellow area*) from station 2L (*green area*). Red and blue indicate arterial and venous structures, respectively.

lobar, and segmental and/or subsegmental lymph nodes. N2 refers to lung cancer spread to ipsilateral mediastinal and/or subcarinal lymph nodes (**Fig. 8**). N3 refers to lung cancer spread to contralateral mediastinal, hilar, interlobar, lobar, segmental, subsegmental lymph nodes and/or to contralateral or ipsilateral low cervical, supraclavicular, or sternal notch lymph nodes. NX refers

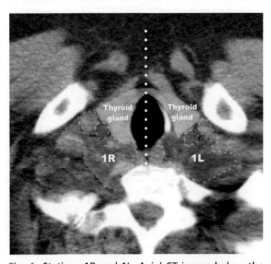

Fig. 1. Stations 1R and 1L. Axial CT image below the level of the cricoid cartilage and above the level of the manubrium. The midline of the trachea (*dotted white line*) separates station 1R (*yellow area*) from station 1L (*green area*). Red and blue indicate arterial and venous structures, respectively.

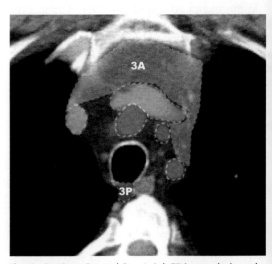

Fig. 3. Stations 3a and 3p. Axial CT image below the level of the apex of the chest and above the level of the carina demonstrates station 3a (*yellow area*) and station 3p (*green area*). Red and blue indicate arterial and venous structures, respectively.

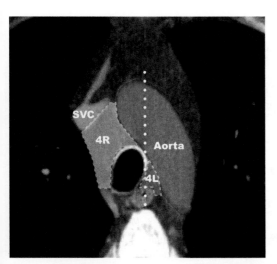

Fig. 4. Stations 4R and 4L. Axial CT image below the level where the caudal margin of the left innominate vein intersects with the trachea and above the level the lower margin of the azygos vein as it crosses over the right main stem bronchus to drain into the superior vena cava. The left lateral wall of the trachea (*dotted white line*) separates station 4R (*yellow area*) from station 4L (*green area*). SVC, superior vena cava.

to inability to assess lung cancer spread to a regional lymph node.

In the current location-based N descriptor categorization, prognosis does not take into consideration the tumor burden in regional lymph nodes. The nN may be a potentially better prognostic indicator in the clinical setting than the location-based nodal classification.[8,9]

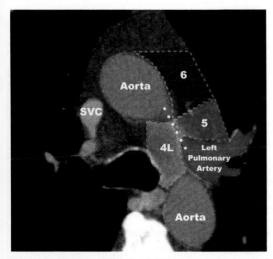

Fig. 5. Stations 5 and 6. Axial CT image at the level of the aorticopulmonary window demonstrates station 5 (*green area*) and station 6 (*purple area*). The ligamentum arteriosum (*white dotted line*) separates station 5 (*green area*) from station 4L (*yellow area*). SVC, superior vena cava.

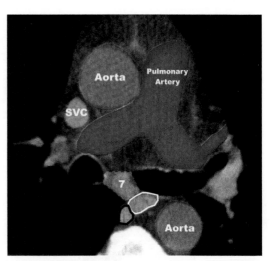

Fig. 6. Station 7. Axial CT image below the level of the carina but above the level of the bronchus intermedius demonstrates station 7 (*yellow area*). SVC, superior vena cava.

In a recent analysis of pathologically staged lung cancers from the IASLC Lung Cancer Staging Project database, it was found that there was a prognostic impact of subcategorizing pN1 and pN2 by the number of involved lymph node stations and by the absence or presence of skip metastasis. The analysis showed survival differences between single vs multiple N1 station involvement, differences between single vs multiple N2 station involvement, but no difference between multiple N1 station involvement and a single N2 station involvement with skip metastasis (no N1 involvement). Because the number of lymph node stations involved has prognostic impact based on pN staging, further classification into the following groups has been suggested: (1) single pN1 station (pN1a) and multiple pN1 stations (pN1b) and (2) single pN2 station (pN2a) and multiple pN2 stations (pN2b). In addition, the presence of skip metastasis should also be denoted with (1) single pN2 node with skip metastasis (no pN1 involvement [pN2a1]) and (2) single pN2 without skip metastasis (pN1 involvement [pN2a2]).[10] In summary, recent analyses suggest that the combination of location of metastatic nodes, number of involved metastatic lymph node stations, and the absence or presence of skip metastasis may be part of future revisions of the TNM staging system for lung cancer.

MEDIASTINAL LYMPH NODE STAGING

In the absence of a distant metastasis, the absence (N0) or location of lung cancer spread to a regional lymph node (N1–N3) determines treatment options and prognosis. For patients

International Association for the Study of Lung Cancer
Nodal Chart

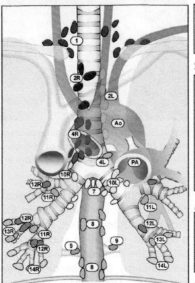

Supraclavicular zone

● 1 Low cervical, supraclavicular, and sternal notch nodes

SUPERIOR MEDIASTINAL NODES

Upper zone

● 2R Upper Paratracheal (right)
○ 2L Upper Paratracheal (left)
● 3a Prevascular
● 3p Retrotracheal
● 4R Lower Paratracheal (right)
○ 4L Lower Paratracheal (left)

AORTIC NODES

AP zone

● 5 Subaortic
○ 6 Para-aortic (ascending aorta or phrenic)

INFERIOR MEDIASTINAL NODES

Subcarinal zone

○ 7 Subcarinal

Lower zone

● 8 Paraesophageal (below carina)
● 9 Pulmonary ligament

N1 NODES

Hilar/Interlobar zone

○ 10 Hilar
● 11 Interlobar

Peripheral zone

● 12 Lobar
○ 13 Segmental
○ 14 Subsegmental

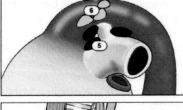

Fig. 7. IASLC nodal chart and nodal definitions. (*From* Rusch VW, Asamura H, Watanabe H, et al. The IASLC lung cancer staging project: a proposal for a new international lymph node map in the forthcoming seventh edition of the TNM classification for lung cancer. J Thorac Oncol 2009;4[5]:568–77; with permission.)

with a pretreatment descriptor of N0M0 or N1M0, surgery may be the only treatment indicated. For patients with pretreatment descriptors of N2M0 or N3M0, treatment options often involve a combination of chemotherapy and/or radiation therapy and/or surgery. Consequently, the clinical determination of the N descriptor is important and is assessed clinically by various imaging modalities and/or invasive procedures.

Modalities Used in Mediastinal Lymph Node Staging

CT, FDG-PET/CT, EBUS, EUS, and mediastinoscopy are the most common modalities used to

International Association for the Study of Lung Cancer
Nodal Definitions

#1 (Left/Right) Low cervical, supraclavicular and sternal notch nodes
Upper border: lower margin of cricoid cartilage
Lower border: clavicles bilaterally and, in the midline, the upper border of the manubrium, 1R designates right-sided nodes, 1L, left-sided nodes in this region.
#L1 and #R1 limited by the midline of the trachea.

#2 (Left/Right) Upper paratracheal nodes
2R: Upper border: apex of the right lung and pleural space and, in the midline, the upper border of the manubrium
Lower border: intersection of caudal margin of innominate vein with the trachea
2L: Upper border: apex of the left lung and pleural space and, in the midline, the upper border of the manubrium
Lower border: superior border of the aortic arch
As for #4, in #2 the oncologic midline is along the left lateral border of the trachea.

#3 Pre-vascular and retrotracheal nodes
3a: Prevascular - On the right
upper border: apex of chest
lower border: level of carina
anterior border: posterior aspect of sternum
posterior border: anterior border of superior vena cava
3a: Prevascular - On the left
upper border: apex of chest
lower border: level of carina
anterior border: posterior aspect of sternum
posterior border: left carotid artery
3p: Retrotracheal
upper border: apex of chest
lower border: carina

#4 (Left/Right) Lower paratracheal nodes
4R: includes right paratracheal nodes, and pretracheal nodes extending to the left lateral border of trachea
upper border: intersection of caudal margin of innominate vein with the trachea
lower border: lower border of azygos vein
4L: includes nodes to the left of the left lateral border of the trachea, medial to the ligamentum arteriosum
upper border: upper margin of the aortic arch
lower border: upper rim of the left main pulmonary artery

MG57591 0409

#5 Subaortic (aorto-pulmonary window)
Subaortic lymph nodes lateral to the ligamentum arteriosum
upper border: the lower border of the aortic arch
lower border: upper rim of the left main pulmonary artery

#6 Para-aortic nodes ascending aorta or phrenic
Lymph nodes anterior and lateral to the ascending aorta and aortic arch
upper border: a line tangential to upper border of aortic arch
lower border: the lower border of the aortic arch

#7 Subcarinal nodes
upper border: the carina of the trachea
lower border: the upper border of the lower lobe bronchus on the left; the lower border of the bronchus intermedius on right

#8 (Left/Right) Para-esophageal nodes (below carina)
Nodes lying adjacent to the wall of the esophagus and to the right or left of the midline, excluding subcarinal nodes
upper border: the upper border of the lower lobe bronchus on the left; the lower border of the bronchus intermedius on right
lower border: the diaphragm

#9 (Left/Right) Pulmonary ligament nodes
Nodes lying within the pulmonary ligament
upper border: the inferior pulmonary vein
lower border: the diaphragm

#10 (Left/Right) Hilar nodes
Includes nodes immediately adjacent to the mainstem bronchus and hilar vessels including the proximal portions of the pulmonary veins and main pulmonary artery
upper border: the lower rim of the azygos vein on the right; upper rim of the pulmonary artery on the left
lower border: interlobar region bilaterally

#11 Interlobar nodes
Between the origin of the lobar bronchi
*#11s: between the upper lobe bronchus and bronchus intermedius on the right
*#11i: between the middle and lower lobe bronchi on the right

#12 Lobar nodes
Adjacent to the lobar bronchi

#13 Segmental nodes
Adjacent to the segmental bronchi

#14 Sub-segmental nodes
Adjacent to the subsegmental bronchi

Fig. 7. (*continued*)

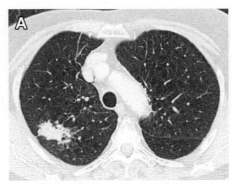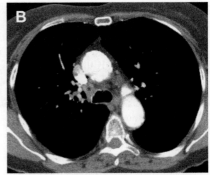

Fig. 8. A 77-year-old woman with lung adenocarcinoma. (*A*) CT shows the right upper lobe primary tumor. (*B*) Contrast-enhanced CT shows a 1.4-cm right lower paratracheal (station 4R) lymph node (*asterisk*). Mediastinoscopy showed adenocarcinoma in the station 4R lymph node (N2). Using a size threshold value of greater than 1-cm short axis diameter for nodal metastatic disease, this node was a true-positive finding on CT.

determine the absence or location of lung cancer spread to a regional mediastinal lymph node prior to the initiation of treatment.

On imaging, nodal size criterion is the only parameter used in the eighth edition of the TNM staging system to identify suspicious lymph nodes (nodal size threshold value of >1-cm short axis diameter) (see **Fig. 8**). The use of size is a major shortcoming in clinical staging because an enlarged lymph node can be enlarged secondary to a non-neoplastic etiology, whereas a nonenlarged lymph node can harbor metastasis. In this regard, Prenzel and colleagues[11] reported that in 2891 resected hilar and mediastinal nodes obtained from 256 patients with lung cancer, 101 of 139 patients (77%) patients with pN0 had at least 1 node greater than 1 cm in diameter and 14 of 117 patients (12%) with pN1/pN2 had no nodes greater than 1 cm. CT, often the first modality obtained, is the least sensitive in detecting nodal involvement when using a size threshold value of greater than 1 cm and has median sensitivity and specificity of 55% and 81%, respectively.[12]

FDG-PET/CT is superior to CT in terms of accuracy for N descriptor of the mediastinum and is increasingly used in staging and management strategies in patients with lung cancer. FDG-PET/CT is more sensitive than CT in detecting mediastinal lymph node metastasis, with median sensitivity and specificity of 77% and 86%, respectively.[12] In nodes less than 1 cm, however, the sensitivity of FDG-PET/CT to detect nodal metastasis is not optimal and has been reported as sensitivity of 32.4% versus 85.3% in nodes greater than or equal to1 cm.[13]

Although FDG-PET/CT reduces the likelihood that a patient with mediastinal nodal metastasis (N3) that precludes surgery undergoes attempted

resection, there are false-positive results due to infectious and inflammatory etiologies (**Fig. 9**). This overlap in the appearance of malignant and benign lymph nodes is a confounding factor in FDG-PET/CT N descriptor determination. Historically, an FDG uptake threshold of maximum standardized uptake value (SUV) of 2.5 has been suggested to indicate malignancy. Numerous factors, however, including the time to imaging after FDG administration and the type of scanner and image reconstruction algorithm used, can affect the thresholds selected. Currently, no prospective multicenter trial has validated an FDG uptake threshold, and visual interpretation tends to be more accurate than SUV quantification.

Because surgical resection and potential use of adjuvant therapy are dependent on a patient's N descriptor, attempts have been made to improve the accuracy of detection of nodal metastases. Point spread function (PSF) reconstruction is commercially available and improves image contrast and reduces image noise. Accordingly, it can be more sensitive in the detection of small-volume nodal metastases.[14] PSF PET has higher sensitivity (97%), negative predictive value (92%), and negative likelihood ratio (0.04) than conventional iterative reconstruction in N descriptor determination in patients with lung cancer.[14] Although there is an increase in false-positive results, significant improvement in sensitivity, negative predictive value, and negative likelihood ratio of PSF potentially allows preoperative invasive nodal evaluation to be omitted when PSF FDG-PET/CT is negative. Artificial neural network (ANN) has the potential to improve N descriptor assessment using 4 FDG-PET/CT–derived input parameters (primary tumor maximum SUV, tumor size, node size, and FDG uptake at N1, N2, and N3 stations).[15]

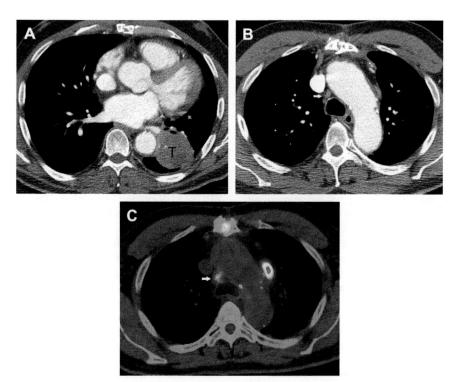

Fig. 9. A 68-year-old man with squamous cell cancer of the left lower lobe. (*A*) CT shows the primary tumor (T) in the left lower lobe. (*B*) Contrast-enhanced CT shows a 7-mm right lower paratracheal (station 4R) lymph node (*arrow*). (*C*) FDG-PET/CT shows FDG-avid left prevascular (station 3a) and right lower paratracheal (station 4R [*arrow*]) lymph nodes suspicious for N2 and N3, respectively. Mediastinoscopy and tissue sampling of the right lower paratracheal lymph node showed no malignant cells. The station 4R lymph node was a true-negative finding on CT and a false-positive finding on FDG-PET/CT. Invasive mediastinal nodal sampling is recommended in a patient with lung cancer with suspicion of N2 and/or N3 involvement on CT and/or PET if this alters patient management.

ANN has been reported to predict the N descriptor in 99.2% of cases compared with 72.4% for an expert reader.[15] In summary, ANN mitigates the subjectivity in the interpretation of PET, can outperform an expert in FDG-PET/CT interpretation, and distinguishes malignant and benign inflammatory lymph nodes with overlapping FDG-PET/CT appearances.

EBUS-guided biopsy, EUS-guided biopsy, and combined EBUS-EUS–guided biopsies are minimally invasive techniques that are increasingly used. These procedures have median sensitivities of 89%, 89%, and 91%, respectively.[12] EBUS is used to sample lymph node stations adjacent to the trachea and proximal bronchi, including stations 2, 3p, 4, and 7, in addition to hilar lymph nodes, whereas EUS allows sampling of periesophageal lymph nodes, including stations 4L, 5, 6, 7, 8, and 9. These 2 techniques are complementary and can be used in combination.[16]

Cervical mediastinoscopy and videomediastinoscopy are more invasive procedures requiring general anesthesia, with median sensitivities of 78% and 89%, respectively.[12] Cervical mediastinoscopy and video mediastinoscopy can be performed to sample mediastinal lymph node stations 2, 3, 4, and 7. Extended cervical mediastinoscopy, video-assisted thoracoscopic surgery, or Chamberlain procedure (left parasternal mediastinotomy) can be performed to sample stations 5 and 6.

The choice of modalities used in N descriptor determination can also be influenced by factors inherent to each modality, such as availability, associated morbidity/mortality, and cost. Patient factors can also influence modality choice, such as patient preference and comorbidities. Therefore, techniques to determine the N descriptor vary among centers.

Algorithms for Mediastinal Lymph Node Staging

The American College of Chest Physicians recommendations for mediastinal lymph node assessment in patients with no evidence of distant metastasis on CT and/or PET/CT vary according to the following 4 clinical scenarios: (1) a peripheral lung cancer (located in the peripheral two-thirds of the hemi-thorax) that is small in size with no suspicion of N1–N3 involvement on CT and PET, (2) a central lung cancer with no suspicion of N2–N3 involvement on CT and PET OR a lung cancer with suspicion of N1 involvement and no suspicion of N2–N3 involvement on CT and/or PET, (3) a lung cancer with suspicion of N2 and/or N3 involvement on CT and/or PET (Figs. 10 and 11), and (4) a lung cancer with extensive mediastinal involvement where a lymph node can longer be discerned or measured on CT or PET/CT.[12] In the first clinical scenario, invasive mediastinal nodal sampling is not recommended. In the second and third clinical scenarios, invasive mediastinal nodal sampling is recommended, with EBUS-guided biopsy, EUS-guided biopsy, or combined EBUS/EUS-guided biopsies recommended over mediastinoscopy. In the fourth clinical scenario, CT assessment of the mediastinal descriptor is usually sufficient without invasive mediastinal nodal sampling. Patients who have a left upper lobe cancer in scenarios 2 or 3 and who are found to have no mediastinal lymph node involvement during mediastinal nodal sampling are recommended to undergo extended cervical mediastinoscopy,

video-assisted thoracoscopic surgery, or Chamberlain procedure to assess lymph node station 5.

The European Society of Thoracic Surgeons recommendations for mediastinal nodal sampling also vary according to the lung cancer clinical scenario.[17] For patients with a suspicious mediastinal lymph node on CT or PET, invasive mediastinal nodal sampling is recommended. EBUS-guided biopsy, EUS-guided biopsy, or combined EBUS/EUS-guided biopsies is the first choice to identify mediastinal lymph node metastasis. If the EBUS-guided biopsy, EUS-guided biopsy, or combined EBUS/EUS-guided biopsies results are negative, then video-assisted mediastinoscopy is the next recommended step. In patients with a left upper lobe cancer, invasive nodal sampling of lymph node station 5 is recommended if positive nodal disease changes treatment strategy. For patients with a peripheral lung cancer, lung cancer size less than or equal to 3 cm, and no suspicious lymph node on CT or PET, direct surgical resection of the tumor without preoperative invasive mediastinal staging is recommended. For patients with a central lung cancer, a lung cancer that is greater than 3 cm, or a lung cancer with suspicion of N1

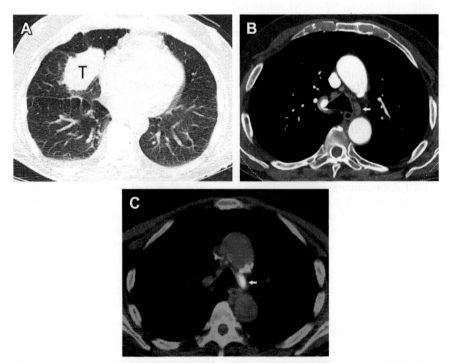

Fig. 10. An 81-year-old man with squamous cell cancer of the right middle lobe. (A) CT shows the right middle lobe tumor (T). (B) Contrast-enhanced CT shows an 8-mm left lower paratracheal (station 4L) lymph node (arrow). (C) FDG-PET/CT shows the node is FDG-avid and biopsy-confirmed N3. The node is a false-negative finding on CT and a true-positive finding on FDG-PET/CT. Due to comorbidities, the patient was not a candidate for systemic chemotherapy and received palliative radiation therapy to the chest.

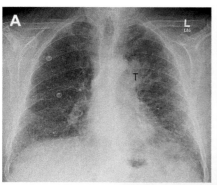
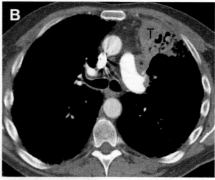
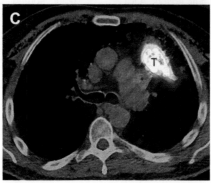

Fig. 11. A 71-year-old man with squamous cell cancer of the left upper lobe and pulmonary fibrosis. (*A*) Chest radiograph shows lobular left upper lobe tumor (T). (*B*) CT shows the left upper lobe tumor (T) and a 2-cm aortopulmonary window (APW) lymph node (*asterisk*) suspicious for N2. (*C*) FDG-PET/CT shows the FDG-avid left upper lobe tumor (T) and the APW (station 5) lymph node (*asterisk*) is not FDG avid. Percutaneous biopsy of the station 5 node showed squamous cell cancer. This was a true-positive finding on CT and a false-negative finding on FDG-PET/CT. Invasive mediastinal nodal sampling is recommended in a patient with lung cancer with suspicion of N2 and/or N3 involvement on CT and/or PET if this alters patient management.

involvement, invasive mediastinal nodal sampling by either EBUS or mediastinoscopy is recommended.

LIMITATIONS AND FUTURE CONSIDERATIONS

Obstacles to the standardization of N descriptor in lung cancer remain.[18–20] The use of lymph node maps other than the IASLC lymph node map continues to exist in many clinical practices around the world.[20] Nodal stations defined by the IASLC are in relation to anatomic structures or boundaries identified optimally during surgery. Thus, when applied to CT imaging, these anatomic definitions can create ambiguity and result in interobserver variability.[18–23] Variability in N1 versus N2, N2 versus N3, and N versus M occur particularly with lymph nodes located about the hilum, carina, thoracic inlet, axilla, internal mammary vessels, and diaphragm.[18–23]

Recent efforts in improving the accuracy of CT in differentiation of malignant from benign lymph nodes have mainly focused on the use of dynamic contrast enhancement and perfusion parameters with diagnostic performance similar to those of FDG-PET/CT demonstrated by a recent study.[24] Studies have also been performed to evaluate the utility of MR imaging, in particular diffusion-weighted imaging (DWI), in characterization of mediastinal lymph nodes in lung cancer. The use of MR imaging in N descriptor evaluation is more comprehensively discussed in the MR imaging review by Mario Ciliberto and colleagues' article, "Update of MR imaging for Evaluation of Lung Cancer." A recent metaanalysis of MR imaging in determining nodal status in patients with non–small cell lung cancer reported sensitivity and specificity of 87% and 88%, respectively.[25] Pauls and colleagues compared the diagnostic accuracy of DWI to that of FDG-PET/CT and showed a tendency for understaging by MR imaging.[26] A separate metaanalysis evaluating the performance of DWI in N descriptor assessment showed sensitivity of 68% and specificity of 92%.[27]

SUMMARY

Regional lymph node classification is an important element in the staging of lung cancer, with implications for treatment planning and prognostication.

According to the eighth edition of the TNM staging system for lung cancer, the IASLC lymph node map should be used for the standardization of N descriptor assessment. CT and FDG-PET/CT are the main imaging modalities used for initial assessment. EBUS, EUS, and mediastinoscopies are frequently performed for tissue confirmation in selected patients without evidence of distant metastases.

REFERENCES

1. Amin MB, Edge SB, Greene FL, et al, editors. AJCC cancer staging manual. 8th edition. New York: Springer; 2017.

2. Naruke T. The spread of lung cancer and its relevance to surgery. Nippon Kyobu Geka Gakkai Zasshi 1967;68:1607–21.

3. Naruke T, Suemasu K, Ishikawa S. Lymph node mapping and curability at various levels of metastasis in resected lung cancer. J Thorac Cardiovasc Surg 1978;76(6):833–9.

4. Tisi GM, Friedman PJ, Peters RM, et al. Clinical staging of primary lung cancer. Am Rev Respir Dis 1983; 127(5):659–64.

5. Mountain CF, Dresler CM. Regional lymph node classification for lung cancer staging. Chest 1997; 111(6):1718–23.

6. Rusch VW, Asamura H, Watanabe H, et al. The IASLC lung cancer staging project: a proposal for a new international lymph node map in the forthcoming seventh edition of the TNM classification for lung cancer. J Thorac Oncol 2009;4(5): 568–77.

7. Watanabe S, Ladas G, Goldstraw P. Inter-observer variability in systematic nodal dissection: comparison of European and Japanese nodal designation. Ann Thorac Surg 2002;73(1):245–8 [discussion: 248–9].

8. Wei S, Asamura H, Kawachi R, et al. Which is the better prognostic factor for resected non-small cell lung cancer: the number of metastatic lymph nodes or the currently used nodal stage classification? J Thorac Oncol 2011;6:310–8.

9. Saji H, Tsuboi M, Shimada Y, et al. A proposal for combination of total number and anatomical location of involved lymph nodes for nodal classification in non-small cell lung cancer. Chest 2013;143: 1618–25.

10. Asamura H, Chansky K, Crowley J, et al. The IASLC lung cancer staging project: proposals for the revisions of the N descriptors in the forthcoming 8th edition of the TNM classification for lung cancer. J Thorac Oncol 2015;10:1675–84.

11. Prenzel KL, Mönig SP, Sinning JM, et al. Lymph node size and metastatic infiltration in non-small cell lung cancer. Chest 2003;123:463–7.

12. Silvestri GA, Gonzalez AV, Jantz MA, et al. Methods for staging non-small cell lung cancer. Diagnosis and management of lung cancer, 3rd ed: American College of Chest Physicians evidence-based clinical practice guidelines. Chest 2013;143:e211S–250.

13. Billé A, Pelosi E, Skanjeti A, et al. Preoperative intrathoracic lymph node staging in patients with non-small-cell lung cancer: accuracy of integrated positron emission tomography and computed tomography. Eur J Cardiothorac Surg 2009;36:440–5.

14. Lasnon C, Hicks RJ, Beauregard JM, et al. Impact of point spread functionreconstruction on thoracic lymph node staging with 18F-FDG PET/CT in non-small cell lung cancer. Clin Nucl Med 2012;37: 971–6.

15. Toney LK, Vesselle HJ. Neural networks for nodal staging of non-small cell lung cancer with FDG PET and CT: importance of combining uptake values and sizes of nodes and primary tumor. Radiology 2014;270:91–8.

16. Gompelmann D, Herth FJ. Role of endobronchial and endoscopic ultrasound in pulmonary medicine. Respiration 2014;87:3–8.

17. De Leyn P, Dooms C, Kuzdzal J, et al. Revised ESTS guidelines for preoperative mediastinal lymph node staging for non-small-cell lung cancer. Eur J Cardiothoracic Surg 2014;45:787–98.

18. Pitson G, Lynch R, Claude L, et al. A critique of the international association for the study of lung cancer lymph node map: a radiation oncology perspective. J Thorac Oncol 2012;7(3):478–80.

19. El-Sherief AH, Lau CT, Wu CC, et al. International Association for the Study of Lung Cancer (IASLC) lymph node map: radiological review with CT illustration. Radiographics 2014;34:1680–91.

20. El-Sherief AH, Lau CT, Obuchowski NA, et al. Cross-disciplinary analysis of lymph node classification in lung cancer on Ct scanning. Chest 2017;151: 776–85.

21. Carter BW, Godoy MC, Wu CC, et al. Current controversies in lung cancer staging. J Thorac Imaging 2016;31:201–14.

22. Rusch VW, Crowley J, Giroux DJ, et al. The IASLC lung cancer staging project: proposals for the revision of the N descriptors in the forthcoming seventh edition of the TNM classifications for lung cancer. J Thorac Oncol 2007;2:603–12.

23. Detterbeck FC, Boffa DJ, Kim AW, et al. The eighth edition lung cancer descriptor classification. Chest 2017;15:193–203.

24. Ohno Y, Fujisawa Y, Sugihara N, et al. Dynamic contrast-enhanced perfusion area-detector ct: preliminary comparison of diagnostic performance for N stage assessment With FDG PET/CT in non-small cell lung cancer. AJR Am J Roentgenol 2017; 20:W1–10.

25. Peerlings J, Troost EG, Nelemans PJ, et al. The diagnostic value of MR imaging in determining the lymph node status of patients with non-small cell lung cancer: a meta-analysis. Radiology 2016;281:86–98.

26. Pauls S, Schmidt SA, Juchems MS, et al. Diffusion-weighted MR imaging in comparison to integrated [^{18}F]-FDG PET/CT for N-staging in patients with lung cancer. Eur J Radiol 2012;81(1):178–82.

27. Shen G, Hu S, Deng H, et al. Performance of DWI in the nodal characterization and assessment of lung cancer: a meta-analysis. AJR Am J Roentgenol 2016;206(2):283–90.

Staging Lung Cancer
Metastasis

Girish S. Shroff, MD*, Chitra Viswanathan, MD, Brett W. Carter, MD,
Marcelo F. Benveniste, MD, Mylene T. Truong, MD, Bradley S. Sabloff, MD

KEYWORDS

• Metastasis • TNM-7 • TNM-8 • Oligometastatic disease • PET/CT

KEY POINTS

• In TNM-8, the M descriptor has been changed. Intrathoracic metastatic disease retains the M1a classification. Extrathoracic metastatic disease is subdivided into M1b (single metastasis) and M1c (multiple extrathoracic metastases) descriptors.
• Preoperative staging with PET/computed tomography identifies more patients with mediastinal and extrathoracic disease than with conventional imaging alone, thereby sparing patients from unnecessary surgery.
• Patients with non–small-cell lung cancer with oligometastatic disease and good performance status can benefit from aggressive local therapy to both primary and metastatic sites.

TNM CLASSIFICATION OF MALIGNANT TUMORS, SEVENTH EDITION

The seventh edition of the tumor, node, metastasis (TNM-7) classification of lung cancer, proposed in 2007 and published in 2009, was based on a retrospective analysis of more than 81,000 patients diagnosed with lung cancer between 1990 and 2000.[1] In TNM-7, metastatic disease (M1) was subdivided into M1a and M1b descriptors. The M1a descriptor included separate tumor nodule(s) in a contralateral lobe and tumor with pleural nodule(s) or malignant pleural (or pericardial) effusion; the M1b descriptor included distant metastatic disease; that is, metastatic disease at sites outside of the thorax.[1]

TNM CLASSIFICATION OF MALIGNANT TUMORS, EIGHTH EDITION

To overcome the limitations of the retrospective nature of the TNM-7 database, the International Staging Committee of the International Association for the Study of Lung Cancer (IASLC) proposed the collection of a large prospective international database that would refine future editions of the TNM classification for lung cancer through the validation of all T, N, and M descriptors.[2] Specific primary study objectives in terms of the M component were to assess the prognostic impact of M-status, especially those descriptors included within the M1a category of the seventh edition, and to assess the prognostic impact of a single metastasis in a single organ, multiple metastases in a single organ, and multiple metastases in several organs.[2]

The new IASLC lung cancer database that was used to form the eighth edition of the TNM classification of lung cancer was composed of retrospective and prospective information on 94,708 new patients who were diagnosed with lung cancer between 1999 and 2010.[3] The final analysis was performed on 1059 cases of non–small-cell lung cancer (NSCLC) with nonresected M1 disease.[4]

Department of Diagnostic Radiology, The University of Texas MD Anderson Cancer Center, 1515 Holcombe Boulevard, Houston, TX 77030, USA
* Corresponding author. Department of Diagnostic Radiology, The University of Texas MD Anderson Cancer Center, 1515 Holcombe Boulevard, Unit 1478, Houston, TX 77030.
E-mail address: gshroff@mdanderson.org

Radiol Clin N Am 56 (2018) 411–418
https://doi.org/10.1016/j.rcl.2018.01.009
0033-8389/18/© 2018 Elsevier Inc. All rights reserved.

radiologic.theclinics.com

Analysis of the M1a descriptors used in TNM-7 revealed similar prognosis among the different descriptors: patients with pleural/pericardial nodules, contralateral/bilateral tumor nodules, pleural/pericardial effusions, and multiple M1a descriptors had a median survival of 14.3, 12.0, 11.4, and 8.9 months, respectively.[4] Furthermore, no prognostic effect of single versus multiple M1a descriptors was determined.[4] As a result of these findings, the recommendation was made to maintain the use of the preexisting M1a category (Figs. 1–3). In terms of patients with distant (extrathoracic) metastatic disease, the site of metastasis was not prognostic for single or multiple lesions in a single organ.[4] Analysis suggested that the number of metastases may be more prognostic than the number of organs involved.[4] Prognosis in patients with a single extrathoracic metastasis (median survival of 11.4 months) was similar to M1a disease (median survival of 11.5 months) and was much better than prognosis in patients with multiple extrathoracic metastases in one or multiple organs (median survival of 6.3 months).[4] As a result, a single extrathoracic metastasis (eg, in brain, liver, bone, distant lymph node, or peritoneum, skin, adrenal) is now categorized as M1b (Fig. 4), whereas multiple metastatic lesions in a single organ and multiple metastatic lesions in multiple organs are categorized as M1c (Fig. 5).[4]

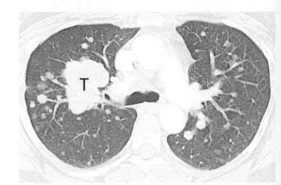

Fig. 2. M1a disease due to contralateral pulmonary metastases. Chest CT shows right upper lobe NSCLC (T) with multiple bilateral discrete lung nodules consistent with hematogenous metastases.

SMALL CELL LUNG CANCER

In 2007, the IASLC, based on analysis of more than 8000 patients in their database who were diagnosed with small cell lung cancer (SCLC) between 1990 and 2000, recommended that the seventh edition of the TNM staging system replace the Veterans Administration Lung Study Group staging system for SCLC.[5] They found that both the T and N descriptors were discriminatory for overall survival in clinically staged patients without hematogenous metastases and overall clinical stage groupings I to IV were also predictive of overall survival.[5,6] Analysis of the new IASLC database (which included more than 5000 patients with SCLC) again confirmed the prognostic value of TNM staging in patients with SCLC and continued usage of the TNM system in SCLC is recommended.[7] In terms of metastatic disease, analysis of

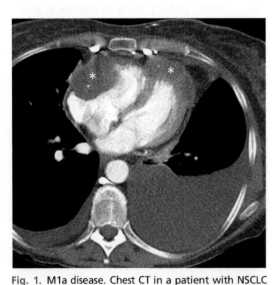

Fig. 1. M1a disease. Chest CT in a patient with NSCLC shows low attenuation metastases involving the myocardium and pericardium (*asterisks*) and a moderate to large left pleural effusion, proven to be malignant. Cases with malignant pleural/pericardial effusions and/ or pleural/pericardial metastases, contralateral pulmonary metastases, or a combination of these findings constitute M1a disease.

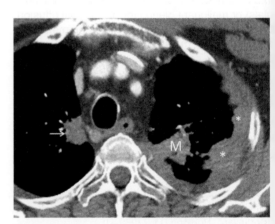

Fig. 3. M1a disease. Chest CT shows the primary tumor in the left upper lobe (M) as well as left pleural lobularity consistent with pleural metastases (*asterisks*) and a right upper lobe metastasis (*arrow*). Intrathoracic metastatic disease is classified as M1a.

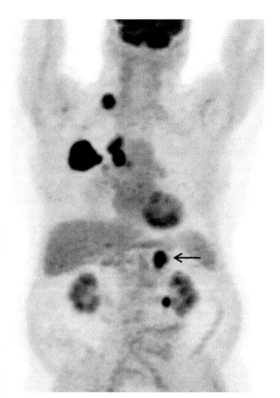

Fig. 4. M1b disease. Whole-body PET shows a right upper lobe primary tumor, nodal metastatic disease at the right paratracheal and right supraclavicular regions, and a solitary extrathoracic metastasis in the left adrenal gland (*arrow*). Extrathoracic metastatic disease, classified as M1b in TNM-7, is now subdivided into M1b for a single metastasis and M1c for multiple extrathoracic metastases.

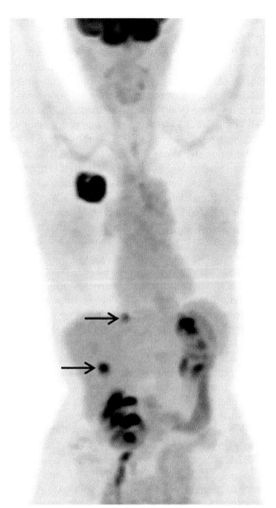

Fig. 5. M1c disease. Whole-body PET shows a right upper lobe primary tumor and 2 hepatic metastases (*arrows*). In TNM-8, multiple metastatic lesions in a single organ and multiple metastatic lesions in multiple organs are categorized as M1c.

the new database showed refinements in the survival data for patients with M1b disease: patients with single-site metastasis (SSM) without pleural effusions and those with brain-only SSM had better prognosis than patients with either multiple-site disease or SSM with a pleural effusion.[7] It was uncertain whether these differences were reflective of ability to treat versus true survival differences based on disease extent, and it was concluded that M descriptors for SCLC should be the same as those for NSCLC.[7]

PET/COMPUTED TOMOGRAPHY

The strength of PET/CT imaging in lung cancer is to detect occult metastatic disease (with common sites including the adrenal glands, liver, brain, and skeleton); detection of metastatic disease usually spares the patient from radical treatment.[8] In this regard, preoperative staging with PET/CT identifies more patients with mediastinal and extrathoracic disease than with conventional imaging

alone, thereby sparing patients from unnecessary surgery.[9,10] Maziak and colleagues[9] found that 13.8% of patients who underwent PET/CT were correctly upstaged (and therefore spared from inappropriate surgery) compared with 6.8% of patients who underwent conventional imaging (consisting of abdominal CT and a whole-body bone scan); patients in both groups had brain imaging. Fischer and colleagues[10] found that the addition of PET/CT to conventional imaging in the preoperative staging of NSCLC improved sensitivity and reduced both the number of thoracotomies and the number of futile thoracotomies; that is, thoracotomies performed for the following: a benign lung lesion, pathologically proven stage IIIA N2 lymph node involvement, stage IIIB or IV disease, inoperable T3 or T4 disease, or recurrent disease or death from any cause within 1 year after randomization.

PET/CT is useful in the differentiation of benign and malignant adrenal lesions in oncology patients (Fig. 6). Metser and colleagues[11] found that when malignant lesions were compared with adenomas, PET data alone using a standardized uptake value (SUV) cutoff of 3.1 yielded a sensitivity, specificity, positive predictive value (PPV), and negative predictive value (NPV) of 98.5%, 92.0%, 89.3%, and 98.9%, respectively; when combined PET/CT data were used (with attenuation values of <10 Hounsfield units for diagnosing an adenoma), sensitivity, specificity, PPV, and NPV were 100%, 98%, 97%, and 100%, respectively. Blake and colleagues[12] retrospectively evaluated the accuracy of PET/CT for characterization of adrenal lesions in patients with proved or suspected malignancy, and found that all malignant lesions had fluorodeoxyglucose (FDG) activity greater than that of the liver with a mean adrenal lesion-liver ratio of 4.04 (range 1.53–17.08). Of the 32 benign lesions, 30 had activity ratios that were less than liver activity (mean adrenal lesion-liver activity ratio of 0.66); maximum adrenal lesion-liver ratio of a benign lesion was 1.47.[12] Boland and colleagues[13] in a meta-analysis concluded that adrenal masses can be characterized with the use of PET/CT, and subsequent imaging is usually unnecessary.

PET/CT is particularly effective for detecting bone metastasis in patients with NSCLC and is superior to 99mTc-methylene-diphosphonate (MDP) bone scintigraphy (Fig. 7).[14,15] Song and colleagues[15] compared the 2 modalities and found that the sensitivity, specificity, PPV, and NPV of PET/CT were 94.3%, 98.8%, 90.0%, and 99.3%, respectively; and those of bone scintigraphy were 78.1%, 97.4%, 75.9%, and 97.4%, respectively. Discordant findings of skeletal metastasis between bone scintigraphy and PET/CT occur in 20% of patients with NSCLC.[14] This discordance is in large part due to the ability of PET to detect early bone metastasis and the failure of 99mTc-MDP scintigraphy to detect early neoplastic infiltration of bone marrow. A meta-analysis of 17 studies demonstrated that the pooled sensitivity and specificity for the detection of bone metastasis were 92% and 98%, respectively, for PET/CT, compared with 86% and 88%, respectively, for bone scintigraphy.[16] As a result, PET/CT has to a large extent replaced bone scintigraphy for the evaluation of possible bone metastasis in patients with NSCLC.[16–18]

PET/CT has limitations in the evaluation of brain metastases because there is physiologic increased metabolic activity of the brain. Brain MR Imaging with contrast is the modality of choice for the evaluation of intracranial metastatic disease; in cases in which brain MR Imaging cannot be done, contrast-enhanced brain CT can be performed.

Although PET/CT improves the detection of metastases compared with CT, focal increased uptake of FDG in extrathoracic lesions that are unrelated to the primary NSCLC can mimic distant metastasis. A prospective study to assess the incidence and diagnosis of a single site of extrapulmonary accumulation of FDG in patients with newly diagnosed NSCLC showed that in 54% of patients this was due to a solitary metastasis, whereas in 46% of patients this was unrelated to the NSCLC (benign tumor, inflammatory lesion, unsuspected second malignancy, or recurrence of a previously diagnosed carcinoma).[19]

TREATMENT

Metastatic disease has historically been considered incurable. Patients with metastatic disease are usually treated with chemotherapy, and

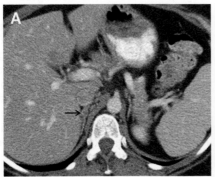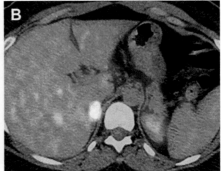

Fig. 6. Utility of PET/CT. (A) CT in a 59-year-old woman with NSCLC shows a small right adrenal nodule (*arrow*). (B) Fused PET/CT shows that the nodule is FDG-avid (SUVmax 9.9) and consistent with an adrenal metastasis. PET/CT is useful in the differentiation of benign and malignant adrenal lesions in oncology patients.

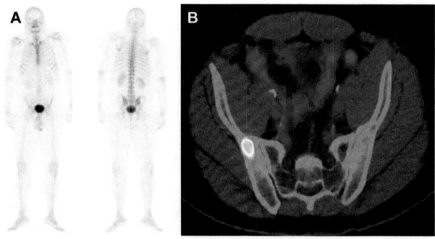

Fig. 7. Bone scintigraphy versus PET/CT in NSCLC. (*A*) Anterior and posterior whole-body bone scintigraphic images in a patient with NSCLC are normal. (*B*) Fused PET/CT image in the same patient shows focal increased FDG uptake in the right iliac bone, biopsy-proven to be a metastasis. PET/CT is superior to bone scintigraphy in the detection of skeletal metastases in patients with NSCLC.

palliative radiation therapy can be administered for symptomatic relief.[20] Patients with NSCLC with oligometastatic disease (defined as a limited number of metastatic lesions in a limited number of organs that is potentially curable with effective local therapy)[21] and good performance status, however, can benefit from aggressive local therapies to both the primary and metastatic sites.[20] Aggressive local therapies include surgery and/or definitive radiation therapy and can be preceded or followed by chemotherapy.[20] Management in these patients is dependent on the location and number of metastases.

BRAIN

Approximately 20% of patients with NSCLC will develop brain metastases.[22] Prognosis in these patients is poor, with median survival ranging from 3.0 months to 14.8 months and is dependent on several factors, including Karnofsky performance score (a scale that classifies patients based on their functional impairment), age, presence of extracranial metastases, and number of brain metastases.[23] Patients with higher numbers of brain metastases have worse overall survival.[23,24] Patients with synchronous brain-only oligometastases benefit from aggressive therapy to known areas of disease.[24] Gray and colleagues[24] showed that patients with NSCLC presenting with synchronous brain-only oligometastases (1–4 metastases) who were treated with aggressive thoracic therapy (defined as resection of the primary disease or chemoradiotherapy, whose total radiation dose exceeded 45 Gy) had improved median overall survival

compared with those who were not treated (26.4 vs 10.5 months).

Treatment options for oligometastatic disease to the brain include (1) stereotactic radiosurgery (SRS, a highly precise form of radiation therapy in which a high dose of radiation is delivered to treat small brain tumors or other neurologic abnormalities) alone, and (2) surgical resection (in cases of symptomatic metastases or when tissue is needed for diagnosis) followed by adjuvant radiation to the resection cavity using SRS or whole-brain radiation therapy (WBRT) (**Fig. 8**).[20] Because patients with NSCLC and brain metastases can have long-term survival and because of the increased risk of neurocognitive deterioration associated with WBRT,[25] the use of WBRT has decreased in patients with limited brain metastases.[20] For multiple (eg, >3) metastases, WBRT is recommended, although in patients with good performance status and low systemic tumor burden, SRS may be preferred.[20]

LUNG

Pulmonary oligometastatic disease can be treated with surgical resection or stereotactic body radiation therapy (SBRT, also known as stereotactic ablative radiation therapy or SABR), whereby short courses of conformal and dose-intensive radiation are precisely delivered to limited-size targets.[20] Benefits of SBRT include its ability to achieve high rates of tumor control with minimal morbidity and its noninvasive nature.[21] SBRT has been shown to be an effective local therapy for the treatment of oligometastases of various primary sites, including the lung.[21,26,27] A multi-institutional trial

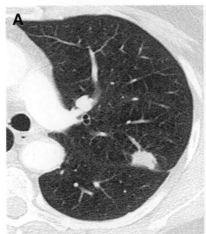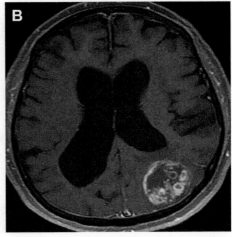

Fig. 8. M1b disease due to solitary brain metastasis. (*A*) Chest CT shows a left upper lobe adenocarcinoma. Lymph node sampling revealed metastases to left hilar and mediastinal nodes (not shown). The patient was treated with chemoradiation. Subsequently, the patient developed confusion, dizziness, and gait disturbance. (*B*) T1-weighted postcontrast MR Imaging revealed a left parietal metastasis. The lesion was resected, and the resection cavity was treated with stereotactic radiosurgery.

done to evaluate the efficacy and tolerability of SBRT for the treatment of patients with 1 to 3 lung metastases found a local control rate at 1 and 2 years after SBRT of 100% and 96%, respectively.[26]

ADRENAL

Adrenal metastases are common and usually accompanied by metastases in other organs, although they can present as oligometastatic disease. It is unclear how often adrenal oligometastatic disease occurs in patients with operable NSCLC. Matthews and colleagues[28] reported that approximately 9% of patients undergoing curative resection of lung cancer had clinically unsuspected metastases to the adrenal at autopsy within 1 month following resection. In cases of a synchronous ipsilateral adrenal metastasis, a combined lung resection and transdiaphragmatic adrenalectomy has been shown to be a safe and effective procedure.[29] Resection of an adrenal oligometastasis from NSCLC has been shown to improve the long-term disease-free survival (**Fig. 9**).[30] Luketich and Burt[30] compared the outcomes of patients with NSCLC with a solitary adrenal metastasis who were treated with chemotherapy alone versus chemotherapy followed by resection. The median survival in the surgical group was significantly greater than in the chemotherapy group (31.0 months vs 8.5 months).[30]

A review of outcomes of adrenalectomy for isolated synchronous or metachronous adrenal metastatic disease in NSCLC found that 5-year survival estimates in both groups were approximately 25%.[31] Median overall survival was shorter for patients with synchronous (defined as ≤6 months from the date of primary lung cancer resection to the date of confirmed diagnosis of adrenal metastasis) metastasis than those with metachronous (defined as ≥6 months from the date of primary lung cancer resection to the confirmed diagnosis of adrenal metastasis) metastasis (12 months vs 31 months, respectively).[31]

Although cases of adrenal resection are usually limited to unilateral adrenal metastasis, bilateral adrenalectomy has been reported in cases of bilateral adrenal metastases from lung cancer.[32,33] Urschel and colleagues[33] reported a patient who was disease-free 9 years after bilateral adrenalectomy for metastatic NSCLC; they postulated that patients with adrenal metastases from lymphatic spread of lung cancer may have a more favorable response than those with adrenal metastases from hematogenous spread.

BONE

Bone metastases, if at risk for pathologic fracture, may undergo orthopedic stabilization and palliative external beam radiation therapy.[20] Pathologic vertebral fractures may be treated with percutaneous vertebral augmentation to relieve pain and increase bone strength. Medical options for patients with bone metastases include denosumab (a monoclonal antibody that inhibits the maturation of osteoclasts) and intravenous bisphosphonate therapy, such as zoledronic acid.[20] Denosumab is associated with improved overall survival compared with zoledronic acid in patients with

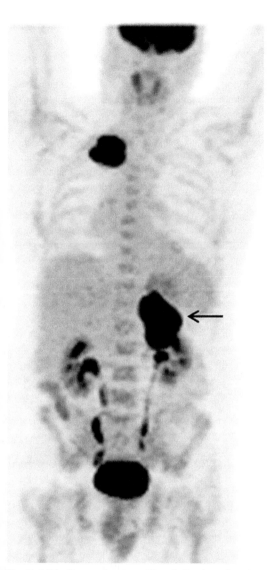

Fig. 9. M1b disease due to solitary left adrenal metastasis. Whole-body PET shows a right upper lobe primary tumor and a left adrenal metastasis (*arrow*). The right upper lobe tumor was treated with chemoradiation. After treatment of the right upper lobe tumor, the patient underwent left adrenalectomy. Resection of an isolated adrenal metastasis from NSCLC has been shown to improve the long-term disease-free survival of such patients.

metastatic lung cancer (8.9 vs 7.7 months).[34] Both denosumab and zoledronic acid are associated with severe hypocalcemia.[20]

SUMMARY

In TNM-8, intrathoracic metastatic disease retains the M1a classification. Extrathoracic metastatic disease is now classified as M1b, in the case of a single metastasis, or M1c, in the case of multiple metastases. The primary goal of extrathoracic imaging in lung cancer is to evaluate for the presence of metastatic disease and avoid futile thoracotomy. PET/CT improves detection of metastatic disease compared with conventional imaging and is useful in determining appropriate management. Patients with metastatic disease are treated with systemic therapy; selected patients with oligometastatic disease, however, may be treated with aggressive local therapy in addition to systemic therapy.

REFERENCES

1. Goldstraw P, Crowley J, Chansky K, et al. The IASLC lung cancer staging project: proposals for the revision of the TNM stage groupings in the forthcoming (seventh) edition of the TNM Classification of malignant tumours. J Thorac Oncol 2007;2:706–14.
2. Giroux DJ, Rami-Porta R, Chansky K, et al. The IASLC lung cancer staging project: data elements for the prospective project. J Thorac Oncol 2009;4: 679–83.
3. Rami-Porta R, Bolejack V, Giroux DJ, et al. The IASLC lung cancer staging project: the new database to inform the eighth edition of the TNM classification of lung cancer. J Thorac Oncol 2014;9: 1618–24.
4. Eberhardt WE, Mitchell A, Crowley J, et al. The IASLC lung cancer staging project: proposals for the revision of the M descriptors in the forthcoming eighth edition of the TNM classification of lung cancer. J Thorac Oncol 2015;10:1515–22.
5. Shepherd FA, Crowley J, Van Houtte P, et al. The International Association for the Study of Lung Cancer lung cancer staging project: proposals regarding the clinical staging of small cell lung cancer in the forthcoming (seventh) edition of the tumor, node, metastasis classification for lung cancer. J Thorac Oncol 2007;2:1067–77.
6. Kalemkerian GP, Gadgeel SM. Modern staging of small cell lung cancer. J Natl Compr Canc Netw 2013;11:99–104.
7. Nicholson AG, Chansky K, Crowley J, et al. The International Association for the Study of Lung Cancer Lung Cancer Staging Project: proposals for the revision of the clinical and pathologic staging of small cell lung cancer in the forthcoming eighth edition of the TNM classification for lung cancer. J Thorac Oncol 2016;11:300–11.
8. Silvestri GA, Gonzalez AV, Jantz MA, et al. Methods for staging non-small cell lung cancer: diagnosis and management of lung cancer, 3rd ed: American College of Chest Physicians evidence-based clinical practice guidelines. Chest 2013;143(5 Suppl): e211S–250.

9. Maziak DE, Darling GE, Inculet RI, et al. Positron emission tomography in staging early lung cancer: a randomized trial. Ann Intern Med 2009;151:221–8.

10. Fischer B, Lassen U, Mortensen J, et al. Preoperative staging of lung cancer with combined PET-CT. N Engl J Med 2009;361:32–9.

11. Metser U, Miller E, Lerman H, et al. 18F-FDG PET/CT in the evaluation of adrenal masses. J Nucl Med 2006;47:32–7.

12. Blake MA, Slattery JM, Kalra MK, et al. Adrenal lesions: characterization with fused PET/CT image in patients with proved or suspected malignancy–initial experience. Radiology 2006;238:970–7.

13. Boland GW, Dwamena BA, Jagtiani Sangwaiya M, et al. Characterization of adrenal masses by using FDG PET: a systematic review and meta-analysis of diagnostic test performance. Radiology 2011; 259:117–26.

14. Ak I, Sivrikoz MC, Entok E, et al. Discordant findings in patients with non-small-cell lung cancer: absolutely normal bone scans versus disseminated bone metastases on positron-emission tomography/computed tomography. Eur J Cardiothorac Surg 2010;37:792–6.

15. Song JW, Oh YM, Shim TS, et al. Efficacy comparison between (18)F-FDG PET/CT and bone scintigraphy in detecting bony metastases of non-small-cell lung cancer. Lung Cancer 2009;65:333–8.

16. Qu X, Huang X, Yan W, et al. A meta-analysis of [18]FDG-PET-CT, [18]FDG-PET, MRI and bone scintigraphy for diagnosis of bone metastases in patients with lung cancer. Eur J Radiol 2012;81:1007–15.

17. Min JW, Um SW, Yim JJ, et al. The role of whole-body FDG PET/CT, Tc 99m MDP bone scintigraphy, and serum alkaline phosphatase in detecting bone metastasis in patients with newly diagnosed lung cancer. J Korean Med Sci 2009;24:275–80.

18. Liu N, Ma L, Zhou W, et al. Bone metastasis in patients with non-small cell lung cancer: the diagnostic role of F-18 FDG PET/CT. Eur J Radiol 2010;74: 231–5.

19. Lardinois D, Weder W, Roudas M, et al. Etiology of solitary extrapulmonary positron emission tomography and computed tomography findings in patients with lung cancer. J Clin Oncol 2005;23:6846–53.

20. NCCN clinical practice guidelines in oncology, non-small cell lung cancer, Version 6.2017-May 12, 2017. Available at: NCCN.org. Accessed June 15, 2017.

21. Shultz DB, Filippi AR, Thariat J, et al. Stereotactic ablative radiotherapy for pulmonary oligometastases and oligometastatic lung cancer. J Thorac Oncol 2014;9:1426–33.

22. Barnholtz-Sloan JS, Sloan AE, Davis FG, et al. Incidence proportions of brain metastases in patients diagnosed (1973 to 2001) in the metropolitan Detroit cancer surveillance system. J Clin Oncol 2004;22: 2865–72.

23. Sperduto PW, Kased N, Roberge D, et al. Summary report on the graded prognostic assessment: an accurate and facile diagnosis-specific tool to estimate survival for patients with brain metastases. J Clin Oncol 2012;30:419–25.

24. Gray PJ, Mak RH, Yeap BY, et al. Aggressive therapy for patients with non-small cell lung carcinoma and synchronous brain-only oligometastatic disease is associated with long-term survival. Lung Cancer 2014;85:239–44.

25. Brown PD, Jaeckle K, Ballman KV, et al. Effect of radiosurgery alone vs radiosurgery with whole brain radiation therapy on cognitive function in patients with 1 to 3 brain metastases: a randomized clinical trial. JAMA 2016;316:401–9.

26. Rusthoven KE, Kavanagh BD, Burri SH, et al. Multi-institutional phase I/II trial of stereotactic body radiation therapy for lung metastases. J Clin Oncol 2009;27:1579–84.

27. Dahele M, Senan S. The role of stereotactic ablative radiotherapy for early-stage and oligometastatic non-small cell lung cancer: evidence for changing paradigms. Cancer Res Treat 2011;43:75–82.

28. Matthews MJ, Kanhouwa S, Pickren J, et al. Frequency of residual and metastatic tumor in patients undergoing curative surgical resection for lung cancer. Cancer Chemother Rep 3 1973;4:63–7.

29. Hunt I, Rankin SC, Lang-Lazdunski L. Combined lung resection and transdiaphragmatic adrenalectomy in patients with non-small cell lung cancer and homolateral solitary adrenal metastasis. Eur J Cardiothorac Surg 2006;30:194–5.

30. Luketich JD, Burt ME. Does resection of adrenal metastases from non-small cell lung cancer improve survival? Ann Thorac Surg 1996;62:1614–6.

31. Tanvetyanon T, Robinson LA, Schell MJ, et al. Outcomes of adrenalectomy for isolated synchronous versus metachronous adrenal metastases in non-small-cell lung cancer: a systematic review and pooled analysis. J Clin Oncol 2008;26:1142–7.

32. Heniford BT, Arca MJ, Walsh RM, et al. Laparoscopic adrenalectomy for cancer. Semin Surg Oncol 1999;16:293–306.

33. Urschel JD, Finley RK, Takita H. Long-term survival after bilateral adrenalectomy for metastatic lung cancer: a case report. Chest 1997;112:848–50.

34. Scagliotti GV, Hirsh V, Siena S, et al. Overall survival improvement in patients with lung cancer and bone metastases treated with denosumab versus zoledronic acid: subgroup analysis from a randomized phase 3 study. J Thorac Oncol 2012;7:1823–9.

Dilemmas in Lung Cancer Staging

Ioannis Vlahos, BSc, MBBS, MRCP, FRCR

KEYWORDS

- TNM8 • Non–small cell lung cancer (NSCLC) • Staging • Limitations • Dilemmas
- Computed tomography (CT) • PET-CT • IASLC

KEY POINTS

- The 8th edition of the non–small cell lung cancer (NSCLC) TNM staging reflects an extremely well-validated evidence-based advance, better stratifying survival than prior staging systems.
- Despite revisions, and several white paper recommendations, the staging system demonstrates residual limitations and dilemmas that relate to the TNM database, the application of radiological staging as well as clinical management.
- Dilemmas arise as to the radiological assignment of T-descriptors in certain clinical scenarios.
- The unchanged imaging staging of nodal disease retains limitations in guiding management of N2 disease.
- Multiple factors impact stage migration and apparent survival differences that also affect backwards compatibility of the staging system with prior staging iterations and management guidance.

INTRODUCTION

The staging of non–small cell lung cancer (NSCLC) is at a juncture; the current 7th edition of the TNM staging system (TNM7) is about to be superseded by the widespread adoption of the 8th edition (TNM8). As with the introduction of TNM7, the TNM8 reclassification of the T, N, M descriptors as well as their associated stage groupings represents a substantial step change for multidisciplinary NSCLC teams and their supporting radiologists.[1–4]

The periodic adjustment of staging systems is a required process to respond to evolution in the natural incidence of disease subtypes, new understandings in the pathology, surgery, and treatment of lung cancer, and advances in staging methodologies. As with all staging systems, the principal purpose of the lung cancer staging system remains to categorize groups of patients with similar disease extent, to accurately prognosticate survival, and to guide best management. The process of staging should be easy to implement, logical, unambiguous, and reproducible, utilizing all current imaging methodologies.

The implementation of TNM7 addressed many limitations of the earlier staging iterations but left several issues unaddressed.[5–8] TNM8 attempts to address many of these, although remaining issues persist, and new issues are raised by staging system changes. This article reviews limitations of the current staging system and dilemmas facing imagers in their interactions with surgical, oncologic, pathologic, and other colleagues managing NSCLC. Unless otherwise specifically stated, the TNM and stage groupings in this article refer to TNM8 as described in the proposal publications of the International Association for the Study of Lung Cancer (IASLC).

STRENGTHS AND WEAKNESSES OF TNM8 PROCESS

The IASLC reclassification of NSCLC represents an unparalleled data-based advancement of the

Disclosures: No pertinent disclosures.
Department of Radiology, St. George's NHS Foundation Trust Hospitals and School of Medicine, St James' Wing, Blackshaw Road, London SW17 0QT, UK
E-mail address: ioannis.vlahos@stgeorges.nhs.uk

Radiol Clin N Am 56 (2018) 419–435
https://doi.org/10.1016/j.rcl.2018.01.010
0033-8389/18/Crown Copyright © 2018 Published by Elsevier Inc. All rights reserved.

radiologic.theclinics.com

accuracy of staging through TNM7 and TNM8. The historical 6th edition (2002) of the TNM classification system, itself unchanged from the 5th edition (1997), was based on only 5319 surgically staged cases, predominantly from a single site.[9] The TNM7 Lung Cancer Project accumulated a database of 68,463 validated NSCLC patients from 46 centers across 20 countries, staged clinically, principally by CT, during 1990 to 2000. A survival analysis of this database supported reclassification of the T, N, and M descriptors and their associated stage groupings in TNM7, adopted by the International Union against Cancer and the American Joint Committee on Cancer in December 2009.

The retrospective nature of the TNM7 database prohibited a detailed analysis of several clinical parameters as well as the validity of existing T parameters. To address these limitations, a prospective study was launched in 2009 in order to create a new database to inform TNM8.[10] This ambitious project incorporated an electronic data capture (EDC) form to record detailed staging information to assess the validity of each of the components of the TNM staging system. The EDC aim was to accumulate extensive clinical, surgical, pathologic, and outcome data that could influence survival. The EDC included demographic data, such as sex, age, and smoking history, and clinical data, such as comorbidities, performance status, serologic and pulmonary function values, and the presence of paraneoplastic syndromes. Pathologic data included histologic subtype, tumor grade, and extent of lymphovascular or visceral pleural invasion (VPI). Where available, biological, molecular, and genetic factors and surgical data relating to resection margins and outcome were recorded. If performed, maximum standardized uptake values from ^{18}F-fludeoxyglucose PET-computed tomography (CT) were solicited.

The finalized TNM8 database comprised new diagnoses of lung cancer between 1999 and 2010.[11] Although of a similar large size to the TNM7 database (70,967 NSCLC validated cases), it is important to recognize several differences between TNM7 and TNM8 databases that have implications for the applicability of the TNM8 staging system and may indicate areas that may change in later TNM versions. Although the TNM8 database was prospectively accrued, most cases were submitted from established databases, with less than 5% submitted by EDC with all the required elements. Hence, in large part the database is lacking in the detailed parameters desired from a prospective evaluation. Although the database remains international, it is now more geographically skewed. Asian cases increased from 11.5% to 44%, almost

exclusively from Japan (93%). Correspondingly, the contribution from North America (5%) and Australia (1.7%) was markedly reduced (previously 21%, 9.3%, respectively). The European contribution to cases was mildly reduced (49% vs 58%), but notably these again were disproportionately from a single nation, Denmark (73%). South America contributed only 0.3% of cases.

The altered geographic distribution is important because overall the cases from Asia, and hence the entire database, were predominantly stage I, whereas European cases were most often stage IV. The Asian cases may have included earlier stage subsolid lesions; however, these data are not recorded. Critically, mutations of epidermal growth factor receptor (EGFR) are also known to be more common in Asian populations; however, these data were also not captured.

The early stage preponderance is reflected in management paradigms and ultimately patient survival profile. As a result, in TNM8, 85% of patients underwent surgery alone, or in combination with chemotherapy or radiotherapy (53% in TNM7). The reduction of advanced stages of disease in the database, and the absence of any chemotherapy trial patients, is reflected in only 9.3% of patients undergoing chemotherapy alone, radiotherapy alone (1.5%), or both (4.7%) compared with TNM7 (23%, 11%, 12%, respectively).

The different constituent characteristics of the current TNM8 database impact on the wider relevance of the new staging system. Arguably the modified staging system descriptors and stages may be more optimized to differentiating survival in early surgically treatable disease than in advanced nonsurgical disease.

IMAGING METHODOLOGIES

A robust staging system must reflect the prevalent imaging modalities available for accurate determination of patient stage. A deficiency of the retrospective TNM7 dataset was that many patients in the acquisition period did not undergo PET-CT. PET-CT functional imaging has proved an invaluable adjunct to CT staging, increasing the diagnostic accuracy of determination of malignancy within primary, nodal, and metastatic sites and providing prognostic information via standardized uptake values.[12–14] Considering the 2 largest contributors of cases, it is likely that a smaller proportion of the earlier stage Japanese cases (submitted earlier in 3 tranches in 1999, 2002, and 2004) underwent PET-CT than the later collected advanced stage Danish cases (submitted gradually over 2001–2010). However, none of the cases from these 2 major contributors were electronically captured, and so no PET-CT data are recorded.[15] As a consequence, the value of PET-CT remains unrepresented in the current staging.

The necessary complex and time-consuming process of planning TNM changes can be inflexible to incorporating technological imaging advances. MR imaging has established value in assessing chest wall invasion, Pancoast tumors, and spinal involvement. However, more recently, perfusion imaging, diffusion-weighted imaging, and PET-MR imaging technical evolutions show promise in lung cancer staging and characterization; however, their incorporation into future TNM classifications may take longer than PET-CT imaging.[16–18]

T DESCRIPTORS

The new TNM8 classification introduces multiple new size cut points for the size T descriptors and a new T category T1c (T1a ≤1 cm, T1b >1 cm ≤2 cm, T1c >2 cm ≤3 cm, T2a >3 cm ≤4 cm, T2b >4 cm ≤5 cm, T3 >5 cm, T4 >7 cm). Morphologic descriptors are also altered with main bronchial involvement, regardless of distance from the carina, and associated partial or total lung atelectasis all assigned as T2 disease. Diaphragmatic involvement is reclassified from T3 to T4 disease, and mediastinal pleural involvement is eliminated from the staging system.[3]

The proliferation of cut points in the TNM8 classification system is justified by survival analysis across clinically and surgically staged cases with better separation of the survival curves of the individual T categories. Although there were less T3

and T4 cases in the current database, the reclassification resulted in statistically significant separation of these groups, which was not evident in TNM7. However, the clinical impact of new surgical advances that permit resection of limited T4 disease (vertebral, central vascular) remains unaddressed.

Central Airways

The reclassification of T2 disease for tumor involvement further or closer to 2 cm was based on only 24 patients with a pathologic staging of T3N0M0 disease solely due to proximal airway involvement.[19] The improved 5-year survival in this group (70%), compared with 25 patients with clinically staged T3N0M0 solely due to proximal airway involvement (59%), may have been related to the lesser involvement of the central airways that permitted surgery, or to T3 extension that was minimal and only determined at surgery. Under the new classification, disease extending to within 1 mm of the carina could technically be determined as T2 disease, whereas more central disease with carinal involvement is T4 disease. It is unlikely that these T descriptors would have survival so disparate. In addition, T2 within 1 mm of the carina and N0M0 disease is unlikely in most centers to be operable despite being as low as stage IB (3-4 cm) or stage IIA (4-5 cm) in TNM8 (Fig. 1).

Visceral Pleural Invasion

The presence of VPI remains a T2 descriptor in the TNM8 classification. In recent years, the pathologic definition of VPI has been standardized by

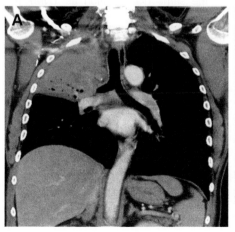
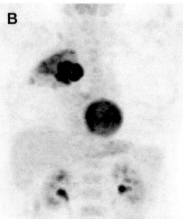

Fig. 1. Right upper lobe central tumor resulting in right upper lobe collapse (T2 descriptor) (A). The tumor size cannot be defined confidently by CT. The extent of central tracheal invasion is at approximately 2 cm; however, invasion proximal to 2 cm is still T2 under TNM8. In practice, PET-CT (B) provides biological functional information as well as delineation of the tumor extent and size >5 cm (T3).

the IASLC to overcome variability in histopathological characterization.[20] Absence of pleural invasion (PL0) represents tumor either within the subpleural lung parenchyma or invading superficially into the pleural connective tissue beneath the elastic layer. VPI is defined as tumor invasion beyond the elastic layer (PL1) or invasion to the pleural surface (PL2), both reflecting T2 disease. Parietal pleural or deeper chest wall invasion is PL3 (T3 disease). Survival is demonstrably stratified by differentiating categories PL0 to PL3.[21,22] Similarly, in the TNM8 database, the greater the depth of VPI (PL2 vs PL1), the worse the prognosis.[3,23]

However, the determination of VPI on CT and other imaging modalities remains problematic. Lesions may abut the pleural surface and yet not result in VPI. The probability of invasion is greater with larger lesions; however, these are already T2 or greater when greater than 3 cm. For lesions less than 3 cm, 3-dimensional (3D) evaluation with calculation of ratios of length and area of interface between tumor and the pleura to tumor size can improve accuracy of determination but are imperfect (**Fig. 2**).[24,25] For subsolid lesions, the likelihood of VPI is less, particularly for pure ground glass lesions.[26] For lesions not abutting the pleural surface but connected via pleural tags, tags associated with thickening at the pleural end demonstrate a moderate association with VPI (sensitivity 36%, specificity 93%) (**Fig. 3**).[27]

The more subtle differentiation of PL2 from PL1 disease is not possible unless there was transfissural extension or there is pleural fluid present. In the latter circumstance, there will almost certainly be pleural disease present indicating more severe M1a disease (minimum stage IVA).

Applying the TNM Classification

In a proportion of cases, it remains difficult to determine the primary site of disease to assign the correct T status. This can occur when there are several lesions present, or both peripheral pulmonary parenchymal disease and central disease infiltrating the hilar or mediastinal regions have similar infiltrative morphology. This difficulty is not addressed in staging manuals and can lead to variability of staging.

Interdependence of T and M Stage

A continuing limitation of TNM8 is that in certain situations the T and M categorization is not independent of each other. A hypothetical 1.5-cm small lesion in the right upper lobe, with no associated nodal or metastatic disease, would be classified as T1bN0M0 (stage IA2). An additional 8-mm nodule within the same lobe would upgrade this lesion to T3 (stage IIB). If the additional nodule is in the right middle lobe, the classification of the primary lesion is upgraded to T4M0 (stage IIIA) whether there is a single nodule or multiple nodules suggestive of metastatic dissemination. If only one additional nodule is present, but in the contralateral lung, the classification of the primary lesion in the right upper lobe is paradoxically downgraded back to T1b; however, the stage is now IVA, unless the additional lesion is considered a synchronous primary in which case the staging could be assigned as 2 primary lesions with stages T1bN0M0 (stage IA2) and T1aN0M0 (stage IA1).

Multiple Lesions

TNM8 database survival analysis has maintained the same classification as TNM7 for additional

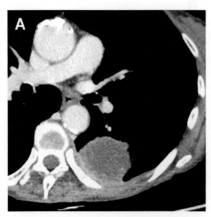
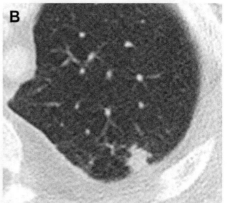

Fig. 2. (A) A 4.3-cm left lower lobe subpleural lesion (T2b by size) demonstrates clear evidence of pleural thickening with loss of extrapleural fat (T3). (B) A 1.4-cm subpleural lesion (T1b by size) with pleural contact is indeterminate for VPI (T2a), a prognostically important factor that may indicate adjuvant chemotherapy in some patients but is challenging to determine in small lesions.

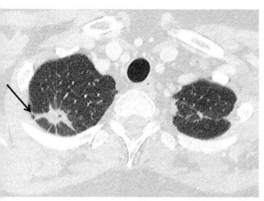

Fig. 3. Spiculated adenocarcinoma. The peripherally thicker spicules (*arrow*) may be indicative of pleural invasion but are not specific. The spiculate morphology also results in variability in measurement and hence T descriptor.

nodules.[28] This classification is intended for nodules that are suspected to be additional nodules of the same subtype as the dominant primary, rather than separate primary lesions or multifocal instances of lepidic predominant tumors. However, this calls for a radiological interpretative opinion, which may lead to variations in staging. The number of cases with additional nodules in the TNM8 database increased after the TNM7 proposals were published; however, survival in these groups remained unaltered.[28] This event suggests that differences were predominantly due to selective reporting rather than incidence. Similarly, the rate of clinically detected additional nodules was only half of that of pathologically detected nodules (1.7% vs 3.5%). The low absolute number of additional nodules and the larger number detected pathologically likely indicate a combination of radiologists underreporting small nodules that they cannot be certain are malignant

as well as pathologists identifying additional incidental nodules in surgical specimens. Because of a paucity of EDC, it remains impossible to determine from current TNM8 data whether the number and size of additional nodules are important prognostic factors (**Fig. 4**).

Clinical staging uncertainty arises from considerations whether additional small nodules are benign or malignant, and if malignant whether they are intrapulmonary metastases or synchronous primary malignancies. Recent IASLC proposals provide a helpful multidisciplinary framework for evaluation of whether 2 or more lesions reflect synchronous primaries or metastatic disease.[29] This situation is a common situation occurring in at least 15% of cases. Although it is easier to prove that 2 histologically dissimilar lesions are separate primaries, proving that a histologically similar lesion is a metastasis of another similar lesion is more complex, particularly as synchronous primary tumors are usually of the same histology. Proposed criteria include reviewing similarities of major and minor histologic subtypes and ideally performing genomic sequencing comparison, although this is unlikely to be ubiquitously available. Biopsy-determined biomarkers, driver mutations, and clonality are also supportive of metastatic disease, but it is recognized that these may differ between the primary and metastases particularly after therapy by targeted or systemic chemotherapy. In clinical practice, it is recommended that the differences or similarities in radiological appearance and growth rate and absence of nodal or systemic metastases be of assistance (**Fig. 5**).

Applicability to Subsolid Lesions

Clinical and study experience has demonstrated significant differences in the growth rates of solid and subsolid malignant lesions. Subsolid lesions

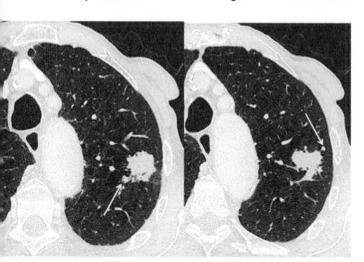

Fig. 4. Satellite nodules (T3) around an adenocarcinoma lesion (*arrows*). Studies suggest the number of satellite nodules may prognosticate poorer survival; however, limited data related to this descriptor in the TNM8 database have resulted in no change of descriptors.

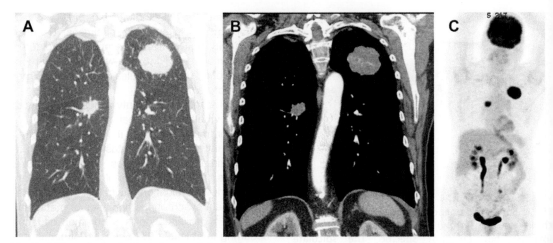

Fig. 5. A 6.2-cm lesion in the left upper lobe and a 2.9-cm lesion in the right lower lobe, both adenocarcinoma at biopsy (*A*). Similar lobular minimally spiculated appearance with similar heterogeneous enhancement (*B*) and the absence of nodal disease (*C*) support that the smaller lesion is a synchronous primary rather than a metastasis.

grow over a period of years, gradually enlarging and becoming more dense or multifocal. In a screening program, the mean volume doubling time of malignant pure ground glass lesions (813 days) was considerably longer than that of malignant part solid (457 days) or solid lesions (149 days).[30] In recognition that these lesions behave differently, a reclassification of adenocarcinoma of the lung introduced the definitions of adenocarcinoma in situ (AIS), minimally invasive adenocarcinoma (MIA), and lepidic predominant adenocarcinoma.[31] In turn, the recognition of the indolence of these lesions has led to an evolution of imaging surveillance recommendations that has become progressively less frequent and longer term.[32,33] Importantly, the imaging characteristics of most TNM8 lesions are unknown, and no differential survival has been ascribed to the histologic subtypes of these subsolid lesions,

which are not discriminated in TNM8. Moreover, the TNM8 revised classification system may potentially underestimate the survival of patients with these earlier categories of disease. This is because survival in TNM8 is measured from the date of clinical diagnosis in nonsurgically managed patients but from the date of surgery in operated patients. Because of the adoption of imaging guidelines, the interval between first appreciation of a subsolid lesion and surgery may be considerably longer than that for solid lesions.

Subsolid Lesion Descriptors

Several studies have suggested that measuring the solid component of subsolid adenocarcinoma lesions, which more closely correlates with the pathologic invasive component, better stratifies survival (**Fig. 6**).[34,35] Although this is also the

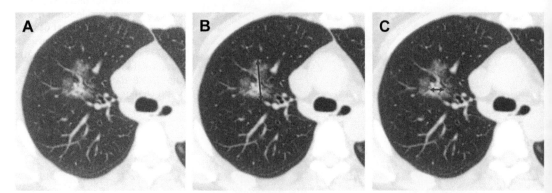

Fig. 6. Subsolid right upper lesion with morphology of lepidic predominant adenocarcinoma (*A*), the ground glass component of which measures 4.2 cm (*B, arrow*), suggesting T2b disease. However, current recommendations are to measure the solid component (*C, arrow*) that better correlates with survival (1.5 cm, T1b).

current recommendation of the IASLC for staging of subsolid lesions, the TNM8 database does not contain data with regards to whether lesions were subsolid and how these were measured clinically or pathologically.[36] In addition, it is unclear that reproducible methods have yet been defined, with reduced interobserver variability, for measuring subsolid lesions that are also dependent on the slice thickness, reconstruction algorithm, and available planes of visualization and not easily amenable to automated measurement (**Fig. 7**).

IASLC proposals have been forwarded to homogenize the application of the TNM staging system for subsolid lesions.[37] These recommendations apply to lesions with at least 10% ground glass or lepidic component. With the exception of pneumonic type adenocarcinoma, for multifocal subsolid lesions, the T stage is determined by the dominant lesion, ignoring T or M descriptors for same lobe, ipsilateral lung, or contralateral additional nodules (**Fig. 8**). An absolute number or the letter "m" is included as a suffix to the T stage to document the multifocality ignoring pure ground glass lesions <5 mm or pathologically confirmed sites of atypical adenomatous hyperplasia (eg, T1b(4) or T1(m)). The solid component of subsolid lesions should be measured as per recent recommendations.[36] AIS should be classified as Tis and MIA as T1a(mi). Nodal and metastatic disease is less common in subsolid lesions, and it is recommended that the "N and M category that applies to all the multiple foci collectively" should be applied. Typically, this is likely to be N0 or N1 disease, although it is likely that some variation in radiologist reporting could occur in the case of bilateral lesions with bilateral hilar adenopathy as to whether this reflected N3 disease or bilateral N1 disease.

Undefined Situations

As the staging system becomes more complex, greater variations in interobserver performance may reasonably be expected. Some variability likely occurs because of unfamiliarity with situations specifically defined in accessory staging manuals but not necessarily repeated in revision articles or radiological summary articles.[9] For example, transfissural extension through 2 layers of visceral pleura reflects T2a disease rather than T3 disease (visceral and parietal pleural involvement) or T4 disease (involvement of 2 lobes) (**Fig. 9**). Variability in staging of main or interlobar arteries invasion is also recognized in determining which anatomy constitutes "great vessel" invasion (T4). In this instance, the great vessels are defined as the aorta, superior and inferior vena cava, the main pulmonary trunk, and the intrapericardial portions of the pulmonary arteries and veins (**Fig. 10**).

However, other situations remain undefined and generate staging quandaries for even the most knowledgeable cancer imager. Lymphangitis carcinomatosa remains a perennial absence from staging systems.[38] When clearly nodular, this can be defined as T3 by virtue of nodules in the same lobe, or M1a disease if there is associated pleural disease. In practice, lymphangitis rarely occurs in isolation but rather when size criteria of the primary, nodal, or other metastatic disease define an advanced overall staging (**Fig. 11**). An exception to this may occur when lymphangitic disease is limited to smooth interlobular septal thickening. This is also a challenging diagnostic issue because radiologists must try to avoid overdiagnosis of lymphangitis compared with obstructive lymphedema. It is hoped that as future electronic capture cases record the extent and distribution of

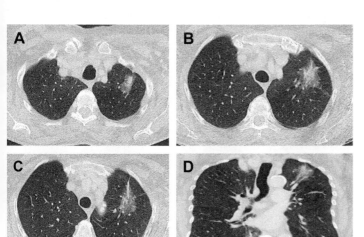

Fig. 7. Lepidic predominant adenocarcinoma. The measurement of the solid component of a subsolid lesion can induce interobserver variation if the morphology of the lesion is irregular and can be influenced by axial slice location (*A–C*), slice thickness, or imaging plane (coronal; *D*).

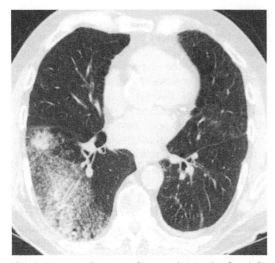

Fig. 8. Pneumonic type adenocarcinoma in the right lower lobe. Measurement of such lesions is subject to variation, because they may contain multiple discrete solid elements. When involving ipsilateral or contralateral other lobes, T4 and M1a apply.

lymphangitis, future staging iterations can address these issues.

NODAL DISEASE

As per the recommendations of the TNM7 classification, the TNM8 nodal classification remains unchanged from earlier staging versions.[1] Although this appears justified by survival analyses, the nodal staging system can be argued to remain deficient for the stratification of patient prognosis and hence optimal disease management.

N2 Disease

A 2007 survey of medical oncologists evaluated the chosen first-line therapy for a hypothetical stage IIIA NSCLC patient based on a 2.6-cm right upper lobe lesion with a single-station 4R mediastinoscopy-proven positive lymph node.[39] Out of 406 respondents, the optimal selected therapy was extremely variable (surgery with adjuvant chemotherapy 19%, surgery with adjuvant chemoradiotherapy 20%, neoadjuvant chemotherapy followed by surgery ± chemotherapy or radiotherapy 20%, induction chemoradiotherapy followed by surgery ± chemotherapy 32%, and nonsurgical chemoradiotherapy 8%). In a similar stage IIIA scenario but with multiple enlarged mediastinal nodes, 52% of respondents elected a nonsurgical approach and 32% still considered induction chemoradiotherapy followed by surgery ± chemotherapy. A comparable survey of the management of IIIA disease by thoracic surgeons identified a similar significant variability of optimal management, based on the extent of microscopic or macroscopic nodal disease.[40]

This lack of consensus reflects the known heterogeneity of N2 disease. Andre and colleagues demonstrated that for surgically treated N2 disease the 5-year survival progressively deteriorated from microscopic single-station N2 disease (34%) through multiple-station N2 microscopic disease (11%), single-station CT evident macroscopic N2 disease (8%), and finally, multistation CT evident macroscopic N2 disease (3%).[41] However, even submicroscopic nodal disease can confer survival differences. In one study of patients with clinical and microscopic N0 disease, the use of immunohistochemical cytokeratin and epithelial markers identified N2 micrometastases in 4.7% of 179 patients with operated stage I or stage II disease operated without induction therapy. These patients had a reduced progression-free survival of 21.5 months compared with 45.3 months in other patients.[42]

CT and PET-CT imaging can routinely determine the size and number of enlarged or metabolically

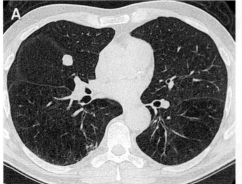
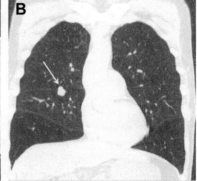

Fig. 9. A 16-mm right middle lobe adenocarcinoma (*A*), T1b by size, demonstrates extension to the right upper lobe, better appreciated on coronal imaging (*B, arrow*). Transfissural extension is defined as T2a disease.

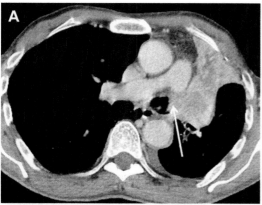 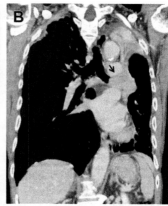

Fig. 10. Left upper lobe central tumor (*A, B*) invades left upper bronchus >2 cm from carina (*long arrow*) (T2) and results in left upper lobe collapse (T2). However, invasion of the main pulmonary artery and the intrapericardial left pulmonary artery (*short arrow*) confirms T4 great vessel invasion.

active mediastinal lymph nodes and morphologically suggest extracapsular extension. These factors are recognized to be adverse parameters with regards to survival, surgical outcome, and recurrence.[43–45] Exploratory analyses in the TNM8 dataset concurred that nodal volume impacts survival, which progressively deteriorated from single-station N1 disease, through multiple-station N1 or single-station N2 disease, to multiple-station N2 disease. Analyses also suggested that patients with single-station N2 disease but no N1 disease (skip disease) may have improved survival compared with single-station N2 disease with N1 disease. However, these exploratory analyses were only possible on the smaller group EDC patients and could not be extended to recommendations for the whole dataset. Analyses were also hampered by differences in recording of the nodal status between the Japanese Naruke system and the Mountain-Dresler modification of the American Thoracic Society before the promulgation of a unified IASLC nodal map in 2009.[46]

As such, the heterogeneity of N2 disease remains a significant clinical and imaging dilemma that impedes the comparison of studies of best management of patients with IIIA disease.[47]

Undefined Situations

Another problematic situation is the presence of lymph node disease in sites not defined in the TNM classification, principally axillary and abdominal adenopathy. Some imagers ascribe this as metastatic disease (M1b in the abdomen, M1a or M1b in the axilla); however, it should be noted that metastatic disease is defined as "non-lymphatic disease." An N3 status can be considered but may perhaps be understating the severity of the disease. However, the N descriptors as defined currently only address nodal metastatic disease in the hilar, mediastinal, and supraclavicular regions. There is a paucity of data published in this regard. Satoh and colleagues[48] suggested that axillary nodes occurred in only 1% of lung cancer cases. However, in the author's personal experience (Ioannis Vlahos, BSc, MBBS, MRCP, FRCR, unpublished data, 2012), abdominal or axillary nodal disease occurred in 13% of 192 cases (Fig. 12). In 40% of these cases, these nodal sites

Fig. 11. Lymphangitic carcinomatosa is not defined in the TNM staging. However, when multinodular, this is at least T3 disease for the same lobe or T4 for involvement of more than one ipsilateral lobe. Commonly, as in this case, effusions are present defining M1a stage IVA disease.

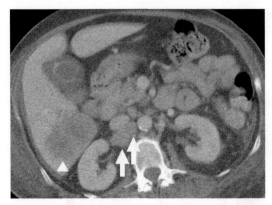

Fig. 12. Retroperitoneal nodes in NSCLC (*arrows*) are not defined in the TNM system but are often termed M1b disease. In this case, further evidence of hepatic metastatic M1b disease is also present (*arrowhead*).

constituted the only site of N3 or M1 disease. Axillary and abdominal adenopathy remain an open issue in lung cancer staging, and it is the personal preference of the author to refer to this disease as M1b disease, although other practitioners operating within their multidisciplinary teams may reasonably adopt an alternative assignment, pending clarity on the issue from international bodies.

METASTATIC DISEASE

The determination of metastatic disease in NSCLC indicates the presence of stage IV disease and historically identified patients in whom palliative therapy was attempted rather than IIIA or IIIB disease, whereby curative intent surgical or chemotherapeutic regimens could be attempted. In recent years, aggressive metastasectomy has been considered for single sites of disease, particularly within the adrenal gland. The TNM8 classification has maintained the prior M1a category (intrathoracic disease) but added the categories of M1b disease (single-site extrathoracic disease) and M1c disease (multiple-site extrathoracic disease). These analyses were based on only a small sample of unresected metastatic disease within the larger database (n = 1025) for which sufficient electronic data were available. Notably, the median survival prognosis of patients with M1a and M1b is similar (11.5 and 11.4 months, respectively), and survival curve separation is dependent on the minority of patients surviving after 2 years. The prognosis of M1c (median survival 6.3 months) is considerably worse. As such, differentiation of the M1 categories, M1a/M1b (stage IVA) and M1c (stage IVB), is not strictly survival based but can be considered exploratory for future TNM iterations to evaluate.

Impact of Diagnostic Rigor on Metastatic Disease Survival

The median survival of TNM8 database patients is improved compared with those of the TNM7 database (M1a 10 months, M1b 6 months).[49] In part, these improvements may relate to improved medical therapy via chemotherapy, targeted therapies, or evolutions in brain stereotactic therapy. However, it is also recognized that some patients, based on imaging findings, may erroneously be initially classified as having metastatic disease, prolonging apparent survival. For example, the presence of pleural or pericardial effusions without nodularity can be radiologically difficult to differentiate from benign disease in patients with cardiac comorbidities. The aggressiveness for biopsy pathologic determination of early metastatic disease varies widely within nations and individual sites (**Fig. 13**).

The corroboration of metastatic disease will be influenced by the variable utilization of PET-CT through 1999 to 2000 in different geographic regions. Certainly PET-CT may aid in dismissing some sites of suspected metastatic disease; however, the overall effect is likely to identify earlier and occult metastatic disease. Earlier detection results in a measurable stage migration of lower metastatic burden disease into the stage IV group and improves metastatic disease survival.[50]

The choice of imaging for brain metastatic disease also likely influences the detection of lower metastatic burden stage IV disease, improving stage IV survival. In recent years, there has been a clear shift from only evaluating patients with clinically symptomatic neurologic disease, likely to have a higher metastatic burden, to screening specific asymptomatic categories for early disease.[51,52] However, recommendations vary widely as do their adoption.[53] In the United States, American College of Radiology appropriateness criteria are that MR brain imaging is indicated if neurologic symptoms are present or in asymptomatic adenocarcinoma greater than 3 cm in size or N2 disease.[54] The UK National Institute for Health and Care Excellence guidelines for asymptomatic patients recommend *considering head MR imaging or CT* in patients treated with curative intent, especially in stage III disease.[55] Based on clinical resources, CT head imaging is usually used in patients with potentially surgically resectable tumors, in particular, adenocarcinoma that has a greater propensity to metastatic disease without local adenopathy.[56] However, brain CT likely underrecognizes metastatic disease. A UK study identified that 6.3% of postoperative NSCLC patients presented with brain recurrence (73% stage I or II),

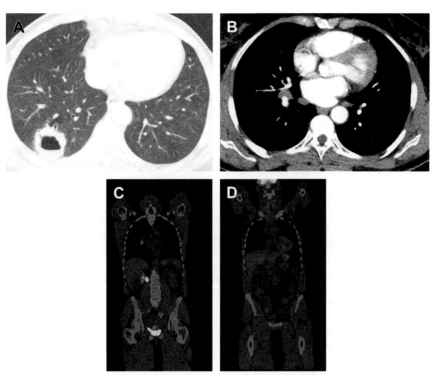

Fig. 13. A 4.1-cm squamous cell carcinoma (T2b) in the right lower lobe (*A*) with right hilar enlarged lymph node (*B*). PET-CT demonstrates increased metabolic activity in the right hilar node (*C*) as well as in <1 cm right axillary and subpectoral nodes (*D*). This would suggest at least N1 disease with axillary/subpectoral nodes not defined in TNM but variably staged as N3 or M1 disease. Axillary nodes were sampled and benign, right hilar nodes reactive at surgical resection (final pT2bN0M0). Variability of PET-CT and biopsy corroboration can influence perceived stage and survival of suspected metastatic disease.

the majority adenocarcinoma, and, projected by volume doubling times, that 71% of these (4.4% of all patients) could have been detected by preoperative MR imaging at the 2- to 5-mm size.[57] Conversely, in the United States, a recent study of stage I patients in the National Lung Screening Trial study suggested that 12% of patients with stage IA tumors (TNM7, T1 [<3 cm] N0M0) underwent CT imaging without detection of metastatic disease, concluding that this was unnecessary and against Choosing Wisely guidelines from the Society of Thoracic Surgeons.[58] However, screening populations may include a larger proportion of indolent tumors, including subsolid lesions, with a reduced propensity to metastatic disease.

Imaging and biopsy sampling variations between sites and nations and over time can lead to earlier detection of advanced or metastatic disease. This "Will Rogers phenomenon of cancer stage migration" results in removal of these lower metastatic burden cases from earlier stages and inclusion in more advanced stages. As a result, the mortality in both groups improves regardless of therapy.[59] Guidelines for optimal imaging strategies to identify metastatic disease will

likely continue to evolve, influenced by new data as well as health care availability. Although there is still variability in imaging for metastases, it is important to be cautious in interpreting variations in outcomes from different geographic regions, according to perceived metastatic burden.

STAGE GROUPINGS

The advent of TNM8 has required the definition of groupings of new T-size descriptors in combination with N and M descriptors. However, TNM8 introduces further complexity with new reclassification of groupings and the introduction of new staging subdivisions of stage I (IA1, IA2, IA3), stage III (IIIC), and stage IV (IVA, IVB).[4]

Increasing the complexity and stratification of staging in TNM8 undoubtedly confers benefits. Within TNM8, there is now better separation of survival curves with the exception of the overlap of stage IIIC and IVA. However, stage groupings also reflect the idiosyncrasies of the database. The overrepresentation of surgically treated cases and the underrepresentation of chemotherapy-treated cases in the TNM8 database are reflected in absolute survival changes from TNM7. Lower-stage disease survival has improved from TNM7, but higher stage survival, particularly stage IIIB, appears to have worsened.

Stage Migration

The TNM7 classification modified 17/48 groupings of the TNM descriptors, including several that impacted the traditional threshold between potential operative management (stage IIIA or less) and nonoperative management (stage IIIB or greater).[60] In practice, data from both the TNM7 database and external sources suggested that between 11% and 17% of patients migrated stage as a result of the TNM classification, and of these, 65% to 70% were upstaged.[61–63]

The TNM8 classification is undoubtedly more complex with changes in stage groupings for 38/60 TNM descriptor combinations. As such, even greater stage migration is to be expected. Stage migration is problematic in that it results in loss of backwards compatibility with reported and ongoing research trials determining the best management of different stages of disease. The substantial change in 2 consecutive iterations of the lung cancer staging system compounds this issue further. In effect, the repeated and substantial reclassification of lung cancer stage groupings can be argued to have the unintended consequence of impairing one of the key aims of a TNM staging system, which is to group patients together in order to define best treatment.

The IASLC correctly highlights that a change in taxonomic classification is not of itself an indication to alter established therapeutic paradigms. In practice, the reality may be different. A survey of 97 clinicians presented with 3 clinical scenarios, where the extent of abnormality was identical but the designated stage shifted between TNM6 and TNM7. A mean of 46% of respondents would change management in each clinical scenario based on the designated stage alone, with 77% of respondents changing management in at least 1 of the 3 scenarios.[64]

Complexity and Reproducibility

Additional T-size cut points in TNM8 increase the granularity of the staging system and result in a better prognostication of multifactorial continuous variables that impact survival. However, in turn this increases the complexity and potentially the time required for staging tumors. At present, CT imaging, supplemented by PET-CT, is reproducible with minor interobserver variability in staging because of differences in interpretation of imaging or the TNM classification system.[65,66]

The increasing number of cut points may increase the interobserver variability of CT size designation, particularly with variation in reconstructed slice thickness and whether imagers use axial, orthogonal multiplanar, or dedicated segmented 3D reconstructions for size determination. These results may indeed vary from those in the TNM8 database because many cases may have been measured on axial sections alone, because thin-section data storage and routing multiplanar reconstructions were not ubiquitous during the acquisition period. In turn, the discrepancy between the clinical and pathologic T descriptors (cT and pT, respectively) in determining stage may be further augmented at the numerous size interfaces now present, particularly for subsolid lesions wherein both radiological and histologic variability increases.

NONANATOMIC STAGING

Although it is clear that anatomic staging of the extent of disease, the basis of the current lung cancer system, fairly reflects survival, it is also abundantly evident that numerous other prognostic factors have been demonstrated to affect survival and influence oncologic management. For example, the presence of VPI[67,68] may indicate value in adjuvant chemotherapy even in node-negative tumors that are 3 to 5 cm in size (TNM7 stage IB). The mitotic index, or presence of microvascular invasion or lymphovascular invasion, appears to be a more important determinant of survival than T1a, T1b, T2a, and T2b size criteria in the TNM7 classification.[69–71] More importantly, the identification of tumor genetics and of driver mutations (eg, EGFR mutations and ALK-EML4 oncogenic fusion genes) that may be selectively treated has become a more important determinant of survival than the anatomic extent of disease. For example, small-molecule inhibitors of the ALK tyrosine kinase inhibitor in patients with ALK rearrangement and stage TNM7 IIIB/IV demonstrated progression-free survival that far exceeded the survival expected for patients with lesser stages of disease (Fig. 14).[72] These observations indicate that a simple anatomic extent of disease is likely insufficient to express the multifactorial knowledge that has been accumulated in the prognostication and treatment planning for NSCLC.

FUTURE DIRECTIONS

The future direction of the lung cancer staging system attracts considerable interest, underpinned by recognition that the anatomic extent

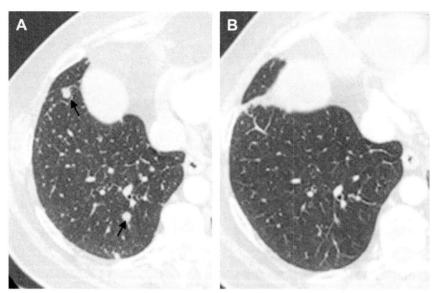

Fig. 14. Metastatic adenocarcinoma with 2 right lower lobe metastases (*A, arrows*). Biopsy demonstrated ALK rearrangement mutation. Six month follow-up following ALK tyrosine kinase inhibitor (Crizotinib) demonstrates complete resolution of metastases (*B*).

of disease is only one of a multitude of factors that govern patient outcome and suitability for therapeutic interventions. Anatomic staging will remain the cornerstone of NSCLC staging for the foreseeable future, periodically revised to reflect changes in knowledge. Aided by increasingly detailed prospectively accumulated data, this may include further size cut points, and further stratification of the pathologic extent of VPI or of the volume and distribution of additional parenchymal nodules or nodal disease. Concomitantly, the prospective accumulation of nonanatomic multifactorial data by the IASLC has commenced and is intended to form a composite prognostic index to be implemented in conjunction with future versions of anatomic staging. This index would incorporate patient demographics, environmental factors, tumor genetics, biology, and functional imaging data as well as information about treatment and outcomes. This prognostic index would be intended to be more fluid, updated regularly as advances in the multidisciplinary fields of NSCLC become available.[73,74]

A future combination of detailed anatomic staging, and prognostic indices, perhaps incorporating functional PET-CT, would be invaluable to addressing significant management issues in NSCLC. For example, is a single-stage system best for subsolid lesions or early screening detected tumors? Can these patients be adequately treated by sublobar anatomic resections?

Currently, the TNM survival analysis process updates staging and descriptors that have evolved from surgical practice. Chemotherapy and radiation treatment criteria are often different, and their applicability is limited by repeated stage migration. It is hopes that further new descriptors or disease subgroupings can also be prospectively coordinated to assess and validate disease subgroups suspected as eliciting differential response in nonsurgical trials.

SUMMARY

The lung cancer stage advances through TNM7 and TNM8, led by the IASLC, are unparalleled in their scientific rigor and have resulted in a staging system that far better reflects its purpose. In addition, a data collection process is now in place to inform detailed changes in anatomic and nonanatomic staging for the future. Despite these advances, some limitations remain. It is important to recognize that no staging system can adequately predict every staging eventuality. For those cases in which there is doubt in the staging, general rule 4 of the TNM classification system provides assistance, stating: "If there is doubt concerning the correct T, N, or M category to which a particular case should be allotted, then the lower (ie, less advanced) category should be chosen. This will also be reflected in the stage grouping."[9] In simplistic summary, radiologists could perhaps recall that when they are in doubt, to give the patients the benefit of the doubt.

REFERENCES

1. Asamura H, Chansky K, Crowley J, et al. The International Association for the Study of Lung Cancer lung cancer staging project: proposals for the revision of the N descriptors in the forthcoming 8th edition of the TNM classification for lung cancer. J Thorac Oncol 2015;10(12):1675–84.

2. Eberhardt WE, Mitchell A, Crowley J, et al. The IASLC lung cancer staging project: proposals for the revision of the M descriptors in the forthcoming eighth edition of the TNM classification of lung cancer. J Thorac Oncol 2015;10(11):1515–22.

3. Rami-Porta R, Bolejack V, Crowley J, et al, IASLC Staging and Prognostic Factors Committee, Advisory Boards and Participating Institutions. The IASLC lung cancer staging project: proposals for the revisions of the T descriptors in the forthcoming eighth edition of the TNM classification for lung cancer. J Thorac Oncol 2015;10(7):990–1003.

4. Goldstraw P, Chansky K, Crowley J, et al. The IASLC lung cancer staging project: proposals for revision of the TNM stage groupings in the forthcoming (eighth) edition of the TNM classification for lung cancer. J Thorac Oncol 2016;11(1):39–51.

5. Boiselle PM, Erasmus JJ, Ko JP, et al. Expert opinion: lung cancer staging. J Thorac Imaging 2011;26(2):85.

6. Goldstraw P. New TNM classification: achievements and hurdles. Transl Lung Cancer Res 2013;2(4):264–72.

7. Nair A, Klusmann MJ, Jogeesvaran KH, et al. Revisions to the TNM staging of non-small cell lung cancer: rationale, clinicoradiologic implications, and persistent limitations. Radiographics 2011;31(1):215–38.

8. Rami-Porta R, Goldstraw P. Strength and weakness of the new TNM classification for lung cancer. Eur Respir J 2010;36(2):237–9.

9. Goldstraw P. International Association for the Study of Lung Cancer: staging manual in thoracic oncology. Orange Park (FL): Editorial Rx Press; 2009.

10. Giroux DJ, Rami-Porta R, Chansky K, et al. The IASLC lung cancer staging project: data elements for the prospective project. J Thorac Oncol 2009; 4(6):679–83.

11. Rami-Porta R, Bolejack V, Giroux DJ, et al. The IASLC lung cancer staging project: the new database to inform the eighth edition of the TNM classification of lung cancer. J Thorac Oncol 2014;9(11): 1618–24.

12. Berghmans T, Dusart M, Paesmans M, et al. Primary tumor standardized uptake value (SUVmax) measured on fluorodeoxyglucose positron emission tomography (FDG-PET) is of prognostic value for survival in non-small cell lung cancer (NSCLC): a systematic review and meta-analysis (MA) by the European Lung Cancer Working Party for the IASLC lung cancer staging project. J Thorac Oncol 2008; 3(1):6–12.

13. Paesmans M, Berghmans T, Dusart M, et al. Primary tumor standardized uptake value measured on fluorodeoxyglucose positron emission tomography is of prognostic value for survival in non-small cell lung cancer: update of a systematic review and meta-analysis by the European Lung Cancer Working Party for the International Association for the Study of Lung Cancer Staging Project. J Thorac Oncol 2010;5(5):612–9.

14. Truong MT, Viswanathan C, Erasmus JJ. Positron emission tomography/computed tomography in lung cancer staging, prognosis, and assessment of therapeutic response. J Thorac Imaging 2011; 26(2):132–46.

15. IASLC Staging and Prognostic Factors Committee. IASLC retrospective database overview. Seattle (WA): IASLC International Staging and Prognostic Factors Committee; 2013. Available at: https://www.iaslc.org/sites/default/files/wysiwyg-assets/staging_slides.pdf.

16. Koyama H, Ohno Y, Seki S, et al. Magnetic resonance imaging for lung cancer. J Thorac Imaging 2013;28(3):138–50.

17. Ohno Y, Koyama H, Lee HY, et al. Magnetic resonance imaging (MRI) and positron emission tomography (PET)/MRI for lung cancer staging. J Thorac Imaging 2016;31(4):215–27.

18. Yoon SH, Goo JM, Lee SM, et al. Positron emission tomography/magnetic resonance imaging evaluation of lung cancer: current status and future prospects. J Thorac Imaging 2014;29(1):4–16.

19. Rami-Porta R, Bolejack V, Crowley J, et al, IASLC Staging and Prognostic Factors Committee, Advisory Boards and Participating Institutions. Supplementary online figures to: the IASLC lung cancer staging project: proposals for the revisions of the T descriptors in the forthcoming eighth edition of the TNM classification for lung cancer. J Thorac Oncol 2015;10(7):990–1003. Available at: http://links.lww.com/JTO/A835.

20. Travis WD, Brambilla E, Rami-Porta R, et al. Visceral pleural invasion: pathologic criteria and use of elastic stains: proposal for the 7th edition of the TNM classification for lung cancer. J Thorac Oncol 2008;3(12):1384–90.

21. Kawase A, Yoshida J, Miyaoka E, et al. Visceral pleural invasion classification in non-small-cell lung cancer in the 7th edition of the tumor, node, metastasis classification for lung cancer: validation analysis based on a large-scale nationwide database. J Thorac Oncol 2013;8(5):606–11.

22. Wang T, Zhou C, Zhou Q. Extent of visceral pleural invasion affects prognosis of resected non-small

cell lung cancer: a meta-analysis. Sci Rep 2017; 7(1):1527.

23. Rami-Porta R, Bolejack V, Crowley J, et al, IASLC Staging and Prognostic Factors Committee, Advisory Boards and Participating Institutions. Supplementary online tables to: the IASLC lung cancer staging project: proposals for the revisions of the T descriptors in the forthcoming eighth edition of the TNM classification for lung cancer. J Thorac Oncol 2015;10(7):990–1003. Available at: http://links.lww.com/JTO/A834.

24. Ebara K, Takashima S, Jiang B, et al. Pleural invasion by peripheral lung cancer: prediction with three-dimensional CT. Acad Radiol 2015;22(3): 310–9.

25. Imai K, Minamiya Y, Ishiyama K, et al. Use of CT to evaluate pleural invasion in non-small cell lung cancer: measurement of the ratio of the interface between tumor and neighboring structures to maximum tumor diameter. Radiology 2013;267(2): 619–26.

26. Ahn SY, Park CM, Jeon YK, et al. Predictive CT features of visceral pleural invasion by T1-sized peripheral pulmonary adenocarcinomas manifesting as subsolid nodules. AJR Am J Roentgenol 2017; 209(3):561–6.

27. Hsu JS, Han IT, Tsai TH, et al. Pleural tags on CT scans to predict visceral pleural invasion of non-small cell lung cancer that does not abut the pleura. Radiology 2016;279(2):590–6.

28. Detterbeck FC, Bolejack V, Arenberg DA, et al. The IASLC lung cancer staging project: background data and proposals for the classification of lung cancer with separate tumor nodules in the forthcoming eighth edition of the TNM classification for lung cancer. J Thorac Oncol 2016;11(5): 681–92.

29. Detterbeck FC, Franklin WA, Nicholson AG, et al. The IASLC lung cancer staging project: background data and proposed criteria to distinguish separate primary lung cancers from metastatic foci in patients with two lung tumors in the forthcoming eighth edition of the TNM classification for lung cancer. J Thorac Oncol 2016;11(5):651–65.

30. Hasegawa M, Sone S, Takashima S, et al. Growth rate of small lung cancers detected on mass CT screening. Br J Radiol 2000;73(876):1252–9.

31. Travis WD, Brambilla E, Noguchi M, et al. International Association for the Study of Lung Cancer/American Thoracic Society/European Respiratory Society international multidisciplinary classification of lung adenocarcinoma. J Thorac Oncol 2011; 6(2):244–85.

32. MacMahon H, Naidich DP, Goo JM, et al. Guidelines for management of incidental pulmonary nodules detected on CT images: from the Fleischner Society 2017. Radiology 2017;284(1):228–43.

33. Naidich DP, Bankier AA, MacMahon H, et al. Recommendations for the management of subsolid pulmonary nodules detected at CT: a statement from the Fleischner Society. Radiology 2013;266(1):304–17.

34. Yanagawa N, Shiono S, Abiko M, et al. New IASLC/ATS/ERS classification and invasive tumor size are predictive of disease recurrence in stage I lung adenocarcinoma. J Thorac Oncol 2013;8(5):612–8.

35. Nakamura S, Fukui T, Taniguchi T, et al. Prognostic impact of tumor size eliminating the ground glass opacity component: modified clinical T descriptors of the tumor, node, metastasis classification of lung cancer. J Thorac Oncol 2013;8(12):1551–7.

36. Travis WD, Asamura H, Bankier AA, et al. The IASLC lung cancer staging project: proposals for coding T categories for subsolid nodules and assessment of tumor size in part-solid tumors in the forthcoming eighth edition of the TNM classification of lung cancer. J Thorac Oncol 2016;11(8):1204–23.

37. Detterbeck FC, Marom EM, Arenberg DA, et al. The IASLC lung cancer staging project: background data and proposals for the application of TNM staging rules to lung cancer presenting as multiple nodules with ground glass or lepidic features or a pneumonic type of involvement in the forthcoming eighth edition of the TNM classification. J Thorac Oncol 2016;11(5):666–80.

38. Raj JV, Coulden R, Entwisle J. IASLC lung cancer staging project–a radiologist perspective. J Thorac Oncol 2008;3(3):318–9 [author reply: 319–20].

39. Tanner NT, Gomez M, Rainwater C, et al. Physician preferences for management of patients with stage IIIA NSCLC: impact of bulk of nodal disease on therapy selection. J Thorac Oncol 2012;7(2):365–9.

40. Veeramachaneni NK, Feins RH, Stephenson BJ, et al. Management of stage IIIA non-small cell lung cancer by thoracic surgeons in North America. Ann Thorac Surg 2012;94(3):922–6 [discussion: 926–8]. [Erratum appears in Ann Thorac Surg 2013;96(4):1532].

41. Andre F, Grunenwald D, Pignon JP, et al. Survival of patients with resected N2 non-small-cell lung cancer: evidence for a subclassification and implications. J Clin Oncol 2000;18(16):2981–9.

42. Herpel E, Muley T, Schneider T, et al. A pragmatic approach to the diagnosis of nodal micrometastases in early stage non-small cell lung cancer. J Thorac Oncol 2010;5(8):1206–12.

43. Liu W, Shao Y, Guan B, et al. Extracapsular extension is a powerful prognostic factor in stage IIA-IIIA non-small cell lung cancer patients with completely resection. Int J Clin Exp Pathol 2015; 8(9):11268–77.

44. Makino T, Hata Y, Otsuka H, et al. Predicted extracapsular invasion of hilar lymph node metastasis by fusion positron emission tomography/computed

tomography in patients with lung cancer. Mol Clin Oncol 2015;3(5):1035–40.

45. Wei S, Asamura H, Kawachi R, et al. Which is the better prognostic factor for resected non-small cell lung cancer: the number of metastatic lymph nodes or the currently used nodal stage classification? J Thorac Oncol 2011;6(2):310–8.

46. Rusch VW, Asamura H, Watanabe H, et al. The IASLC lung cancer staging project: a proposal for a new international lymph node map in the forthcoming seventh edition of the TNM classification for lung cancer. J Thorac Oncol 2009;4(5):568–77.

47. Yamaguchi M, Sugio K. Current status of induction treatment for N2-stage III non-small cell lung cancer. Gen Thorac Cardiovasc Surg 2014;62(11):651–9.

48. Satoh H, Ishikawa H, Kagohashi K, et al. Axillary lymph node metastasis in lung cancer. Med Oncol 2009;26(2):147–50.

49. Postmus PE, Brambilla E, Chansky K, et al. The IASLC Lung Cancer Staging Project: proposals for revision of the M descriptors in the forthcoming (seventh) edition of the TNM classification of lung cancer. J Thorac Oncol 2007;2(8):686–93.

50. Dinan MA, Curtis LH, Carpenter WR, et al. Stage migration, selection bias, and survival associated with the adoption of positron emission tomography among medicare beneficiaries with non-small-cell lung cancer, 1998-2003. J Clin Oncol 2012;30(22):2725–30.

51. Tanaka K, Kubota K, Kodama T, et al. Extrathoracic staging is not necessary for non-small-cell lung cancer with clinical stage T1-2 N0. Ann Thorac Surg 1999;68(3):1039–42.

52. Yohena T, Yoshino I, Kitajima M, et al. Necessity of preoperative screening for brain metastasis in non-small cell lung cancer patients without lymph node metastasis. Ann Thorac Cardiovasc Surg 2004;10(6):347–9.

53. Backhus LM, Farjah F, Varghese TK, et al. Appropriateness of imaging for lung cancer staging in a national cohort. J Clin Oncol 2014;32(30):3428–35.

54. American College of Radiology. ACR appropriateness criteria: non-invasive staging of bronchogenic carcinoma. American College of Radiology; 2013. Available at: https://acsearch.acr.org/docs/69456/Narrative/.

55. The National Institute for Health and Care Excellence. Lung cancer: diagnosis and management. Clinical guideline [CG121]. National Institute for Health and Care Excellence; 2011. Available at: https://www.nice.org.uk/guidance/cg121/chapter/1-Guidance#diagnosis-and-staging.

56. Shi AA, Digumarthy SR, Temel JS, et al. Does initial staging or tumor histology better identify asymptomatic brain metastases in patients with non-small cell lung cancer? J Thorac Oncol 2006;1(3):205–10.

57. O'Dowd EL, Kumaran M, Anwar S, et al. Brain metastases following radical surgical treatment of non-small cell lung cancer: is preoperative brain imaging important? Lung Cancer 2014;86(2):185–9.

58. Balekian AA, Fisher JM, Gould MK. Brain imaging for staging of patients with clinical stage IA non-small cell lung cancer in the National Lung Screening Trial: adherence with recommendations from the choosing wisely campaign. Chest 2016;149(4):943–50.

59. Feinstein AR, Sosin DM, Wells CK. The Will Rogers phenomenon. Stage migration and new diagnostic techniques as a source of misleading statistics for survival in cancer. N Engl J Med 1985;312(25):1604–8.

60. Goldstraw P, Crowley J, Chansky K, et al. The IASLC Lung Cancer Staging Project: proposals for the revision of the TNM stage groupings in the forthcoming (seventh) edition of the TNM classification of malignant tumours. J Thorac Oncol 2007;2(8):706–14 [Erratum appears in J Thorac Oncol 2007;2(10):985].

61. Lyons G, Quadrelli S, Jordan P, et al. Clinical impact of the use of the revised International Association for the Study of Lung Cancer staging system to operable non-small-cell lung cancers. Lung Cancer 2011;74(2):244–7.

62. Van Meerbeeck JP, Chansky K, Goldstraw P. The impact of stage migration on survival after resection in the UICC 7 TNM classification of lung cancer. J Clin Oncol 2010;28(15_suppl):7022.

63. Strand TE, Rostad H, Wentzel-Larsen T, et al. A population-based evaluation of the seventh edition of the TNM system for lung cancer. Eur Respir J 2010;36(2):401–7.

64. Boffa DJ, Detterbeck FC, Smith EJ, et al. Should the 7th edition of the lung cancer stage classification system change treatment algorithms in non-small cell lung cancer? J Thorac Oncol 2010;5(11):1779–83.

65. Hofman MS, Smeeton NC, Rankin SC, et al. Observer variation in FDG PET-CT for staging of non-small-cell lung carcinoma. Eur J Nucl Med Mol Imaging 2009;36(2):194–9.

66. Webb WR, Sarin M, Zerhouni EA, et al. Interobserver variability in CT and MR staging of lung cancer. J Comput Assist Tomogr 1993;17(6):841–6.

67. Jiang L, Liang W, Shen J, et al. The impact of visceral pleural invasion in node-negative non-small cell lung cancer: a systematic review and meta-analysis. Chest 2015;148(4):903–11.

68. Park SY, Lee JG, Kim J, et al. Efficacy of platinum-based adjuvant chemotherapy in T2aN0 stage IB non-small cell lung cancer. J Cardiothorac Surg 2013;8:151.

69. Matsumura Y, Hishida T, Shimada Y, et al. Impact of extratumoral lymphatic permeation on postoperative

survival of non-small-cell lung cancer patients. J Thorac Oncol 2014;9(3):337–44.

70. Ruffini E, Asioli S, Filosso PL, et al. Significance of the presence of microscopic vascular invasion after complete resection of Stage I-II pT1-T2N0 non-small cell lung cancer and its relation with T-Size categories: did the 2009 7th edition of the TNM staging system miss something? J Thorac Oncol 2011;6(2): 319–26.

71. Duhig EE, Dettrick A, Godbolt DB, et al. Mitosis trumps T stage and proposed International Association for the Study of Lung Cancer/American Thoracic Society/European Respiratory Society classification for prognostic value in resected

stage 1 lung adenocarcinoma. J Thorac Oncol 2015;10(4):673–81.

72. Kwak EL, Bang YJ, Camidge DR, et al. Anaplastic lymphoma kinase inhibition in non-small-cell lung cancer. N Engl J Med 2010;363(18):1693–703 [Erratum appears in N Engl J Med 2011;364(6):588].

73. Detterbeck F. Stage classification and prediction of prognosis: difference between accountants and speculators. J Thorac Oncol 2013;8(7):820–2.

74. Rami-Porta R, Asamura H, Goldstraw P. Predicting the prognosis of lung cancer: the evolution of tumor, node and metastasis in the molecular age-challenges and opportunities. Transl Lung Cancer Res 2015;4(4):415–23.

Update of MR Imaging for Evaluation of Lung Cancer

Mario Ciliberto, MD[a,b,c], Yuji Kishida, MD[d], Shinichiro Seki, MD, PhD[a,b], Takeshi Yoshikawa, MD, PhD[a,b], Yoshiharu Ohno, MD, PhD[a,b],*

KEYWORDS

• Lung cancer • MR imaging • Functional imaging • Pulmonary nodules • Staging

KEY POINTS

- Since MR imaging was introduced for the assessment of thoracic and lung diseases, various limitations have hindered its widespread adoption in clinical practice.
- Since 2000, however, various techniques have demonstrated the usefulness of MR imaging for lung cancer evaluation, and it is now reimbursed by health insurance companies in many countries.
- This article reviews recent advances in lung MR imaging, focusing on its use for lung cancer evaluation.

INTRODUCTION

Since MR imaging was introduced for the assessment of thoracic and lung diseases, various limitations, mostly related to the relatively low proton density of lung parenchyma, the presence of cardiac and respiratory motion artifacts, and long acquisition time, have hampered the clinical application of this technique. In the last few decades, technical advancements in MR systems, sequence, and reconstruction methods, including parallel imaging techniques as well as postprocessing software, and adjustments in the clinical protocol for gadolinium contrast media administration have addressed many of these limitations.

Since 1996, pulmonary functional MR techniques, such as non–contrast-enhanced (non-CE) and contrast-enhanced (CE) perfusion MR imaging,[1] hyperpolarized noble gas MR imaging,[2] and oxygen (O_2)-enhanced MR imaging[3,4] have been available to assess various cardiopulmonary diseases, and these techniques continue to be evaluated clinically. Moreover, new sequences such as ultrashort echo time (UTE) provide images that resemble computed tomography (CT) and show promise in pulmonary nodule detection and characterization.[5]

Since 2000, various MR imaging techniques have been developed that have usefulness in lung cancer evaluation. These techniques include: (1) CE MR angiography for T descriptor evaluation,[6] (2) short tau inversion recovery (STIR) turbo spin echo (SE) sequence as well as diffusion-weighted imaging (DWI) for N descriptor evaluation,[7–10] (3) whole-body MR imaging with and without DWI and PET

Disclosure Statement: Drs S. Seki, T. Yoshikawa, and Y. Ohno have received a research grant from Toshiba Medical Systems Corporation. Drs T. Yoshikawa and Y. Ohno have received a research grant from Philips Electronics Japan. Dr Y. Ohno has received research grants from Bayer Pharma, Guerbet Japan, Fuji Pharma, Daiichi-Sankyo, Co, Ltd, and Eizai, Co Ltd.

[a] Division of Functional and Diagnostic Imaging Research, Department of Radiology, Kobe University Graduate School of Medicine, 7-5-2 Kusunoki-cho, Chuo-ku, Kobe, Hyogo 650-0017, Japan; [b] Advanced Biomedical Imaging Research Center, Kobe University Graduate School of Medicine, 7-5-2 Kusunoki-cho, Chuo-ku, Kobe, Hyogo 650-0017, Japan; [c] Department of Radiology, Catholic University of the Sacred Heart, A. Gemelli Hospital, Largo F. Vito 1, Roma, Rome 00168, Italy; [d] Division of Radiology, Department of Radiology, Kobe University Graduate School of Medicine, 7-5-2 Kusunoki-cho, Chuo-ku, Kobe, Hyogo 650-0017, Japan
* Corresponding author. Division of Functional and Diagnostic Imaging Research, Department of Radiology, Kobe University Graduate School of Medicine, 7-5-2 Kusunoki-cho, Chuo-ku, Kobe, Hyogo 650-0017, Japan.
E-mail addresses: yosirad@kobe-u.ac.jp; yosirad@med.kobe-u.ac.jp; yoshiharuohno@aol.jp

fused with MR imaging (PET/MR imaging) for M descriptor and overall TNM stage evaluation as well as assessment for tumor recurrence,[11–14] and (4) STIR turbo SE imaging, DWI and dynamic CE MR imaging using the dynamic CE perfusion MR technique for nodule management.[15–20] As a result, MR imaging for lung cancer is now reimbursed by health insurance companies in many countries in North America, Eastern Asia and Europe.

This article will review recent advances in lung MR imaging focusing on its application in lung cancer evaluation, especially with regard to (I) pulmonary nodule detection, (II) pulmonary nodule and mass assessment, (III) lung cancer staging and recurrence evaluation, (IV) postoperative lung function prediction, and (V) therapeutic response evaluation and prediction.

PULMONARY NODULE DETECTION

A pulmonary nodule is a rounded or irregular opacity, well or poorly defined, measuring up to 3 cm in diameter, and surrounded by aerated lung on radiologic imaging.[21] An opacity smaller than 3 mm is referred to as a micronodule and one larger than 3 cm as a mass.[21] The incidence of small indeterminate pulmonary nodules detected by imaging in clinical practice as well as lung cancer screening programs has increased.[22] Owing to its high spatial resolution, CT is optimal for evaluation of small lung nodules although radiation dose is a limiting factor. Small size has historically been a limitation in the use of MR in nodule detection and morphologic evaluation. However, advances in MR techniques together with the revised Fleischner Society Guidelines[23] that have increased the size threshold for nodules that require follow-up evaluation as well as prolonged surveillance, have created a potential clinical role for MR in the evaluation of indeterminate lung nodules.[24–26] In this regard, MR imaging is particularly useful in patients with subsolid nodules requiring prolonged surveillance. The new guidelines of the National Comprehensive Cancer Network (NCCN) recommend a threshold value of 6 mm for solid and part-solid nodules, and for 20 mm for non-solid nodules that require further evaluation[27] and this matches the sensitivity of MR imaging for nodule detection. In this clinical context, MR imaging using UTE imaging has a potential role in the detection and evaluation of pulmonary nodules.

Pulmonary MR Imaging Without Ultrashort Echo Time

Since the early 1990s, various MR imaging sequences have been used to detect and evaluate pulmonary nodules (Table 1).[15,28–43] Non-CE MR techniques have been used since 1992 for nodule detection mostly to evaluate the usefulness of SE, turbo SE, single-shot T2-weighted (T2W) turbo SE, and STIR turbo SE sequences to detect pulmonary nodules. Detection rates using these techniques range from 46% to 100%.[15,28–39] Schroeder and colleagues[33] showed a detection rate of 73% for lesions less than 3 mm, 84% for those 3 to 5 mm, 95% for those 6 to 10 mm, and 100% for those greater than 10 mm in the 1102 pulmonary nodules evaluated. T2W MR imaging using the periodically rotated overlapping parallel lines with enhanced reconstruction (PROPELLER) technique has been shown to be superior to classical FSE, with an overall detection rate of 56% to 59% compared with 50% to 53% for nodules less than 8 mm.[40]

Three-dimensional (3D) gradient echo (GRE) sequence has also been used to evaluate nodules in a large number of studies. Nodule detection rates range from 52% to 100% for 3D GRE sequences without significant differences between non-CE and CE 3D GRE sequences.[30,32,34–36,38,41] Recently, Dewes and colleagues[41] performed a study concerning 3D GRE on a 3T system with CT as reference standard and reported a detection rate of 77% for lesions less than 5 mm, 87% for lesions from 5 to 10 mm, and 100% for lesions greater than 10 mm.

In terms of detection of pulmonary nodules, DWI is inferior to 3D GRE sequences and further technical improvements are required for this technique to have clinical usefulness.[37,42] In this regard, a metaanalysis of the use of DWI for malignant nodule detection reported pooled weighted estimates of sensitivity, specificity, positive likelihood ratio, and negative likelihood ratio were 0.828 (95% confidence interval [CI], 0.801–0.853), 0.801 (95% CI, 0.753–0.843), 4.01 (95% CI, 2.78–5.80), and 0.20 (95% CI, 0.15–0.27), respectively.[43]

Pulmonary MR Imaging With Ultrashort Echo Time

A challenge concerning lung MR imaging is the inhomogeneous magnetic susceptibility of lung parenchyma resulting from its air/soft tissue interfaces.[44,45] This factor results in a very short $T2^*$ relaxation times compared with other tissues.[46,47] $T2^*$ values of lung parenchyma on a 3T system are shorter than those on 1.5T,[48] even though 3T scanners can obtain images with higher spatial resolution and increased signal-to-noise-ratio than 1.5T scanners.[49–54] The drawbacks of the shorter $T2^*$ from lung parenchyma have been mitigated by recent advances in gradient hardware, 3D GRE sequences and reconstruction methods. 3D GRE pulse sequences with UTE of less than

Table 1
Studies using different MR imaging sequences to assess detection rate of pulmonary nodules

Author, Year	Magnet (T)	No. of Nodules	Sequence(s)	Detection (%)
Feuerstein et al,[28] 1992	0.5	33	STIR	82
			T2W-SE	71
			T1W-SE	33
			T1W-SE + CM	52
Kersjes et al,[29] 1997	1.5	340	T2W-turbo SE	84
Biederer et al,[30] 2003	1.5	366	2D GRE	40 (1.4 mm), 84 (5.2 mm), 98 (>7 mm)
			3D GRE	49 (1.4 mm), 88 (5.2 mm), 98 (>7 mm)
			T2W-turbo SE	12 (1.4 mm), 69 (5.2 mm), 97 (>7 mm)
			T2W-ssTSE	0 (1.4 mm), 0.05 (5.2 mm), 98 (>7 mm)
Vogt et al,[31] 2004	1.5	226	HASTE	93
Both et al,[32] 2005	1.5	15	VIBE	80
			T2W-turbo SE	60
			HASTE	46.7
Schroeder et al,[33] 2005	1.5	1102	HASTE	73.6 (<3 mm), 84.3 (3–5 mm), 95.7 (6–10 mm), 100 (>10 mm)
Bruegel et al,[34] 2007	1.5	225	HASTE	47.1–48.4
			IR-HASTE	44–47.1
			T2-turbo SE	68–69.8
			STIR	60–66.2
			Triggered-STIR	70.2–73.3
			VIBE	52–55.6
			VIBE + CM	48.9–52.4
Regier et al,[35] 2007	3	67	3D GRE	73.3–82.7 (2–5 mm), 88–96 (6–10 mm), 100 (>10 mm)
			HASTE	46.7–60 (2–5 mm), 76–88 (6–10 mm), 92.6–96.3 (>10 mm)
Koyama et al,[15] 2008	1.5	200	Triggered T1W-SE	82.5
			T2W-turbo SE	82.5
			STIR	82.5
Frericks et al,[36] 2008	1.5	268	T2W-turbo SE	90.8
			STIR	91.1–92.5
			VIBE	87.3
Koyama et al,[37] 2010	1.5	33	STIR	100
			DWI	85
Regier et al,[42] 2011	1.5	71	DWI	53 (<5 mm), 86.4 (6–9 mm), 97 (>10 mm)
Heye et al,[38] 2012	1.5	108	True FISP	53
			HASTE	49
			VIBE	57
			VIBE + CM	59
Meier-Schroers et al,[40] 2016	1.5	41	T2W-PROPELLER	58.8–55.9 (4–8 mm), 100 (>8 mm)
			T2W-FSE	50–52.9 (4–8 mm), 100 (>8 mm)
Dewes et al,[41] 2016	3	137	CAIPIRINHA-VIBE	88% (all lesions), 77.2 (<5 mm), 87.2 (5–10 mm), 100 (>10 mm)

(continued on next page)

Table 1 (continued)				
Author, Year	**Magnet (T)**	**No. of Nodules**	**Sequence(s)**	**Detection (%)**
Cieszanowski et al,[39] 2016	1.5	113	T2W-turbo SE	48.7 (all lesions), 40.6 (4–8 mm), 85.7 (>8 mm)
			T2W-STIR	54.9 (all lesions), 51.6 (4–8 mm), 82.1 (>8 mm)
			T2W-SPIR	45.1 (all lesions), 35.9 (4–8 mm), 78.6 (>8 mm)
			T2W-HASTE	25.7 (all lesions), 20.3 (4–8 mm), 50 (>8 mm)
			T1W-out of phase	48.7 (all lesions), 37.5 (4–8 mm), 92.9 (>8 mm)
			VIBE	69 (all lesions), 64.1 (4–8 mm), 100 (>8 mm)

Abbreviations: 2D, 2-dimensional; 3D, 3-dimensional; CAIPIRINHA, controlled aliasing in parallel imaging results in higher acceleration; CM, contrast media; DWI, diffusion weighted imaging; FISP, fast imaging with steady-state free precession; GRE, gradient echo; HASTE, half-Fourier acquisition single-shot turbo spin echo; PROPELLER, periodically rotated overlapping parallel lines with enhanced reconstruction; ssTSE, single-shot turbo spin echo; STIR, short-tau inversion recovery; T1W-SE, T1-weighted spin echo; T2W-SE, T2-weighted spin echo; T2W-FSE, T2-weighted fast spin echo; T2W-SPIR, T2-weighted spectral presaturation with inversion recovery; T2W-STIR, T2-weighted short-tau inversion recovery; VIBE, volumetric interpolated breath-hold examination.

200 μsec reduce the effects of signal dephasing caused by the heterogeneous magnetic susceptibility at the air/tissue interface in lung parenchyma. This technique uses radial k-space sampling from free induction decay to shorten the echo times, thus, reducing signal decay caused by T2* of lung parenchyma and provides MR images with proton density contrast that resemble CT images. Therefore, this sequence has been extensively used for quantitative and qualitative assessment of pulmonary nodules and diseases such as emphysema and interstitial lung disease.[5,55–63]

In a study comparing thoracic 3T MR imaging with UTE, low-dose CT and standard dose CT, intermethod agreements between pulmonary MR imaging and standard dose and low-dose CTs were all significant and either substantial or almost perfect ($0.67 \leq \kappa \leq 0.98$; $P<.0001$).[5] In addition, there were no significant differences among the 3 methods in terms of detection of pulmonary abnormalities such as micronodules, ground glass opacities, and consolidation, although areas under the curve for emphysema or bullae, bronchiectasis or traction bronchiectasis, and reticular opacity were significantly greater for standard dose CT than those for low-dose CT ($P<.05$) or pulmonary MR imaging ($P<.05$).[5] More recently, Ohno and colleagues[63] compared the detection and assessment of nodule morphology on 3D pulmonary MR imaging with UTE on a 3T system with standard dose and low-dose CT. Two hundred forty-three nodules were evaluated and there was no significant difference in nodule detection and nodule morphologic

assessment of UTE compared with those of standard dose and low-dose CT (**Figs. 1–3**). Furthermore, another study, which assessed the detection capability of UTE with 80μs of a 3T PET/MR imaging system in comparison with that of dual-echo GRE sequence, established a higher detection rate of UTE than of dual-echo GRE for both nodules smaller than 4 mm (89% vs 34%) and between 4 and 8 mm (79% vs 21%).[64] Pulmonary MR imaging with UTE can be expected to have a role in routine clinical practice in the near future, especially for nodule detection and evaluation in screening studies, as well as in surveillance of lung metastases in oncology patients.

DIAGNOSIS OF PULMONARY NODULE AND MASS

After a lung nodule is detected, it is important to determine the risk for malignancy to avoid unnecessary diagnostic or therapeutic procedures. Risk factors for malignancy have been investigated extensively.[65–67] Nodule size and growth rate are the most commonly used features to assess the probability of malignancy and to determine management.[22,23,68,69]

MR imaging owing to its multiparametric capability provides not only morphologic but also functional and pathophysiologic information about pulmonary nodules. In this section, current applications of MR imaging for the assessment of pulmonary nodules are reviewed including DWI, dynamic CE perfusion MR imaging, and CEST imaging.

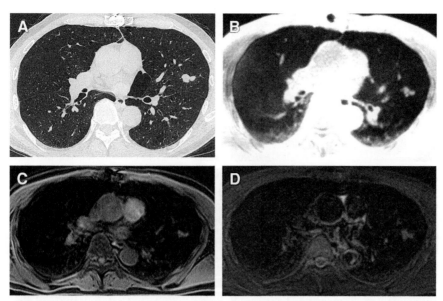

Fig. 1. An 83-year-old man with a 13-mm solid nodule in the left upper lobe. (*A*) Computed tomography scan, (*B*) MR imaging with ultra-short echo time, (*C*) 3-dimensional gradient echo, and (*D*) short-tau inversion recovery imaging all show the nodule. Pathology revealed invasive adenocarcinoma.

Non–Contrast-Enhanced MR Imaging and Conventional Contrast–Enhanced MR Imaging

Many MR imaging sequences have been evaluated for the detection and characterization of pulmonary nodules. Although malignant lung nodules typically have a low to intermediate signal intensity (SI) on T1-weighted (T1W) imaging and slightly high intensity on T2W imaging, benign nodules can have similar imaging features (**Table 2**).[70–81] Accordingly, standard T1W and T2W sequences as well as CE

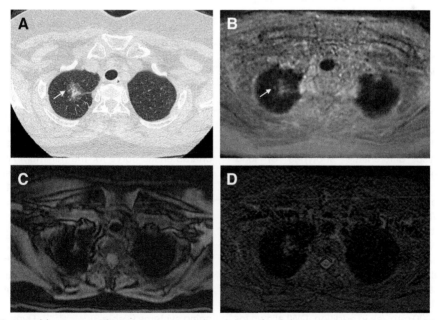

Fig. 2. A 62-year-old woman with a 26-mm part solid nodule in the right upper lobe. (*A*) computed tomography (CT), (*B*) MR imaging with ultra-short echo time (UTE), (*C*), 3-dimensional gradient echo (3D GRE), and (*D*) short-tau inversion recovery (STIR) imaging show the nodule. CT scan and MR imaging with UTE show the sub-solid portion of the nodule (*arrow*) in contradistinction to 3D GRE imaging and STIR imaging. Pathology revealed invasive adenocarcinoma.

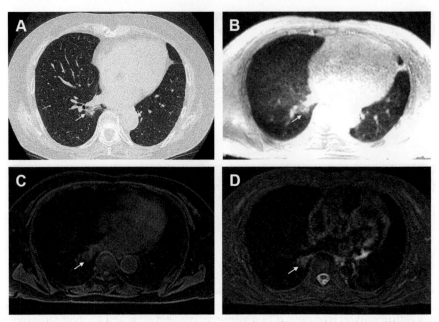

Fig. 3. A 78-year-old woman with a 23-mm ground glass nodule in the right lower lobe. (*A*) Computed tomography (CT), (*B*) MR imaging with ultra-short echo time (UTE), (*C*) 3-dimensional gradient echo (3D GRE), (*D*) and short-tau inversion recovery (STIR) imaging all show the nodule. The ground glass morphology of the nodule (*arrow*) was identified on CT, MR imaging with UTE and 3D GRE. However, this nodule seemed to be solid on STIR imaging. Pathology revealed minimally invasive adenocarcinoma.

T1W sequences have had limited clinical usefulness in differentiating malignant from benign nodules.[74] However, STIR turbo SE imaging and DWI, together with other sequences, can be used clinically to differentiate malignant and benign pulmonary nodules. In this regard, because STIR turbo SE imaging is sensitive to changes in T1 and T2 relaxation times, a component of T1-dependent decay can be subordinated to T2-dependent decay, resulting in an improvement in tissue contrast.[7,82] STIR turbo SE imaging is not only superior to non-CE T1W or T2W imaging in differentiating malignant from benign nodules with a sensitivity, specificity, and accuracy of 83%, 61%, and 75%, respectively, but can also differentiate subtypes of lung adenocarcinoma.[15,37]

Diffusion-weighted MR imaging is useful in the evaluation of lung nodules and the staging of lung cancer. DWI exploits the random motion of water protons in biologic tissue. This motion results in signal loss with the use of diffusion-sensitive sequences and can be quantified by calculating the apparent diffusion coefficient (ADC). DWI is useful in the detection pulmonary nodules because of the high lesion-to-background ratio on high b-value images (500–1000 mm²/s). In addition, DWI allows for a quantitative evaluation of diffusion of water molecules by calculating the ADC, and this can be used for the characterization of pulmonary nodules.[83] A metaanalysis reported a pooled sensitivity and

specificity of 83% and 80%, respectively, in the differentiation of malignant and benign nodules.[43] In addition, subgroup analyses showed that the diagnostic performance of retrospectively designed studies (sensitivity, 0.88 [95% CI, 0.82–0.92]; specificity, 0.89 [95% CI, 0.79–0.96]) was significantly higher than that of prospectively designed studies. The lesion-to-spinal cord SI ratio at high b-values has been reported to be more accurate and practical than ADC in the quantitative differentiation of solitary pulmonary nodules.[16,84] However, Çakmak and colleagues[85] showed that the minimum ADC performed better than the lesion-to-spinal cord SI ratio, with an area under the receiving operating characteristic curve for the minimum ADC (0.931; 95% CI, 0.868–0.993), which was greater than that for lesion-to-spinal cord SI ratio (0.801; 95% CI, 0.675–0.926; $P = .029$).

Dynamic Contrast-Enhanced MR Imaging

Dynamic CE-enhanced MR imaging with 2-dimensional, multislice or 3D SE, turbo SE, and/or GRE sequences has been used for differentiating malignant from benign nodules with 1.5T and 3T MR imaging systems (**Table 3**).[17–20,86–91] Dynamic CE MR imaging has been reported to have a sensitivity, specificity, and accuracy ranging from 55% to 100%, 54% to 100%, and 75% to 96%, respectively, in differentiating malignant from benign

Table 2
Pulmonary nodules characterization with different MR imaging sequences

	T1W	T2W	Fat-Sat (Eg, STIR)	Post CM (Eg, T1W CE Turbo SE)	DWI[a]
Lung carcinoma/lung metastasis	Low-intensity and/or focal areas of high-intensity owing to mucinous component or hemorrhage	High/very high intensity Adenocarcinoma can show central low-intensity (central scar) Mucinous adenocarcinoma can show focal areas of high-intensity (proteinaceous material)	High/very high intensity	Diffuse/focal/heterogeneous enhancement Small cell carcinoma can show "angiogram sign"	Usually high intensity (low ADC values)
Carcinoid	Isointense	High intensity	Very high intensity	Pronounced enhancement (>arterial phase)	
Hamartoma	Isointense Can show focal high signal owing to fat	Isointense/high intensity (cartilaginous tissue/fat)	Can show foci of low intensity in chemical-shift T1W opposed-phase GRE	Low heterogeneous enhancement of mesenchymal component and septa	
Granuloma	Homogeneous low intensity/isointense	Isointense/high intensity	Isointense/high intensity	Low-to-moderate homogeneous enhancement	Low to high intensity
Tuberculoma	Homogeneous low intensity/isointense Can show cavitation	Homogeneous low intensity/isointense Capsule can show high intensity Can show cavitation		Thin peripheral contrast enhancement (fibrous capsule), no central enhancement (necrotic material)	Low to high intensity
Aspergilloma	Homogeneous low intensity/isointense	Homogeneous high intensity with hyperintense center (targetlike) after 10 d from infection		Homogeneous enhancement (early infection), rim enhancement after 10 d (late infection)	
Organizing pneumonia	Homogeneous low intensity/isointense	Isointense/high intensity	Isointense/high intensity	Moderate homogeneous enhancement	Low to high intensity

Abbreviations: ADC, apparent diffusion coefficient; CE, contrast enhanced; CM, contrast media; DWI, diffusion-weighted imaging; Fat-Sat, fat saturated; SE, spin echo; STIR, short-tau inversion recovery; T1W, T1-weighted; T2W, T2-weighted.
[a] Also assessed quantitatively with lesion-to-spinal cord ratio (LSR).

Table 3
Dynamic CE perfusion MR imaging for differentiating benign and malignant pulmonary lesions

Author, Year	Field Strength	Sequence	Image Analysis	No. of Lesions	Sensitivity (%)	Specificity (%)	Accuracy (%)
Hittmair et al,[86] 1995	1.5	2D-GRE	Relative SI increase (%)	21	100	67	90
Gückel et al,[87] 1996	1.5	2D turbo fast imaging with steady-state precession	Slope of enhancement	28	100	88	96
Ohno et al,[17] 2002	1.5	3D GRE	Maximum relative enhancement ratio; slope of enhancement	58	100	70	95
Schaefer et al,[88] 2004	1.0	2D-GRE	Maximum peak enhancement, slope of enhancement, washout	51	96 (maximum peak) 96 (slope) 52 (washout)	88 (maximum peak) 75 (slope) 100 (washout)	92 (maximum peak) 86 (slope) 75 (washout)
Kim et al,[89] 2004	1.5	3D GRE	Peak enhancement	81	100	76	85
Kono et al,[90] 2007	0.5	T1W SE	Maximum enhancement ratio, slope of time enhancement ratio curves	202	63 (maximum enhancement ratio) 55 (slope)	84 (maximum enhancement ratio) 71 (slope)	NR
Ohno et al,[19] 2008	1.5	3D GRE (TE = 0.6 ms)	Maximum relative enhancement, slope of enhancement ratio	202	96 (maximum relative enhancement) 96 (slope of enhancement ratio)	54 (maximum relative enhancement) 64 (slope of enhancement ratio)	85.6 (maximum relative enhancement) 88.1 (slope of enhancement ratio)
Zou et al,[91] 2008	1.5	T1W turbo SE	Steepest slope in time–SI curve combined with enhancement of SI	68	93	89	93
Ohno et al,[20] 2015	1.5	3D GRE (TE = 0.6 ms)	Maximum relative enhancement ratio, slope of enhancement	218	92 (maximum relative enhancement ratio) 93 (slope of enhancement)	49 (maximum relative enhancement ratio) 49 (slope of enhancement)	76 (maximum relative enhancement ratio) 76 (slope of enhancement)

Abbreviations: 2D, 2-dimensional; 2D-GRE, 2-dimensional gradient echo; 3D GRE, 3-dimensional gradient echo; ADC, apparent diffusion coefficient; CE, contrast enhanced; CM, contrast media; DWI, diffusion-weighted imaging; Fat-Sat, fat saturated; NR, not reported; SI, signal intensity; STIR, short-tau inversion recovery; TE, echo time; T1W, T1-weighted; T1W SE, T1-weighted spin echo; T1W turbo SE, T1-weighted turbo spin echo; T2W, T2-weighted.

nodules.[17–20,86–91] A meta-analysis in the diagnostic performance of dynamic CE CT, dynamic CE MR imaging, PET with fluorine-18 fluorodeoxyglucose (FDG-PET), and single-photon emission CT (SPECT) with technetium 99m depreotide reported no significant differences among these 4 modalities in the evaluation of pulmonary nodules. Sensitivities, specificities, positive predictive values, and negative predictive values were 0.93, 0.76, 0.80, and 0.95 for dynamic CE CT, 0.94, 0.79, 0.86, and 0.93 for dynamic CE MR imaging, 0.95, 0.82, 0.91, and 0.90 for FDG-PET, and 0.95, 0.82, 0.90, and 0.91 for technetium 99m depreotide SPECT.[92] However, importantly, the diagnostic performance of dynamic CE MR imaging was determined from the results of prior studies using older techniques.[92] Advances in dynamic CE MR imaging, for instance using a 3D GRE sequence and a UTE of 600 µs or greater allow improved differentiation of malignant from benign nodules.[18–20] Moreover, pulmonary arterial, parenchymal, pulmonary venous, and systemic arterial phases can be evaluated on these images.[93] In addition, this technique is superior to dynamic CE CT and FDG-PET/CT, with a sensitivity, specificity, and accuracy of 96%, 64%, 88% for dynamic MR imaging, 93%, 52%, and 82% for dynamic CT, and 93%, 54%, 84% for FDG-PET/CT, respectively.[19] In contrast, in a more recent study by Ohno and colleagues semi-quantitatively assessed dynamic CE MR imaging with first-pass CE perfusion MR technique is slightly inferior to quantitatively assessed dynamic first-pass CE perfusion area-detector CT scanning and superior to FDG-PET/CT scanning for differentiating malignant and benign nodules with a sensitivity, specificity, and accuracy of 93%, 49%, and 76% for dynamic CE MR imaging, 92%, 71%, and 84% for dynamic first-pass CE perfusion area-detector CT scanning, and 89%, 31%, and 67% for FDG-PET/CT, respectively.[20] Nevertheless, for routine clinical practice, dynamic CE MR imaging has the potential to be used as a complementary or alternative study to dynamic CE area-detector CT and FDG-PET/CT scanning for the characterization of pulmonary nodules (Fig. 4).

Chemical Exchange Saturation Transfer Imaging on a 3T MR Imaging System

When using intravenous contrast, high concentrations of contrast media are required on MR imaging. CEST imaging is a relatively new MR imaging contrast technique that overcomes this limitation. In CEST imaging, compounds containing either exchangeable protons or exchangeable molecules are selectively saturated and, after transfer of this saturation, become visible on the water signal, allowing the presence of low-concentration compounds to be imaged indirectly.[94–97] CEST imaging provides an indirect quantification of the proton in the target compound through the negative imaging contrast produced by the reduction in bulk water SI.[98–101] Amide proton transfer imaging, a subset of CEST imaging, is applied specifically to the chemical exchange between protons of bulk water and amide groups of endogenous mobile proteins and peptides. These amide groups are more abundant in tumors than in normal tissues.[102] Tumor evaluation, based on amide proton transfer imaging, can differentiate between normal tissues and different types of lung cancer cell lines.[98] In a prospective study, Ohno and colleagues[103] tested amide proton transfer–weighted CEST imaging on a 3T system and demonstrated that the difference in magnetization transfer asymmetry of 3.5 ppm was significantly higher for malignant tumors than for benign lesions ($P = .008$), as well as for other thoracic malignancies than for lung cancer ($P = .005$), and for adenocarcinoma than for squamous cell carcinoma ($P = .02$). Although further investigations are warranted, this MR-based metabolic imaging has the potential for differentiation and characterization of thoracic nodules and masses (Figs. 5 and 6).

LUNG CANCER STAGING

Lung cancer is the leading cause of tumor-related deaths worldwide,[104] with non–small cell lung cancer (NSCLC) accounting for 80% to 85% of all lung malignancies.[105] Historically, MR imaging has been used in various clinical settings to clarify imaging dilemmas.[106] However, recent advancements in MR imaging now allow imaging of intrathoracic diseases without initial CT evaluation. In this section, we discuss the MR imaging techniques used for TNM staging of lung cancer with both dedicated chest MR imaging as well as whole-body MR imaging and whole-body PET/MR imaging. Suggested protocols for dedicated chest MR imaging and whole-body MR imaging are provided in Table 4.

Dedicated Chest MR Imaging

T descriptor
Many authors have investigated the usefulness of chest MR imaging for assessing the primary lung cancer for resectability (Table 5).[6,106–111] Historically, there was no difference in the accuracy of CT scanning compared with T1W MR imaging for the diagnosis of bronchial involvement or chest wall invasion, although MR imaging was significantly more accurate than CT scanning for the diagnosis of mediastinal invasion ($P = .047$).[106] Consequently, MR imaging was widely used for

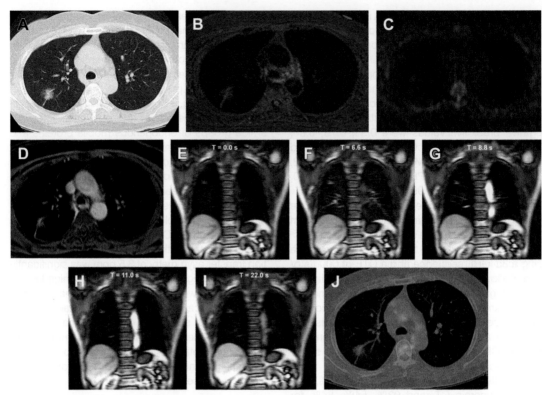

Fig. 4. A 64-year-old man with biopsy-proven adenocarcinoma. (*A*) Computed tomography (CT) shows a 20-mm, part solid nodule in the right upper lobe. (*B*) Short-tau inversion recovery imaging shows the nodule as an area of high signal intensity, suspicious for malignancy (true positive). (*C*) Diffusion-weighted imaging shows high signal intensity, favoring malignancy (true positive). (*D*) Contrast-enhanced (CE) T1-weighted imaging with fat suppression (CE-quick 3-dimensional imaging with double fat suppression) technique shows contrast enhancement consistent with malignancy (true positive). (*E–I*) Dynamic CE MR imaging with ultrashort echo time (TE) shows the nodule (T = 0 seconds), well-defined nodule enhancement in the late pulmonary parenchymal phase (T = 6.6 seconds), and continuing enhancement in the systemic circulation phases (T = 8.8, 11, and 22 seconds). These findings suggest the nodule is malignant (true positive). (*J*) PET/CT shows the nodule is not fluorine-18 fluorodeoxyglucose avid (false negative).

assessing mediastinal invasion until thin section multiplanar reconstructed images on multidetector row CT scanning became available.[112]

More recently, Sakai and colleagues[108] evaluated the accuracy of dynamic cine MR imaging for the detection of pleural invasion by assessing the movement of the primary tumor and the adjacent partial pleura during respiration. They reported the sensitivity, specificity, and accuracy of dynamic cine MR imaging for the detection of chest wall invasion as 100%, 70%, and 76%, respectively, whereas the corresponding values for conventional CT scanning and MR imaging were 80%, 65%, and 68%, respectively.[108]

More advanced techniques have been used recently to evaluate for cardiovascular or mediastinal invasion. Cardiac-gated CE MR angiography has a sensitivity, specificity, and accuracy for detection of mediastinal and hilar invasion that ranges from 78% to 90%, 73% to 87%, and

75% to 88%, respectively, and is superior to CT scanning, T1W turbo SE imaging, and conventional CE MR angiography.[6] More recently, dynamic CE MR imaging on a 3T MR system was found to be slightly superior to multidetector row CT scanning in the preoperative assessment of the T descriptor in 45 patients with NSCLC, particularly those with more advanced tumors (T3, T4) with pleural and mediastinal invasion.[111] However, currently, multidetector row CT scanning remains the primary modality in determining the T descriptor in patients with NSCLC, with the exception of patients with superior sulcus tumors where assessment of the brachial plexus is ideally performed with MR imaging.

N descriptor
Historically, when using CT and MR imaging to assess the N descriptor, size criterion was the only method to differentiate between metastatic and

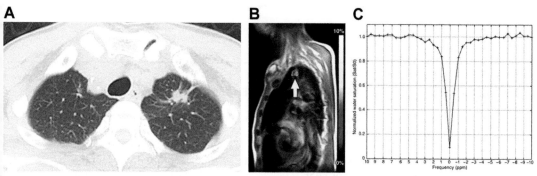

Fig. 5. Organizing pneumonia in a 68-year-old man. (*A*) Computed tomography scanning shows a spiculated left upper lobe nodule with pleural indentation and notching. (*B*) Sagittal amide proton transfer (APT)-weighted chemical exchange saturation transfer (CEST) MR map generated as fused CEST information within a region of interest (ROI), and displayed in a heat scale on an image with the first frequency offset at 210 ppm and displayed as a gray-scale image shows nodule (*arrow*) with low (0.6%) difference in magnetization transfer asymmetry (MTR_{asym}; at 3.5 ppm). Using a threshold for malignancy of greater than 0.6% for APT-weighted CEST MR images, this nodule was benign and a true negative. Note the heat scale with different colors, such as red, yellow, and white, assigned to progressively higher temperatures. (*C*) Z-spectrum (S/S0 vs the frequency for the 210 to 10 ppm range) within the ROI. The MTR_{asym} (at 3.5 ppm) was automatically determined as 0.6% by the software. The x-axis represents frequency, y-axis is normalized water saturation calculated as S_{sat}/S_0, and S_{sat} and S_0 are the signal intensities when MT pulses are applied to each frequency offset with the farthest frequency offset at +10 or 210 ppm. (*From* Ohno Y, Yui M, Koyama H, et al. Chemical exchange saturation transfer MR imaging: preliminary results for differentiation of malignant and benign thoracic lesions. Radiology 2016;279:578–89; with permission.)

nonmetastatic lymph nodes.[106,113] Accordingly, earlier reports showed MR imaging with its multiplanar capability allowed the improved detection of lymph nodes in areas such as the aortopulmonary window and subcarinal regions. Currently, STIR turbo SE imaging and DWI are promising

techniques for the determination of the N descriptor in patients with NSCLC (**Fig. 7**, **Table 6**).[7–9,114–121]

In addition to nodal size, the addition of increased T1 and T2 relaxation times in STIR turbo SE imaging yields a significantly higher net tissue contrast for malignant lymph nodes than for

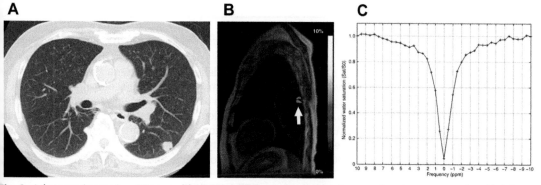

Fig. 6. Adenocarcinoma in a 71-year-old man. (*A*) Computed tomography scanning shows a speculated left lower lobe nodule with pleural indentation and notching. (*B*) Sagittal amide proton transfer (APT)-weighted chemical exchange saturation transfer (CEST) MR map shows nodule (*arrow*) with high (3.63%) difference in magnetization transfer asymmetry (MTR_{asym}; at 3.5 ppm). Using a threshold for malignancy of greater than 0.6% for APT-weighted CEST MR images, this nodule was malignant and a true positive. Note a threshold less than 1.1% is used to distinguish lung cancer from other thoracic malignancies. A threshold of 1.0% or greater is used to differentiate adenocarcinoma from squamous cell carcinoma. (*C*) Z-spectrum (S/S_0 vs frequency for the 210 to 10 ppm range) within the region of interest. The MTR_{asym} (at 3.5 ppm) was automatically determined as 3.63% by the software. The x-axis represents frequency, and the y-axis is normalized water saturation, calculated as S_{sat}/S_0. S_{sat} and S_0 are the signal intensities when MT pulses are applied to each frequency offset with the farthest frequency offset at +10 or 210 ppm. (*From* Ohno Y, Yui M, Koyama H, et al. Chemical exchange saturation transfer MR imaging: preliminary results for differentiation of malignant and benign thoracic lesions. Radiology 2016;279:578–89; with permission.)

Table 4
Dedicated chest MR imaging and whole-body MR imaging protocols in TNM staging

	Sequence(s)	Comments
Dedicated chest MR imaging		
T descriptor	Axial and coronal STIR FASE or turbo SE	Can detect mediastinal and/or thoracic wall invasion owing to fat suppression
	Axial and coronal 3D T1W GRE with and without gadolinium contrast media administration	Useful for assessing vascular invasion and size of primary tumor
N descriptor	Axial and coronal STIR FASE or turbo SE Axial DWI using EPI or FASE (b = 0–1000 s/mm^2)	High-accuracy detection and characterization of hilar and mediastinal lymph node metastasis
M descriptor	Axial and/or coronal UTE Axial and coronal 3D T1W GRE with and without gadolinium contrast media administration	Detection of contralateral lung nodules Can detect pleural metastasis
Whole-body MR imaging		
T descriptor	Coronal (and axial) STIR FASE or turbo SE	Can detect mediastinal and/or thoracic wall invasion owing to fat suppression
	Coronal (and axial) 3D T1W GRE with and without gadolinium contrast media administration	Useful for assessing vascular invasion
N descriptor	Coronal (and axial) STIR FASE or turbo SE Coronal (and axial) DWI using EPI or FASE (b = 0–1000 s/mm^2)	High accuracy for detection and characterization of hilar and mediastinal lymph node metastasis
M descriptor	Coronal and sagittal STIR FASE or turbo SE Coronal and sagittal T1W GRE in-phase/ out-phase Coronal (and axial) DWI using EPI or FASE (b = 0–1000 s/mm^2) Coronal and sagittal 3D T1W GRE with and without gadolinium contrast media administration	Detection of distant metastases (eg, cerebral, adrenal, skeletal)

Abbreviations: 3D, 3-dimensioanl; DWI, diffusion weighted imaging; EPI, echo-planar imaging; FASE, fast advanced spin echo; GRE, gradient echo; SE, spin echo; STIR, short-tau inversion recovery; T1W, T1-weighted; UTE, ultra-short echo time.

benign lymph nodes. Previous studies reported a range for the sensitivity of quantitatively and qualitatively assessed STIR turbo SE imaging, on a per-patient basis, from 83.7% to 100%, for specificity from 74.4% to 96%, and for accuracy from 83% to 92%, and these values were equal to or higher than those for CE CT, FDG-PET, or PET/CT scanning.[7–9,114] Another study, however, found that the quantitatively and qualitatively assessed sensitivity, specificity, and accuracy of STIR turbo SE imaging were not significantly different from those of FDG-PET/CT.[117] In contrast, the combination of FDG-PET/CT scanning with STIR turbo SE imaging was found to be significantly more effective for detecting nodal involvement on a per-patient basis (97% specificity, 90% accuracy) than FDG PET/CT scanning alone (66% specificity, 82% accuracy).[117] These results indicate that STIR turbo SE imaging may be the best MR imaging technique for

differentiating between metastatic and nonmetastatic lymph nodes in initial staging.

DWI is useful for quantitative and qualitative differentiation of metastatic from nonmetastatic lymph nodes with reported range of sensitivity, specificity, and accuracy from 38% to 82.8%, 88.5% to 100%, and 75% to 98%, respectively, and are equal to or better than those for FDG-PET or PET/CT scanning.[10,115,116,122] In a comparison of STIR turbo SE imaging, DWI and PET/CT scanning for detecting lymph node metastasis on a per-node and a per-patient basis, the sensitivity (82.8%) and accuracy (86.8%) of quantitatively assessed STIR turbo SE imaging are significantly higher than those of ADC on DWI (sensitivity 74.2%, accuracy 84.4%) and maximum standardized uptake value on PET/CT scanning (sensitivity 74.2%). In addition, sensitivity of qualitatively assessed STIR turbo SE imaging (77.4%) was significantly higher than that of qualitatively

Table 5
CT and MR imaging in assessment of T descriptor

Author, Year	Field Strength	Sequence	Image Analysis	MR Imaging			CT		
				Sensitivity	Specificity	Accuracy	Sensitivity	Specificity	Accuracy
Webb et al,[106] 1991	0.35 and 1.50	ECG-gated T1- and T2-weighted	Distinction between T0-T2 from T3-T4	80	56	73	84	63	78
Sakai et al,[108] 1997	1.5	Free-breathing cine GRASS	Chest-wall invasion	10	70	76	80	65	68
Ohno et al,[6] 2001	1.5	Dynamic ECG-triggered 3D GRE	Tumor invasion of pulmonary vessels	78–90	73–87	75–88	67–70	60–64	68–71
Tang et al,[111] 2015	3.0	Breath-hold dynamic CE 2D-GRE	T-stage	NR	NR	82.2	NR	NR	84.4

Abbreviations: 2D, 2-dimensional; 3D, 3-dimensional; CE, contrast enhanced; CT, computed tomography; ECG, electrocardiography; GRASS, gradient recalled acquisition in steady state; GRE, gradient echo; NR, not reported.

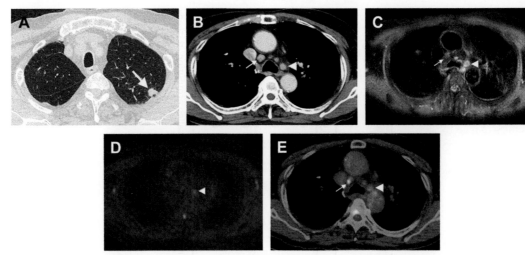

Fig. 7. A 73-year-old man with a left upper lobe lung cancer. Sampling of the mediastinal lymph nodes was negative for malignancy except for N2-positive disease in a left lower paratracheal node. (*A*) Computed tomography (CT) scanning shows primary lung cancer (*large arrow*) in the left upper lobe. (*B*) Contrast-enhanced CT scanning shows an 11-mm right lower paratracheal node (*arrow*) suspicious for nodal metastasis (false positive). The 8-mm left lower paratracheal node (*arrowhead*) is normal using a 1-cm short axis threshold for malignancy (false negative). (*C*) Short-tau inversion recovery (STIR) turbo spin echo, and (*D*) diffusion-weighted imaging (DWI) show the left lower paratracheal node (*arrowhead*) has a high signal intensity suspicious for malignancy (true positive). The enlarged right lower paratracheal node (*arrow*) has low signal intensity on STIR imaging, and is not detected on DWI (true negative). (*E*) PET/CT scanning shows increased fluorine-18 fluorodeoxyglucose (FDG) uptake in the right lower paratracheal node (*arrow*), a false positive, whereas the left lower paratracheal node (*arrowhead*) is not FDG avid, a false negative.

assessed DWI (71%) and FDG-PET/CT scanning (69.9%).[9] Two meta-analyses compared diagnostic performance between of DWI and PET/CT scanning for detecting mediastinal nodal metastasis in NCSLC. There was no statistically significant difference between the 2 imaging modalities. The first meta-analysis reported a pooled sensitivity and specificity of 0.72 and 0.95 for DWI and 0.75 and 0.89 for FDG-PET/CT scanning.[123] The second meta-analysis reported a pooled sensitivity and specificity of 0.72 and 0.97 for DWI and 0.65 and 0.93 respectively, for PET/CT scanning.[124] Although DWI is similar to PET/CT scanning for the diagnosis of lymph node metastasis in patients with NSCLC, a drawback is image distortion, severe susceptibility, and motion artifacts, because DWI is frequently obtained by using the echo-planar imaging sequence. In addition, image degradation owing to these artifacts is more severe on the 3T MR than the 1.5T MR imaging system owing to the increased inhomogeneity of static B field as well as shorter T2* value and severe motion artifacts within the lung and mediastinum. To overcome this limitation, it has been suggested that DWI should be performed with the fast advantage SE sequence rather than the echo-planar imaging sequence with a 3T MR imaging system because sensitivity

and accuracy of STIR fast advantage SE imaging (sensitivity, 82.1%; accuracy, 90.4%) and fast advantage SE DWI sequence (sensitivity, 82.1%; accuracy, 90.4%) were reportedly significantly higher than those of the echo-planar imaging DWI sequence (sensitivity, 60.3%; accuracy, 79.5%) and PET/CT scanning (sensitivity, 57.7%; accuracy, 77.6%).[10]

Whole-Body MR Imaging and PET/MR Imaging

Whole-body MR imaging and PET/MR imaging are new imaging methods that have potential in the TNM staging of oncology patients.[11,125] Whole-body MR imaging can be more effective in staging than CT scanning and nuclear medicine studies owing to the improvements in whole-body MR imaging temporal resolution by using newly developed parallel imaging techniques, a moving table technique, and/or multiple body array coils.[11,125,126] More recently, whole-body PET/MR imaging has been introduced as a new whole-body imaging technique. The capabilities of whole-body MR imaging and PET/MR imaging for TNM staging are shown in **Tables 7–9.** In addition, the accuracy of whole-body MR imaging (97%) and of PET/MR imaging with SI assessment based on STIR turbo SE-

Table 6
PET/CT or CT compared with chest MR imaging in assessment of N descriptor

Author, Year	Field Strength	Sequence	Reference Standard	MR Imaging			FDG-PET/CT (or CT)		
				Sensitivity	Specificity	Accuracy	Sensitivity	Specificity	Accuracy
Takenaka et al,[114] 2002	1.5	ECG-triggered T1W turbo SE	Histology	52	91	83	52	91	83
		STIR		100	96	96			
Ohno et al,[7] 2004	1.5	STIR	Histology	93	87	89	53	83	72
Ohno et al,[8] 2007	1.5	STIR	Histology and/or follow-up	83.7 (qualitative), 90.1 (quantitative)	74.4 (qualitative), 76.7 (quantitative)	87.8 (qualitative), 92.2 (quantitative)	87.5 (qualitative), 87.5 (quantitative)	90.3 (qualitative), 93.1 (quantitative)	82.6 (qualitative), 83.5 (quantitative)
Hasegawa et al,[115] 2008	1.5	DWI	Histology	80	97	95	—	—	—
Nomori et al,[116] 2008	1.5	DWI	Histology and/or follow-up	67	99	98	72	97	96
Morikawa et al,[117] 2009	1.5	STIR	Histology	93.9 (qualitative), 96.3 (quantitative)	70.9 (qualitative), 67.3 (quantitative)	84.7 (qualitative), 84.7 (quantitative)	90.2	65.5	80.3
Nakayama et al,[118] 2010	1.5	DWI	Histology	69	100	94	—	—	—

(continued on next page)

Table 6
(continued)

Author, Year	Field Strength	Sequence	Reference Standard	MR Imaging			FDG-PET/CT (or CT)		
				Sensitivity	Specificity	Accuracy	Sensitivity	Specificity	Accuracy
Usuda et al,[119] 2011	1.5	T1W SE, T2-W FSE, SS-EPI-SPAIR	Histology	59	93	81	33	90	71
Ohno et al,[9] 2011	1.5	STIR, DWI	Histology	82.8 (quantitative-STIR), 74.2 (quantitative-DWI), 77.4 (qualitative-STIR), 71 (qualitative-DWI)	89.2 (quantitative-STIR), 90.4 (quantitative-DWI), 88.5 (qualitative-STIR), 89.8 (qualitative-DWI)	86.8 (quantitative-STIR), 84.4 (quantitative-DWI), 84.4 (qualitative-STIR), 82.8 (qualitative-DWI)	74.2 (quantitative), 69.9 (qualitative)	92.4 (quantitative), 91.7 (qualitative)	85.6 (quantitative), 83.6 (qualitative)
Ohno et al,[10] 2015	3.0	STIR-FASE, EPI-DWI, FASE-DWI	Histology	82.1 (FASE-DWI), 60.3 (EPI-DWI), 82.1 (STIR-FASE)	98.7 (FASE-DWI), 98.7 (EPI-DWI), 98.7 (STIR-FASE)	90.4 (FASE-DWI), 79.5 (EPI-DWI), 90.4 (STIR-FASE)	57.7	97.4	77.6
Usuda et al,[120] 2015	1.5	SE-T1W, FSE-T2W, DWI	Histology and/or follow-up	71	100	91	86	31	48
Nomori et al,[121] 2016	1.5	DWI	Histology	38–79	92–94	75	33–58	89–90	67

Abbreviations: CT, computed tomography; DWI, diffusion-weighted imaging; ECG, electrocardiograph; EPI, echo-planar imaging; FASE, fast advantage spin echo; FDG, fluorine-18 fluorodeoxyglucose; FSE, fast spin echo; SE, spin echo; SPAIR, spectral attenuated inversion recovery; STIR, short-tau inversion recovery; T1W, T1-weighted.

Table 7
Whole-body MR imaging, PET/MR imaging and FDG-PET/CT in the assessment of T descriptor

Author, Year	Whole-Body MR Imaging			FDG-PET/MR Imaging			FDG-PET/CT		
	Sensitivity	Specificity	Accuracy	Sensitivity	Specificity	Accuracy	Sensitivity	Specificity	Accuracy
Yi et al,[125] 2008	—	—	86	—	—	—	—	—	82
Sommer et al,[126] 2012	—	—	63	—	—	—	—	—	56
Heusch et al,[127] 2014	—	—	—	—	—	100	—	—	100
Ohno et al,[11] 2015	100	55.6	94.3	100 (with and without SI assessment)	55.6 (with SI assessment) 33.3 (without SI assessment)	94.3 (with SI assessment) 91.4 (without SI assessment)	100	33.3	91.4
Huellner et al,[128] 2016	—	—	—	—	—	69	—	—	81
Lee et al,[129] 2016	—	—	—	—	—	80	—	—	80

Abbreviations: FDG, fluorine-18 fluorodeoxyglucose; SI, s gnal intensity.

Table 8
Whole-body MR imaging, PET/MR imaging and FDG-PET/CT in the assessment of N descriptor

Author, Year	Whole-Body MR Imaging			FDG-PET/MR Imaging			FDG-PET/CT		
	Sensitivity	Specificity	Accuracy	Sensitivity	Specificity	Accuracy	Sensitivity	Specificity	Accuracy
Yi et al,[125] 2008	—	—	78	—	—	—	—	—	80
Sommer et al,[126] 2012	—	—	66	—	—	—	—	—	71
Heusch et al,[127] 2014	—	—	—	—	—	91	—	—	82
Xu et al,[131] 2014	75 (DWI)	90.9 (DWI)	87.8 (DWI)	—	—	—	—	—	—
Ohno et al,[11] 2015	100	92.9	98.6	100 (with SI assessment) 93.8 (without SI assessment)	92.9 (with SI assessment) 85.7(without SI assessment)	98.6 (with SI assessment) 92.1 (without SI assessment)	93.8	95.7	92.1
Huellner et al,[128] 2016	—	—	—	—	—	79	—	—	88
Lee et al,[129] 2016	—	—	—	—	—	57.1	—	—	52.4

Abbreviations: CT, computed tomography; DWI, diffusion-weighted imaging; FDG, fluorine-18 fluorodeoxyglucose; SI, signal intensity.

Table 9
Whole-body MR imaging, PET/MR imaging and FDG-PET/CT in the assessment of M descriptor

Author, Year	Whole-Body MR Imaging			FDG-PET/MR Imaging			FDG-PET/CT		
	Sensitivity	Specificity	Accuracy	Sensitivity	Specificity	Accuracy	Sensitivity	Specificity	Accuracy
Ohno et al,[12] 2007	—	—	80	—	—	—	—	—	73.3
Yi et al,[125] 2008	—	—	86	—	—	—	—	—	86
Ohno et al,[13] 2008	57.5 (DWI) 60 (WB-MR imaging without DWI) 70 (WB-MR imaging with DWI)	87.7 (DWI) 92 (WB-MR imaging without DWI) 92 (WB-MR imaging with DWI)	81.8 (DWI) 85.7 (WB-MR imaging without DWI) 87.7 (WB-MR imaging with DWI)	—	—	—	62.5	94.5	88.2
Takenaka et al,[135] 2009	95.5 (DWI) 73.1 (WB-MR imaging without DWI) 95.5 (WB-MR imaging with DWI)	93.7 (DWI) 96.4 (WB-MR imaging without DWI) 96.1 (WB-MR imaging with DWI)	93.9 (DWI) 94.8 (WB-MR imaging without DWI) 96.1 (WB-MR imaging with DWI)	—	—	—	97	95.4	95.5
Ohno et al,[11] 2015	100	87.5	98.6	100 (with SI assessment) 92.7 (without SI assessment)	87.5 (with SI assessment) 81.3 (without SI assessment)	98.6 (with SI assessment) 91.4 (without SI assessment)	92.7	75	90.7
Huellner et al,[128] 2016	—	—	—	—	—	81	—	—	83

Abbreviations: CT, computed tomography; DWI, diffusion-weighted imaging; FDG, fluorine-18 fluorodeoxyglucose; SI, signal intensity; WB-MR imaging, whole-body MR imaging.

based sequence (97%) is significantly higher than that of PET/MR imaging without SI assessment (85%; $P<.001$) and integrated FDG PET/CT (85%; $P<.001$).[11]

T descriptor

Only a few studies have compared the diagnostic performance of whole-body MR imaging with that of PET/CT scanning in T descriptor determination. The accuracy of these 2 techniques is not significantly different, ranging from 63% to 86% and 56% to 86% for whole-body-MR imaging and FDG-PET/CT scanning, respectively.[125,126] The reported accuracy of whole-body PET/MR imaging and PET/CT scanning for the assessment of T descriptor in NSCLC ranges from 69% to 100% and 56% to 100%, respectively.[11,127–129] These studies concluded that there were no significant differences between the 2 modalities. In addition, Ohno and colleagues[11] reported the accuracy of whole-body MR imaging is similar to that of PET/MR imaging and PET/CT scanning. Schaarschmidt and colleagues[130] compared CE-PET/MR and PET/CT and concluded that, despite differences between these modalities for assessment of the T descriptor, there was no impact on patient management. In summary, there is no significant difference among whole-body MR imaging, PET/MR imaging, and PET/CT scanning in the determination of the T descriptor in patients with NSCLC.

N descriptor

The function of whole-body MR imaging for assessing the N descriptor has been evaluated, on both 1.5T and 3T MR imaging, with and without DWI.[11,125,126,131] The accuracy of whole-body MR imaging is not significantly different from that of PET/CT scanning, and there is no advantage of whole-body DWI.[122] However, a recent study that compared N descriptor evaluation among whole-body MR imaging, PET/MR imaging, and PET/CT scanning reported the sensitivity and accuracy of whole-body MR imaging (sensitivity, 100%; accuracy, 98.6%) and PET/MR imaging with SI assessment (sensitivity, 100%; accuracy, 98.6%) were significantly higher than those of PET/MR imaging without SI assessment (sensitivity, 93.8%; accuracy, 92.1%) and PET/CT scanning (sensitivity, 93.8%; accuracy, 92.1%). There was no significant difference between PET/MR imaging without SI assessment and PET/CT scanning.[11] There are studies that show that whole-body PET/MR and PET/CT scanning in NSCLC had similar accuracies, which ranged from 57.1% to 91% and 52.1% to 88%, respectively.[127–129] An advantage of PET/MR imaging

was dose reduction of 31% compared with that of PET/CT scanning.[129]

In summary, relaxation time–dependent information based on STIR turbo SE imaging in PET/MR imaging and whole-body MR imaging improves the assessment of N descriptor and shows potential in routine clinical practice.

M descriptor

Currently, CE CT scanning, brain CE MR imaging, and PET/CT scanning are the imaging modalities routinely used in clinical practice for the evaluation of distant metastases in patients with lung cancer.[132–134] However, as a result of technical advances, whole-body MR imaging is an additional modality with clinical usefulness in patients with lung cancer.[12,13,125,135,136] In terms of M descriptor determination, whole-body MR imaging without DWI (sensitivity, 60%–73.1%; specificity, 92%–96.4%; accuracy, 85.7%–94.8%) was equal to slightly lower than FDG-PET/CT (sensitivity, 62.5%–97%, specificity, 94.5%–95.4%, accuracy, 73.3%–95.5%).[12,13,135] In contrast, whole-body MR imaging with DWI was not significantly different from PET/CT scanning (sensitivity, specificity, and accuracy ranging from 70%–95.5%, 92%–96.1%, and 87.7%–96.1%, respectively).[13,135] Consequently, DWI should be used as a component of whole-body MR examination in routine clinical practice. However, although the addition of DWI improved the sensitivity and accuracy of whole-body MR imaging, whole-body DWI alone had a significantly lower sensitivity and accuracy than whole-body MR imaging with and without DWI and PET/CT scanning.[13,135]

More recently, hybrid PET/MR imaging was compared with PET/CT scanning in M descriptor assessment in patients with lung cancer. The accuracy of PET/MR imaging was equal to or higher than PET/CT scanning, ranging from 57.1% to 79% and 52.4% to 88%, respectively (Fig. 8).[128,129] Despite the limited number of published studies, whole-body MR imaging and whole-body PET/MR imaging have promise in M descriptor evaluation in patients with lung cancer in routine clinical practice.

Postoperative recurrence assessment

Despite advances in diagnosis, staging, and treatment, NSCLC recurrence rates range between 30% and 75%, even after complete resection.[137] In the last few years, the use of whole-body MR imaging and PET/MR imaging to assess the postoperative recurrence of NSCLC has been compared with CT and FDG-PET/CT scanning.[14,138,139] Lee and colleagues[138] compared the diagnostic performance of 3T whole-body

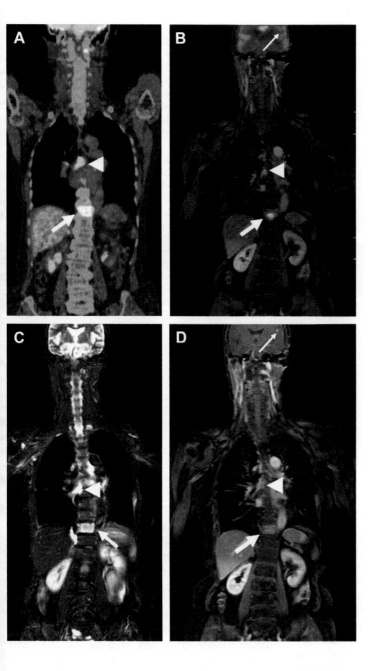

Fig. 8. An 80-year-old woman with adenocarcinoma of the lung with lymph node, bone, and cerebral metastases. (*A*) PET/computed tomography scan shows fluorine-18 fluorodeoxyglucose (FDG)-avid subcarinal lymph node metastasis (*arrowhead*) and T11 vertebral metastasis (*thick arrow*). (*B*) Whole-body PET/MR imaging (CE-Quick 3-dimensional [3D] imaging with the double-fat suppression technique) shows increased FDG uptake and contrast enhancement in subcarinal lymph node metastasis (*arrowhead*) and T11 vertebral metastasis (*thick arrow*). In addition, there is a brain metastasis manifesting as an FDG-avid, contrast-enhanced nodule in the left temporal lobe (*arrow*). (*C*) Whole-body short-tau inversion recovery fast advantage spin echo imaging shows high signal intensity in subcarinal lymph node metastasis (*arrowhead*) and T11 vertebral metastasis (*thick arrow*). (*D*) Whole-body CE-Quick 3D imaging with a double fat suppression radiofrequency pulse technique shows contrast enhancement in the subcarinal lymph node metastasis (*arrowhead*), T11 vertebral metastasis (*thick arrow*), and left temporal lobe brain metastasis (*thin arrow*).

MR imaging with PET/CT scanning for detection of NSCLC recurrence in 62 patients after curative treatment and found that the 2 modalities had the same sensitivity (86%), but that whole-body MR imaging had a higher specificity than PET/CT scanning (56% and 47%, respectively). More recently, Ohno and colleagues[14] compared PET/MR, whole-body MR imaging with and without DWI, FDG-PET/CT scanning with brain CE MR imaging, and routine radiologic examinations for assessment of postoperative recurrence in patients with NSCLC. They reported a better diagnostic performance of PET/MR and whole-body MR imaging with and without DWI (Az = 0.99) than that of PET/CT (Az = 0.92; $P<.05$) and radiologic examinations (Az = 0.91), although whole-body MR imaging with and without DWI showed slightly lower sensitivity than PET/CT (88% and 100%, respectively).[14] Whole-body MR imaging and PET/MR imaging have the potential as alternative imaging modalities to CT and FDG-PET/CT scanning for assessing postoperative recurrence of NSCLC in routine clinical practice (**Fig. 9**).

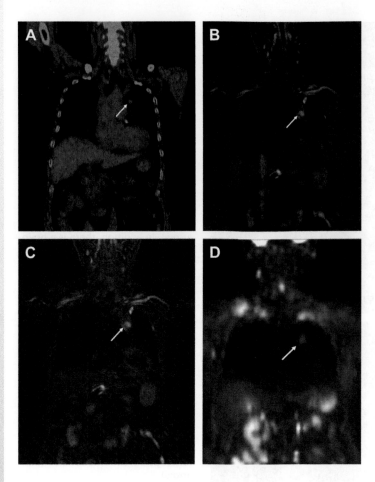

Fig. 9. An-80 year-old man with mediastinal lymph node recurrence after surgical resection of lung adenocarcinoma. (*A*) PET/computed tomography scanning shows fluorine-18 fluorodeoxyglucose (FDG)-avid mediastinal lymph node recurrence (*arrow*). (*B*) PET/MR imaging (short-tau inversion recovery fast advantage spin echo [STIR FASE] image) shows mediastinal lymph node recurrence (*arrow*) has increased FDG uptake and high signal intensity. (*C*) Wholebody STIR FASE imaging and (*D*) whole-body diffusion-weighted imaging show mediastinal lymph node recurrence (*arrow*) has high signal intensity.

POSTTHERAPY LUNG FUNCTION PREDICTION

Primary lung cancer is frequently associated with chronic obstructive pulmonary disease and other cardiopulmonary diseases, especially in heavy smokers.[140] Because surgical resection in these patients is associated with high rates of morbidity and mortality, the selection of patients suitable for surgery is important. Standard lung function tests, such as spirometry, plethysmography, and carbon monoxide diffusing capacity, CT, and/or nuclear medicine examinations are currently used to evaluate respiratory function in the preoperative evaluation of patients with lung cancer.[141–145] Pulmonary functional MR imaging can be used for this purpose and its efficacy is comparable with that of CT scanning, perfusion scan, perfusion SPECT scanning, and/or SPECT/CT scanning (Table 10). Currently, various MR imaging techniques are available for the prediction of postoperative lung function, including 3D dynamic CE perfusion MR imaging,[146–148] non-CE perfusion MR imaging,[149] and oxygen (O_2)-enhanced MR imaging.[150]

Dynamic CE perfusion MR imaging is the most useful new technique in the prediction of postoperative lung function.[147,148] When compared with thin-section CT, perfusion scan (PS), SPECT scanning, and SPECT/CT scanning, the predictive capability of quantitatively assessed 3D CE perfusion MR imaging is superior to qualitatively assessed thin-section CT, PS, and perfusion SPECT scanning, and almost the same as that of quantitatively assessed thin-section CT and perfusion SPECT/CT.[147,148] In addition, 3D CE perfusion MR imaging has a less than 10% discrepancy between actual and predicted postoperative lung function, making its use feasible in clinical practice.[147,148] In addition, this technique does not require further examination time in routine clinical practice because it uses the same dataset as dynamic CE MR imaging with ultrashort TE. Therefore, when appropriate software as well as workstations are available, 3D CE perfusion MR imaging can replace PS, SPECT, and SPECT/CT for perfusion-based prediction of postoperative lung function in routine clinical practice.

Table 10
Prediction of postoperative lung function/radiated lung function

Author, Year	Field Strength	Method	Image/Data Analysis	Outcome
Iwasawa et al,[146] 2002	1.5	Dynamic CE perfusion MR imaging (3D GRE)	Correlation between perfusion ratios derived from MR and radionuclide perfusion scan	$r = 0.92$ ($P<.05$)
			Correlation between MR perfusion ratio and FEV_1	$r = 0.68$ ($P<.05$)
Ohno et al,[147] 2004	1.5	Dynamic CE perfusion MR imaging (3D GRE)	Correlation and Loa between predicted FEV_1-MR imaging and postoperative FEV_1	$r = 0.93$ ($P<.05$); Loa: (0.9% ± 10.4%)
			Correlation and Loa between predicted FEV_1-PS and postoperative FEV_1	$r = 0.89$ ($P<.05$); Loa: (2.1% ± 13.2%)
Ohno et al,[150] 2005	1.5	O_2-enhanced MR imaging (single-shot T1W turbo SE)	Correlation and Loa between predicted FEV_1-MR imaging and postoperative FEV_1	$r = 0.81$ ($P<.05$); Loa: (−9.9% to 10.9%)
			Correlation Loa between predicted FEV_1-qualitative CT and postoperative FEV_1	$r = 0.76$ ($P<.05$); Loa: (−10.7% to 12.9%)
			Correlation and Loa between predicted FEV_1-quantitative CT and postoperative FEV_1	$r = 0.81$ ($P<.05$); Loa: (−10.3% to 11.7%)
			Correlation and Loa between predicted FEV_1-PS and postoperative FEV_1	$r = 0.77$ ($P<.05$); Loa: (−11.9% to 10.9%)
Ohno et al,[148] 2007	1.5	Dynamic CE perfusion MR imaging (3D GRE)	Correlation and Loa between predicted FEV_1-MR imaging and postoperative FEV_1	$r = 0.87$ ($P<.05$); Loa: (5.3% ± 11.8%)
			Correlation and Loa between predicted FEV_1-CT and postoperative FEV_1	$r = 0.88$ ($P<.05$); Loa: (6.8% ± 14.4%)
			Correlation and Loa between predicted FEV_1-PS and postoperative FEV_1	$r = 0.83$ ($P<.05$); Loa: (5.1% ± 14.0%)
Mathew et al,[161] 2010	3.0	Static ^3He MR imaging ventilation	Comparison of ^3He percent ventilated volume between radiation therapy treated and untreated lung: At baseline (35.1 ± 12.2 wk after radiation therapy)	Treated lung: 55 ± 29%; untreated lung: 88 ± 5%
			After 22 wk	Treated lung: no change; untreated lung: 16% ± 6%, ($P = .012$)

(continued on next page)

Table 10
(continued)

Author, Year	Field Strength	Method	Image/Data Analysis	Outcome
Ohno et al,[149] 2015	3.0	Non-CE perfusion MR imaging (3D-ECG-gated non–CE-FBI) and dynamic perfusion MR imaging (3D CE-GRE)	Correlation and Loa between predicted FEV_1– non-CE MR imaging and postoperative FEV_1	r = 0.98 (P<.05); Loa: (−0.3% ± 4.7%)
			Correlation and Loa between predicted FEV_1- CE MR imaging and postoperative FEV_1	r = 0.98 (P<.05); Loa: (−0.3% ± 5.2%)
			Correlation and Loa between predicted FEV_1- CT and postoperative FEV_1	r = 0.98 (P<.05); Loa: (0.3% ± 4.9%)
			Correlation and Loa between predicted FEV_1- PS and postoperative FEV_1	r = 0.94 (P<.05); Loa: (0.6% ± 10.1%)

Abbreviations: 3D, 3-dimensional; CE, contrast enhanced; CT, computed tomography; ECG, electrocardiograph; FBI, fresh blood imaging; FEV_1, forced expiratory volume in 1 second; Loa, limits of agreement; PS, perfusion scan; SE, spin echo; T1W, T1-weighted.

In addition to dynamic CE perfusion MR imaging, non-CE perfusion MR imaging on a 3T system using the fresh blood imaging technique may have a role in respiratory function assessment.[149] In a comparison study evaluating postoperative respiratory function in 60 patients with NSCLC, respiratory and cardiac electrocardiography-gated non-CE and dynamic CE perfusion MR imaging was superior to thin-section CT in the prediction of postoperative percent FEV_1.[149] Non-CE and dynamic perfusion MR imaging was more accurate than qualitative assessment with CT (limits of agreement with actual postoperative percent FEV_1: non-CE MR imaging, 0.3 + 10.0%; dynamic CE perfusion MR imaging, 1.0 + 10.8%; quantitative CT, 1.2 + 9.0%; qualitative CT, 1.5 + 10.2%).[149] Non-CE perfusion MR imaging is an alternative technique in the evaluation of respiratory function in patient with lung cancer with contraindication to gadolinium contrast media.

Oxygen-enhanced MR imaging is another potentially promising method to evaluate respiratory function. In a study evaluating postoperative lung function prediction, O_2-enhanced MR imaging is superior to quantitative and qualitative thin-section CT and perfusion scanning.[150] This study reported excellent correlation between estimated and actual postoperative lung function (r = 0.81; P<.001) when using O_2-enhanced MR imaging or quantitatively assessed thin-section CT. The correlation coefficients for both techniques were better than the result for qualitatively assessed thin-section CT (r = 0.76, P<.001) and PS (r = 0.77; P<.0001).[150] In addition, O_2-enhanced MR imaging can be useful to evaluate regional respiration based on ventilation, oxygen diffusion through the membrane and perfusion, and disease severity in patients with chronic obstructive pulmonary disease[151,152] and interstitial lung disease.[153] However, for O_2-enhanced MR imaging to replace other imaging modalities in the prediction of postoperative lung function, further technical advances in sequencing and imaging processing tools are needed.

Hyperpolarized noble gas (^{3}He, ^{129}Xe) MR imaging is an emerging technique that enables a novel, quantitative analysis of pulmonary physiology and has been evaluated for assessing various pulmonary diseases, including lung cancer.[154–157] With the nonradioactive isotope helium-3 (^{3}He), MR images of in vivo lung ventilation and oxygen sensitivity can be obtained with excellent spatial and temporal resolutions. The technique shows great promise in radiation therapy planning and monitoring lung function after radiation therapy in patients with lung cancer.[158–161] In addition, ^{3}He MR imaging provides information that can be useful in understanding the regional distribution and the functional and structural nature of changes that accompany the decline in pulmonary function after radiation therapy. In this regard, in a pilot study, there was a significant increase in ^{3}He percent ventilated volume (16 ± 6%; P = .012) in the contralateral lung 22 weeks after radiation therapy and none in the treated lung, suggesting a functional compensatory change occurred in the untreated lung.[161] Although further investigation is needed, pulmonary functional MR imaging is a promising tool and potential alternative to CT and nuclear medicine examinations for assessment of respiratory function before and after radiation therapy in patients with lung cancer.

THERAPEUTIC EFFECT PREDICTION AND ASSESSMENT

Currently, the evaluation of treatment response in oncology relies on the response evaluation criteria in solid tumors (RECIST), based on changes in size.[162] CE T1W imaging, dynamic CE MR imaging including perfusion MR imaging technique and DWI are alternative and effective in predicting and evaluating treatment response in patients with lung cancer (Table 11).[163–171]

The therapeutic effect prediction and evaluation was initially performed in 2000 with CE T1W imaging to assess the importance of tumor necrosis on prognosis. In a study of 90 patients with NSCLC, changes in tumor necrosis, and/or cavity size together with a reduction in tumor size showed better correlation with prognosis than did a reduction in size.[163] Dynamic CE MR imaging to evaluate tumor angiogenesis is another technique potentially useful in patients with NSCLC. In a study by Fujimoto and colleagues,[164] a statistically significant difference was established between the slope value of vascular endothelial growth factor (VEGF)-positive and VEGF-negative tumors ($P<.01$); moreover, overall survival of patients with VEGF-positive tumors was significantly shorter than that of patients with VEGF-negative tumors ($P<.01$).

A recent study by Huang and colleagues[167] evaluated the role of dynamic CE MR imaging in a hybrid 3T PET/MR imaging system to assess response in patients with NSCLC receiving radiation therapy. The authors reported that the percentage reduction in K_{trans} mean 6 weeks after stereotactic body radiation therapy correlated with the percentage reduction in tumor size 3 months after stereotactic body radiation therapy.

Dynamic CE MR imaging also has a potential role in the detection of tumor recurrence.[165] In a study of 114 patients with NSCLC treated with chemoradiotherapy, Ohno and colleagues[165] found that the values of the maximum relative enhancement ratio and of the slope of enhancement for the local control group were significantly lower than those for the local failure group ($P<.05$). Using 0.08/s as the threshold value for the slope of enhancement, the sensitivity and specificity for differentiation between the 2 groups were 90.9% and 91.3%, respectively. In addition, when the slope of enhancement was used to estimate prognosis after therapy, the mean survival period of patients whose slope of enhancement of 0.08/s or greater was significantly longer than patients with a slope of enhancement of greater than 0.08/s ($P<.01$).[165]

DWI with quantitative evaluation with ADC may also be useful to evaluate response to therapy and prognosis.[168–171] In fact, early changes in ADC after therapy correlated with tumor size reduction at the end of treatment ($P<.05$). Furthermore, the patients with an increase in ADC showed longer median progression-free and overall survivals ($P<.05$).[168] These results have been recently confirmed in another study by Weiss and colleagues[171]; these authors found that, after serial DWI performed during chemoradiotherapy, the increase in ADC for patients with overall survival less than 12 months was lower than that for patients with longer survival ($P<.05$). In addition, a study reported that the performance of ADC to distinguish partial response from stable disease or disease progression in NSCLC was better than that of standard uptake value in PET/CT scanning. The application of feasible threshold values resulted in specificity (44.4%) and accuracy (76.6%) of DWI becoming significantly higher than those of PET/CT scanning (specificity, 11.1% [$P<.05$] and accuracy, 67.2% [$P<.05$]). In addition, overall survival and progression-free survival of the 2 groups divided by ADC at 2.1×10^{-3} mm^2/s and maximum standardized uptake value at 10 showed a significant difference ($P<.05$).[169] Currently, DWI together with dynamic CE MR imaging, show promise in the evaluation of treatment response as well as tumor recurrence in patients with NSCLC.

SUMMARY

Recent advances in MR imaging enable unprecedented tissue contrast with and without contrast media, together with quantitative and qualitative analysis, expand the role of MR imaging in the evaluation of patients with lung cancer. Technical improvements in gradients and coils systems and new MR imaging techniques such as short time inversion recovery turbo SE sequence, DWI, and whole-body MR imaging with and without DWI, dynamic CE MR imaging, and PET/MR imaging have usefulness in pulmonary nodule detection, nodule characterization, lung cancer staging, therapeutic

Table 11
Prediction and assessment of response to therapy

Author, Year	Field Strength	Method	Data Analysis	Outcome
Ohno et al,[163] 2000	1.5	T1W CE SE	Comparison between RRT and RRVT evaluated by T1W CE MR and CE CT; Comparison between RFS and OS evaluated with RRT and RRVT	Excellent interobserver agreement for RRT ($\kappa = 0.98$) and RRVT ($\kappa = 0.98$) between the 2 methods. PR of RRVT showed significant difference between the 2 methods ($P = .04$). RFS and OS correlated better with RRVT than with RRT.
Ohno et al,[165] 2005	1.5	Dynamic CE perfusion MR imaging (3D GRE)	Differences in maximum relative enhancement ratio and slope of enhancement between local control and local failure; mean survival period	Significant difference between values for the 2 groups ($P<.05$); slope of enhancement correlated with prognosis ($P<.05$)
de Langen et al,[166] 2011	1.5	Dynamic CE perfusion MR imaging (3D GRE)	Correlation of tumor size (CT), and k-trans (dynamic CE MR imaging) with PFS	An increase of more than 15% in the SD of K-trans values after 3 wk correlated with shorter PFS ($P<.05$) and performance was better than CT
Yabuuchi et al,[168] 2011	1.5	Dynamic CE MR imaging (T1W CE turbo SE) DWI-EPI	Correlation of time to peak enhancement, maximum enhancement ratio, and washout ratio ADC with final tumor size reduction, PFS and OS	Significant correlation between early changes in ADC and final tumor size reduction ($r_2 = 0.41$; $P<.05$); increase in ADC correlated with longer OS ($P<.05$)
Ohno et al,[169] 2012	1.5	DWI-EPI	Diagnostic accuracy of DW-MR imaging and FDG-PET/CT for assessing response to therapy (RECIST); correlation of ADC and SUV with PFS and OS	Accuracy of DWI was higher than that of PET-CT (76.6% vs 67.2%; $P<.05$). PFS and OS of 2 groups divided by ADC of 2.1 and SUV_{max} of 10 showed a significant difference ($P<.05$)
Chang et al,[170] 2012	3.0	DWI-EPI	Evaluation of changes in ADC values after therapy between responders and nonresponders	Responders showed significant increases in ADC value compared with pretreatment values (1.12 ± 0.27 to 1.82 ± 0.27; $P<.05$); mean percentage increase in ADC of responders was $67.7\% \pm 33.5\%$
Weiss et al,[171] 2016	1.5	DWI-EPI	Correlation of ADC values during therapy (3–6 wk) with changes in tumor volume and OS	ADC value increase was smaller than tumor volume regression; lower increase in ADC correlated with overall survival <12 mo ($P = .008$)

Abbreviations: 3D, 3-dimensional; ADC, apparent diffusion coefficient; CT, computed tomography; DWI, diffusion weighted imaging; EPI, echo planar imaging; FDG, fluorine-18 fluorodeoxyglucose; GRE, gradient echo; OS, overall survival; PFS, progression-free survival; PR, partial response; RFS, relapse-free survival; RRT, reduction ration of tumor size; RRVT, reduction ratio of viable tumor size; SUV, standardized uptake value; SUV_{max}, maximum standardized uptake value; T1W, t1-weighted; TSE, turbo spin echo.

response evaluation, prediction of prognosis, detection of recurrence, and postoperative lung function prediction. MR imaging has the potential to be an alternative imaging modality to CT and FDG-PET/CT scanning in the management of patients with lung cancer. Further development and standardization of protocols will ensure an important role for MR imaging in the imaging evaluation of patients with lung cancer.

REFERENCES

1. Hatabu H, Tadamura E, Levin DL, et al. Quantitative assessment of pulmonary perfusion with dynamic contrast-enhanced MRI. Magn Reson Med 1999; 42:1033–8.
2. Albert MS, Balamore D. Development of hyperpolarized noble gas MRI. Nucl Instrum Methods Phys Res A 1998;402:441–53.
3. Edelman RR, Hatabu H, Tadamura E, et al. Noninvasive assessment of regional ventilation in the human lung using oxygen-enhanced magnetic resonance imaging. Nat Med 1996;2:1236–9.
4. Hatabu H, Tadamura E, Chen Q, et al. Pulmonary ventilation: dynamic MRI with inhalation of molecular oxygen. Eur J Radiol 2001;37:172–8.
5. Ohno Y, Koyama H, Yoshikawa T, et al. Pulmonary high-resolution ultrashort TE MR imaging: comparison with thin-section standard- and low-dose computed tomography for the assessment of pulmonary parenchyma diseases. J Magn Reson Imaging 2016;43:512–32.
6. Ohno Y, Adachi S, Motoyama A, et al. Multiphase ECG-triggered 3D contrast-enhanced MR angiography: utility for evaluation of hilar and mediastinal invasion of bronchogenic carcinoma. J Magn Reson Imaging 2001;13:215–24.
7. Ohno Y, Hatabu H, Takenaka D, et al. Metastases in mediastinal and hilar lymph nodes in patients with non-small cell lung cancer: quantitative and qualitative assessment with STIR turbo spin-echo MR imaging. Radiology 2004;231:872–9.
8. Ohno Y, Koyama H, Nogami M, et al. STIR turbo SE MR imaging vs. coregistered FDG-PET/CT: quantitative and qualitative assessment of N-stage in non-small-cell lung cancer patients. J Magn Reson Imaging 2007;26:1071–80.
9. Ohno Y, Koyama H, Yoshikawa T, et al. N stage disease in patients with non-small cell lung cancer: efficacy of quantitative and qualitative assessment with STIR turbo spin-echo imaging, diffusion-weighted MR imaging, and fluorodeoxyglucose PET/CT. Radiology 2011;261:605–15.
10. Ohno Y, Koyama H, Yoshikawa T, et al. Diffusion-weighted MR imaging using FASE sequence for 3T MR system: preliminary comparison of capability for N-stage assessment by means of diffusion-weighted MR imaging using EPI sequence, STIR FASE imaging and FDG PET/CT for non small cell lung cancer patients. Eur J Radiol 2015;84:2321–31.
11. Ohno Y, Koyama H, Yoshikawa T, et al. Three-way comparison of whole-body MR, coregistered whole-body FDG PET/MR, and integrated whole-body FDG PET/CT imaging: TNM and stage assessment capability for non-small cell lung cancer patients. Radiology 2015;275:849–61.
12. Ohno Y, Koyama H, Nogami M, et al. Whole-body MR imaging vs. FDG-PET: comparison of accuracy of M-stage diagnosis for lung cancer patients. J Magn Reson Imaging 2007;26:498–509.
13. Ohno Y, Koyama H, Onishi Y, et al. Non-small cell lung cancer: whole-body MR examination for M-stage assessment–utility for whole-body diffusion-weighted imaging compared with integrated FDG PET/CT. Radiology 2008;248:643–54.
14. Ohno Y, Yoshikawa T, Kishida Y, et al. Diagnostic performance of different imaging modalities in the assessment of distant metastasis and local recurrence of tumor in patients with non-small cell lung cancer. J Magn Reson Imaging 2017. https://doi.org/10.1002/jmri.25726.
15. Koyama H, Ohno Y, Kono A, et al. Quantitative and qualitative assessment of non-contrast-enhanced pulmonary MR imaging for management of pulmonary nodules in 161 subjects. Eur Radiol 2008;18:2120–31.
16. Koyama H, Ohno Y, Seki S, et al. Value of diffusion-weighted MR imaging using various parameters for assessment and characterization of solitary pulmonary nodules. Eur J Radiol 2015;84:509–15.
17. Ohno Y, Hatabu H, Takenaka D, et al. Solitary pulmonary nodules: potential role of dynamic MR imaging in management initial experience. Radiology 2002;224:503–11.
18. Ohno Y, Hatabu H, Takenaka D, et al. Dynamic MR imaging: value of differentiating subtypes of peripheral small adenocarcinoma of the lung. Eur J Radiol 2004;52:144–50.
19. Ohno Y, Koyama H, Takenaka D, et al. Dynamic MRI, dynamic multidetector-row computed tomography (MDCT), and coregistered 2-[fluorine-18]-fluoro-2-deoxy-D-glucose-positron emission tomography (FDG-PET)/CT: comparative study of capability for management of pulmonary nodules. J Magn Reson Imaging 2008;27:1284–95.
20. Ohno Y, Nishio M, Koyama H, et al. Solitary pulmonary nodules: comparison of dynamic first-pass contrast-enhanced perfusion area-detector CT, dynamic first-pass contrast-enhanced MR imaging, and FDG PET/CT. Radiology 2015;274:563–75.
21. Hansell DM, Bankier AA, MacMahon H, et al. Fleischner society: glossary of terms for thoracic imaging. Radiology 2008;246:697–722.

22. Callister ME, Baldwin DR, Akram AR, et al. British Thoracic Society guidelines for the investigation and management of pulmonary nodules. Thorax 2015;70:1–54.

23. MacMahon H, Naidich DP, Goo JM, et al. Guidelines for management of incidental pulmonary nodules detected on CT images: from the Fleischner society 2017. Radiology 2017;23:161659.

24. Horeweg N, van Rosmalen J, Heuvelmans MA, et al. Lung cancer probability in patients with CT-detected pulmonary nodules: a prespecified analysis of data from the NELSON trial of low-dose CT screening. Lancet Oncol 2014;15: 1332–41.

25. Yankelevitz DF, Yip R, Smith JP, et al. CT screening for lung cancer: nonsolid nodules in baseline and annual repeat rounds. Radiology 2015;277:555–64.

26. National Lung Screening Trial Research Team, Aberle DR, Adams AM, Berg CD, et al. Reduced lung-cancer mortality with low-dose computed tomographic screening. N Engl J Med 2011;365: 395–409.

27. The National Comprehensive Cancer Network (NCCN). Lung cancer screening. Version 1.2017. Available at: https://www.nccn.org/patients/guidelines/lung_screening/files/assets/common/downloads/files/lung_screening.pdf.

28. Feuerstein IM, Jicha DL, Pass HI, et al. Pulmonary metastases: MR imaging with surgical correlation–a prospective study. Radiology 1992; 182:123–9.

29. Kersjes W, Mayer E, Buchenroth M, et al. Diagnosis of pulmonary metastases with turbo-SE MR imaging. Eur Radiol 1997;7:1190–4.

30. Biederer J, Schoene A, Freitag S, et al. Simulated pulmonary nodules implanted in a dedicated porcine chest phantom: sensitivity of MR imaging for detection. Radiology 2003;227:475–83.

31. Vogt FM, Herborn CU, Hunold P, et al. HASTE MRI versus chest radiography in the detection of pulmonary nodules: comparison with MDCT. AJR Am J Roentgenol 2004;183:71–8.

32. Both M, Schultze J, Reuter M, et al. Fast T1- and T2-weighted pulmonary MR-imaging in patients with bronchial carcinoma. Eur J Radiol 2005;53: 478–88.

33. Schroeder T, Ruehm SG, Debatin JF, et al. Detection of pulmonary nodules using a 2D HASTE MR sequence: comparison with MDCT. AJR Am J Roentgenol 2005;185:979–84.

34. Bruegel M, Gaa J, Woertler K, et al. MRI of the lung: value of different turbo spin-echo, single-shot turbo spin-echo, and 3D gradient-echo pulse sequences for the detection of pulmonary metastases. J Magn Reson Imaging 2007;25:73–81.

35. Regier M, Kandel S, Kaul MG, et al. Detection of small pulmonary nodules in high-field MR at 3 T: evaluation of different pulse sequences using porcine lung explants. Eur Radiol 2007;17:1341–51.

36. Frericks BB, Meyer BC, Martus P, et al. MRI of the thorax during whole-body MRI: evaluation of different MR sequences and comparison to thoracic multidetector computed tomography (MDCT). J Magn Reson Imaging 2008;27:538–45.

37. Koyama H, Ohno Y, Aoyama N, et al. Comparison of STIR turbo SE imaging and diffusion-weighted imaging of the lung: capability for detection and subtype classification of pulmonary adenocarcinomas. Eur Radiol 2010;20:790–800.

38. Heye T, Ley S, Heussel CP, et al. Detection and size of pulmonary lesions: how accurate is MRI? A prospective comparison of CT and MRI. Acta Radiol 2012;53(2):153–60.

39. Cieszanowski A, Lisowska M, Dabrowska, et al. MR imaging of pulmonary nodules: detection rate and accuracy of size estimation in comparison to computed tomography. PLoS One 2016;11: e0156272.

40. Meier-Schroers M, Kukuk G, Homsi R, et al. MRI of the lung using the PROPELLER technique: artifact reduction, better image quality and improved nodule detection. Eur J Radiol 2016; 85:707–13.

41. Dewes P, Frellesen C, Al-Butmeh F, et al. Comparative evaluation of non-contrast CAIPIRINHA-VIBE 3T-MRI and multidetector CT for detection of pulmonary nodules: In vivo evaluation of diagnostic accuracy and image quality. Eur J Radiol 2016; 85:193–8.

42. Regier M, Schwarz D, Henes FO, et al. Diffusion-weighted MR-imaging for the detection of pulmonary nodules at 1.5 Tesla: intraindividual comparison with multidetector computed tomography. J Med Imaging Radiat Oncol 2011;55:266–74.

43. Li B, Li Q, Chen C, et al. A systematic review and meta-analysis of the accuracy of diffusion-weighted MRI in the detection of malignant pulmonary nodules and masses. Acad Radiol 2014;21: 21–9.

44. Bergin CJ, Glover GM, Pauly J. Magnetic resonance imaging of lung parenchyma. J Thorac Imaging 1993;8:12–7.

45. Puderbach M, Hintze C, Ley S, et al. MR imaging of the chest: a practical approach at 1.5 T. Eur J Radiol 2007;64:345–55.

46. Hatabu H, Alsop DC, Listerud J, et al. T2* and proton density measurement of normal human lung parenchyma using submillisecond echo time gradient echo magnetic resonance imaging. Eur J Radiol 1999;9:245–52.

47. Stock KW, Chen Q, Hatabu H, et al. Magnetic resonance T2* measurements of the normal lung in vivo with ultra-short echo times. Magn Reson Imaging 1999;7:997–1000.

48. Yu J, Xue Y, Song HK. Comparison of lung T2* during free-breathing at 1.5 T and 3.0 T with ultrashort echo time imaging. Magn Reson Med 2011;6:248–54.

49. Ramalho M, Herédia V, Tsurusaki M, et al. Quantitative and qualitative comparison of 1.5 and 3.0 Tesla MRI in patients with chronic liver diseases. J Magn Reson Imaging 2009;29:869–79.

50. Lee VS, Hecht EM, Taouli B, et al. Body and cardiovascular MR imaging at 3.0 T. Radiology 2007;244:692–705.

51. Merkle EM, Dale BM. Abdominal MRI at 3.0 T: the basics revisited. AJR 2006;186:1524–32.

52. Barth MM, Smith MP, Pedrosa I, et al. Body MR imaging at 3.0 T: understanding the opportunities and challenges. Radiographics 2007;27:1445–62.

53. van den Bergen B, Stolk CC, Berg JB, et al. Ultra fast electromagnetic field computations for RF multi-transmit techniques in high field MRI. Phys Med Biol 2009;54:1253–64.

54. Soher BJ, Dale BM, Merkle EM. A review of MR physics: 3T versus 1.5T. Magn Reson Imaging Clin N Am 2007;15:277–90.

55. Johnson KM, Fain SB, Schiebler ML, et al. Optimized 3D ultrashort echo time pulmonary MRI. Magn Reson Med 2013;70:1241–50.

56. Ohno Y, Koyama H, Yoshikawa T, et al. T2* measurements of 3-T MRI with ultrashort TEs: capabilities of pulmonary function assessment and clinical stage classification in smokers. AJR Am J Roentgenol 2011;197:W279–85.

57. Ohno Y, Nishio M, Koyama H, et al. Pulmonary MR imaging with ultra-short TEs: utility for disease severity assessment of connective tissue disease patients. Eur J Radiol 2013;82:1359–65.

58. Ohno Y, Nishio M, Koyama H, et al. Pulmonary 3 T MRI with ultrashort TEs: influence of ultrashort echo time interval on pulmonary functional and clinical stage assessments of smokers. J Magn Reson Imaging 2014;39:988–97.

59. Kruger SJ, Fain SB, Johnson KM, et al. Oxygen enhanced 3D radial ultrashort echo time magnetic resonance imaging in the healthy human lung. NMR Biomed 2014;27:1535–41.

60. Bauman G, Johnson KM, Bell LC, et al. Three-dimensional pulmonary perfusion MRI with radial ultrashort echo time and spatial-temporal constrained reconstruction. Magn Reson Med 2015;73:555–64.

61. Ma W, Sheikh K, Svenningsen S, et al. Ultra-short echo-time pulmonary MRI: evaluation and reproducibility in COPD subjects with and without bronchiectasis. J Magn Reson Imaging 2015;41:1465–74.

62. Bell LC, Johnson KM, Fain SB, et al. Simultaneous MRI of lung structure and perfusion in a single breathhold. J Magn Reson Imaging 2015;41:52–9.

63. Ohno Y, Koyama H, Yoshikawa T, et al. Standard-, reduced-, and no-dose thin-section radiologic examinations: comparison of capability for nodule detection and nodule type assessment in patients suspected of having pulmonary nodules. Radiology 2017;161037. https://doi.org/10.1148/radiol.2017161037.

64. Burris NS, Johnson KM, Larson PEZ, et al. Detection of small pulmonary nodules with ultrashort echo time sequences in oncology patients by using a PET/MR system. Radiology 2016;278:239–46.

65. Swensen SJ, Silverstein MD, Ilstrup DM, et al. The probability of malignancy in solitary pulmonary nodules. Application to small radiologically indeterminate nodules. Arch Intern Med 1997;157:849–55.

66. Gould MK, Ananth L, Barnett PG. A clinical model to estimate the pretest probability of lung cancer in patients with solitary pulmonary nodules. Chest 2007;131:383–8.

67. Soardi GA, Perandini S, Larici AR, et al. Multicentre external validation of the BIMC model for solid solitary pulmonary nodule malignancy prediction. Eur Radiol 2017;27:1929–33.

68. MacMahon H, Austin JH, Gamsu G, et al. Guidelines for management of small pulmonary nodules detected on CT scans: a statement from the Fleischner Society. Radiology 2005;237:395–400.

69. Naidich DP, Bankier AA, MacMahon H, et al. Recommendations for the management of subsolid pulmonary nodules detected at CT: a statement from the Fleischner society. Radiology 2013;266:304–17.

70. Ohno Y, Koyama H, Dinkel J, et al. Lung cancer. In: Kauczor HU, editor. MRI of the lung. Springer; 2008. p. 180–216.

71. Sakai F, Sone S, Maruyama A, et al. Thin-rim enhancement in Gd-DTPA-enhanced magnetic resonance images of tuberculoma: a new finding of potential differential diagnostic importance. J Thorac Imaging 1992;7:64–9.

72. Sakai F, Sone S, Kiyono K, et al. MR of pulmonary hamartoma: pathologic correlation. J Thorac Imaging 1994;9:51–5.

73. Chung MH, Lee HG, Kwon SS, et al. MR imaging of solitary pulmonary lesion: emphasis on tuberculomas and comparison with tumors. J Magn Reson Imaging 2000;11:629–37.

74. Fujimoto K, Meno S, Nishimura H, et al. Aspergilloma within cavitary lung cancer: MR imaging findings. AJR Am J Roentgenol 1994;163:565–7.

75. Blum U, Windfuhr M, Buitrago-Tellez C, et al. Invasive pulmonary aspergillosis. MRI, CT, and plain radiographic findings and their contribution for early diagnosis. Chest 1994;106:1156–61.

76. Gaeta M, Minutoli F, Ascenti G, et al. MR white lung sign: incidence and significance in pulmonary consolidations. J Comput Assist Tomogr 2001;25:890–6.

77. Gaeta M, Vinci S, Minutoli F, et al. CT and MRI findings of mucin-containing tumors and pseudotumors of the thorax: pictorial review. Eur Radiol 2002;12:181–9.

78. Kono M, Adachi S, Kusumoto M, et al. Clinical utility of Gd-DTPA-enhanced magnetic resonance imaging in lung cancer. J Thorac Imaging 1993;8:18–26.

79. Kusumoto M, Kono M, Adachi S, et al. Gadopentetate- dimeglumine-enhanced magnetic resonance imaging for lung nodules. Differentiation of lung cancer and tuberculoma. Invest Radiol 1994;29: S255–6.

80. Kurihara Y, Matsuoka S, Yamashiro T, et al. MRI of pulmonary nodules. AJR Am J Roentgenol 2014; 202:W210–6.

81. Leutner CC, Gieseke J, Lutterbey G, et al. MR imaging of pneumonia in immunocompromised patients: comparison with helical CT. AJR Am J Roentgenol 2000;175:391–7.

82. Walker R, Kessar P, Blanchard R, et al. Turbo STIR magnetic resonance imaging as a whole-body screening tool for metastases in patients with breast carcinoma: preliminary clinical experience. J Magn Reson Imaging 2000;11:343–50.

83. Matoba M, Tonami H, Kondou T, et al. Lung carcinoma: diffusion-weighted MR imaging–preliminary evaluation with apparent diffusion coefficient. Radiology 2007;243:570–7.

84. Uto T, Takehara Y, Nakamura Y, et al. Higher sensitivity and specificity for diffusion-weighted imaging of malignant lung lesions without apparent diffusion coefficient quantification. Radiology 2009;252: 247–54.

85. Çakmak V, Ufuk F, Karabulut N. Diffusion-weighted MRI of pulmonary lesions: comparison of apparent diffusion coefficient and lesion-to-spinal cord signal intensity ratio in lesion characterization. J Magn Reson Imaging 2017;45:845–54.

86. Hittmair K, Eckersberger F, Klepetko W, et al. Evaluation of solitary pulmonary nodules with dynamic contrast-enhanced MR imaging: a promising technique. Magn Reson Imaging 1995;13:923–33.

87. Gückel C, Schnabel K, Deimling M, et al. Solitary pulmonary nodules: MR evaluation of enhancement patterns with contrast-enhanced dynamic snapshot gradient-echo imaging. Radiology 1996; 200:681–6.

88. Schaefer JF, Vollmar J, Schick F, et al. Solitary pulmonary nodules: dynamic contrast-enhanced MR imaging—perfusion differences in malignant and benign lesions. Radiology 2004;232:544–53.

89. Kim JH, Kim HJ, Lee KH, et al. Solitary pulmonary nodules: a comparative study evaluated with contrast-enhanced dynamic MR imaging and CT. J Comput Assist Tomogr 2004;28:766–75.

90. Kono R, Fujimoto K, Terasaki H, et al. Dynamic MRI of solitary pulmonary nodules: comparison of enhancement patterns of malignant and benign small peripheral lung lesions. AJR 2007;188:26–36.

91. Zou Y, Zhang M, Wang Q, et al. Quantitative investigation of solitary pulmonary nodules: dynamic contrast-enhanced MRI and histopathologic analysis. AJR 2008;191:252–9.

92. Cronin P, Dwamena BA, Kelly AM, et al. Solitary pulmonary nodules: meta-analytic comparison of cross-sectional imaging modalities for diagnosis of malignancy. Radiology 2008;246:772–82.

93. Ohno Y, Koyama H, Lee HY, et al. Contrast-enhanced CT- and MRI-based perfusion assessment for pulmonary diseases: basics and clinical applications. Diagn Interv Radiol 2016;22:407–21.

94. van Zijl PC, Yadav NN. Chemical exchange saturation transfer (CEST): what is in a name and what isn't? Magn Reson Med 2011;65:927–48.

95. Wu B, Warnock G, Zaiss M, et al. An overview of CEST MRI for non-MR physicists. EJNMMI Phys 2016;3:19.

96. Ward KM, Aletras AH, Balaban RS. A new class of contrast agents for MRI based on proton chemical exchange dependent saturation transfer (CEST). J Magn Reson 2000;143:79–87.

97. Vinogradov E, Sherry AD, Lenkinski RE. CEST: from basic principles to applications, challenges and opportunities. J Magn Reson 2013;229:155–72.

98. Togao O, Kessinger CW, Huang G, et al. Characterization of lung cancer by amide proton transfer (APT) imaging: an in vivo study in an orthotopic mouse model. PLoS One 2013;8:e77019.

99. Togao O, Yoshiura T, Keupp J, et al. Amide proton transfer imaging of adult diffuse gliomas: correlation with histopathological grades. Neuro-oncology 2014;16:441–8.

100. Sagiyama K, Mashimo T, Togao O, et al. In vivo chemical exchange saturation transfer imaging allows early detection of a therapeutic response in glioblastoma. Proc Natl Acad Sci U S A 2014; 111:4542–7.

101. Ren J, Trokowski R, Zhang S, et al. Imaging the tissue distribution of glucose in livers using a PARACEST sensor. Magn Reson Med 2008;60: 1047–55.

102. Zhou J, Lal B, Wilson DA, et al. Amide proton transfer (APT) contrast for imaging of brain tumors. Magn Reson Med 2003;50:1120–6.

103. Ohno Y, Yui M, Koyama H, et al. Chemical exchange saturation transfer MR imaging: preliminary results for differentiation of malignant and benign thoracic lesions. Radiology 2016;279:578–89.

104. World Health Organization. International Agency for Research on Cancer. GLOBOCAN 2012: estimated cancer incidence, mortality and prevalence worldwide in 2012. Lung cancer. Available at: http:// globocan.iarc.fr/Pages/fact_sheets_cancer.aspx. Accessed July 3, 2015.

105. U.S. National Institutes of Health. National Cancer Institute: SEER cancer statistics review, 1975-2012. Available at: http://seer.cancergov/csr/1975_2012/browse_csr.php?sectionSEL=15&pageSEL=sect_15_table.28.html. Accessed July 3, 2015.

106. Webb WR, Gatsonis C, Zerhouni EA, et al. CT and MR imaging in staging non-small cell bronchogenic carcinoma: report of the radiologic diagnostic oncology group. Radiology 1991;178: 705–13.

107. White CS. MR evaluation of the pericardium and cardiac malignancies. Magn Reson Imaging Clin N Am 1996;4:237–51.

108. Sakai S, Murayama S, Murakami J, et al. Bronchogenic carcinoma invasion of the chest wall: evaluation with dynamic cineMRI during breathing. J Comput Assist Tomogr 1997;21:595–600.

109. Murata K, Takahashi M, Mori M, et al. Chest wall and mediastinal invasion by lung cancer: evaluation with multisection expiratory dynamic CT. Radiology 1994;191:251–5.

110. Takahashi K, Furuse M, Hanaoka H, et al. Pulmonary vein and left atrial invasion by lung cancer: assessment by breath-hold gadolinium-enhanced three-dimensional MR angiography. J Comput Assist Tomogr 2000;24:557–61.

111. Tang W, Wu N, OuYang H, et al. The presurgical T staging of non-small cell lung cancer: efficacy comparison of 64-MDCT and 3.0 T MRI. Cancer Imaging 2015;15:14.

112. Higashino T, Ohno Y, Takenaka D, et al. Thin-section multiplanar reformats from multidetector-row CT data: utility for assessment of regional tumor extent in non-small cell lung cancer. Eur J Radiol 2005;56:48–55.

13. Boiselle PM, Patz EF Jr, Vining DJ, et al. Imaging of mediastinal lymph nodes: CT, MR, and FDG PET. Radiographics 1998;18:1061–9.

14. Takenaka D, Ohno Y, Hatabu H, et al. Differentiation of metastatic versus non-metastatic mediastinal lymph nodes in patients with non-small cell lung cancer using respiratory-triggered short inversion time inversion recovery (STIR) turbo spin-echo MR imaging. Eur J Radiol 2002;44:216–24.

15. Hasegawa I, Boiselle PM, Kuwabara K, et al. Mediastinal lymph nodes in patients with non-small cell lung cancer: preliminary experience with diffusion-weighted MR imaging. J Thorac Imaging 2008;23: 157–61.

16. Nomori H, Mori T, Ikeda K, et al. Diffusion-weighted magnetic resonance imaging can be used in place of positron emission tomography for N staging of non-small cell lung cancer with fewer false-positive results. J Thorac Cardiovasc Surg 2008; 135:816–22.

17. Morikawa M, Demura Y, Ishizaki T, et al. The effectiveness of 18F-FDG PET/CT combined with STIR MRI for diagnosing nodal involvement in the thorax. J Nucl Med 2009;50:81–7.

118. Nakayama J, Miyasaka K, Omatsu T, et al. Metastases in mediastinal and hilar lymph nodes in patients with non-small cell lung cancer: quantitative assessment with diffusion-weighted magnetic resonance imaging and apparent diffusion coefficient. J Comput Assist Tomogr 2010;34:1–8.

119. Usuda K, Zhao XT, Sagawa M, et al. Diffusion-weighted imaging is superior to positron emission tomography in the detection and nodal assessment of lung cancers. Ann Thorac Surg 2011;91:1689–95.

120. Usuda K, Maeda S, Motono N, et al. Diagnostic performance of diffusion-weighted imaging for multiple hilar and mediastinal lymph nodes with FDG accumulation. Asian Pac J Cancer Prev 2015;16:6401–6.

121. Nomori H, Cong Y, Sugimura H, et al. Diffusion-weighted imaging can correctly identify false-positive lymph nodes on positron emission tomography in non-small cell lung cancer. Surg Today 2016;46:1146–51.

122. Pauls S, Schmidt SA, Juchems MS, et al. Diffusion-weighted MR imaging in comparison to integrated [18F]-FDG PET/CT for N-staging in patients with lung cancer. Eur J Radiol 2012;81:178–82.

123. Wu LM, Xu JR, Gu HY, et al. Preoperative mediastinal and hilar nodal staging with diffusion-weighted magnetic resonance imaging and fluorodeoxyglucose positron emission tomography/computed tomography in patients with non-small-cell lung cancer: which is better? J Surg Res 2012;178: 304–14.

124. Shen G, Lan Y, Zhang K, et al. Comparison of 18F-FDG PET/CT and DWI for detection of mediastinal nodal metastasis in non-small cell lung cancer: a meta-analysis. PLoS One 2017;12:e0173104.

125. Yi CA, Shin KM, Lee KS, et al. Non-small cell lung cancer staging: efficacy comparison of integrated PET/CT versus 3.0-T whole-body MR imaging. Radiology 2008;248:632–42.

126. Sommer G, Wiese M, Winter L, et al. Preoperative staging of non-small-cell lung cancer: comparison of whole-body diffusion-weighted magnetic resonance imaging and 18F-fluorodeoxyglucose-positron emission tomography/computed tomography. Eur Radiol 2012;22:2859–67.

127. Heusch P, Buchbender C, Köhler J, et al. Thoracic staging in lung cancer: prospective comparison of 18F-FDG PET/MR imaging and 18F-FDG PET/CT. J Nucl Med 2014;55:373–8.

128. Huellner MW, de Galiza Barbosa F, Husmann L, et al. TNM staging of non-small cell lung cancer: comparison of PET/MR and PET/CT. J Nucl Med 2016;57:21–6.

129. Lee SM, Goo JM, Park CM, et al. Preoperative staging of non-small cell lung cancer: prospective

comparison of PET/MR and PET/CT. Eur Radiol 2016;26:3850–7.

130. Schaarschmidt BM, Grueneisen J, Metzenmacher M, et al. Thoracic staging with 18F-FDG PET/MR in non-small cell lung cancer - does it change therapeutic decisions in comparison to 18F-FDG PET/CT? Eur Radiol 2017;27:681–8.

131. Xu L, Tian J, Liu Y, et al. Accuracy of diffusion-weighted (DW)MRI with background signal suppression (MR-DWIBS) in diagnosis of mediastinal lymph node metastasis of non small cell lung cancer (NSCLC). J Magn Reson Imaging 2014;40:200–5.

132. Silvestri GA, Gould MK, Margolis ML, et al, American College of Chest Physicians. Noninvasive staging of non-small cell lung cancer: ACCP evidenced-based clinical practice guidelines (2nd edition). Chest 2007;132:178S–201S.

133. Samson DJ, Seidenfeld J, Simon GR, et al, American College of Chest Physicians. Evidence for management of small cell lung cancer: ACCP evidence-based clinical practice guidelines (2nd edition). Chest 2007;132:314S–23S.

134. Silvestri GA, Gonzalez AV, Jantz MA, et al. Methods for staging non-small cell lung cancer: diagnosis and management of lung cancer, 3rd ed: American College of Chest Physicians evidence-based clinical practice guidelines. Chest 2013;143:e211S–5S.

135. Takenaka D, Ohno Y, Matsumoto K, et al. Detection of bone metastases in non-small cell lung cancer patients: comparison of whole-body diffusion-weighted imaging (DWI), whole-body MR imaging without and with DWI, whole-body FDG-PET/CT, and bone scintigraphy. J Magn Reson Imaging 2009;30:298–308.

136. Ciliberto M, Maggi F, Treglia G, et al. Comparison between whole-body MRI and Fluorine-18-Fluorodeoxyglucose PET or PET/CT in oncology: a systematic review. Radiol Oncol 2013;47:206–18.

137. Martini N, Bains MS, Burt ME, et al. Incidence of local recurrence and second primary tumors in resected stage I lung cancer. J Thorac Cardiovasc Surg 1995;109:120–9.

138. Lee MH, Kim SR, Park SY, et al. Application of whole-body MRI to detect the recurrence of lung cancer. Magn Reson Imaging 2012;30:1439–45.

139. Ohno Y, Nishio M, Koyama H, et al. Comparison of the utility of whole-body MRI with and without contrast-enhanced Quick 3D and double RF fat suppression techniques, conventional whole-body MRI, PET/CT and conventional examination for assessment of recurrence in NSCLC patients. Eur J Radiol 2013;82:2018–27.

140. Durham AL, Adcock IM. The relationship between COPD and lung cancer. Lung Cancer 2015;90:121–7.

141. Pierce RJ, Copland JM, Sharpe K, et al. Preoperative risk evaluation for lung cancer resection: predicted postoperative product as a predictor of surgical mortality. Am J Respir Crit Care Med 1994;150:947–55.

142. Bolliger CT, Jordan P, Solèr M, et al. Exercise capacity as a predictor of postoperative complications in lung resection candidates. Am J Respir Crit Care Med 1995;151:1472–80.

143. Wyser C, Stulz P, Soler M, et al. Prospective evaluation of an algorithm for the functional assessment of lung resection candidates. Am J Respir Crit Care Med 1999;159:1450–6.

144. Mazzone PJ, Arroliga AC. Lung cancer: preoperative pulmonary evaluation of the lung resection candidate. Am J Med 2005;118:578–83.

145. Colice GL, Shafazand S, Griffin JP, et al, American College of Chest Physicians. Physiologic evaluation of the patient with lung cancer being considered for resectional surgery: ACCP evidenced-based clinical practice guidelines (2nd edition). Chest 2007;132:161S–77S.

146. Iwasawa T, Saito K, Ogawa N, et al. Prediction of postoperative pulmonary function using perfusion magnetic resonance imaging of the lung. J Magn Reson Imaging 2002;15:685–92.

147. Ohno Y, Hatabu H, Higashino T, et al. Dynamic perfusion MRI versus perfusion scintigraphy: prediction of postoperative lung function in patients with lung cancer. AJR Am J Roentgenol 2004; 182:73–8.

148. Ohno Y, Koyama H, Nogami M, et al. Postoperative lung function in lung cancer patients: comparative analysis of predictive capability of MRI, CT, and SPECT. AJR Am J Roentgenol 2007;189: 400–8.

149. Ohno Y, Seki S, Koyama H, et al. 3D ECG- and respiratory-gated non-contrast-enhanced (CE) perfusion MRI for postoperative lung function prediction in non-small-cell lung cancer patients: A comparison with thin-section quantitative computed tomography, dynamic CE-perfusion MRI, and perfusion scan. J Magn Reson Imaging 2015;42:340–53.

150. Ohno Y, Hatabu H, Higashino T, et al. Oxygen enhanced MR imaging: correlation with postsurgical lung function in patients with lung cancer. Radiology 2005;236:704–11.

151. Ohno Y, Nishio M, Koyama H, et al. Asthma: comparison of dynamic oxygen-enhanced MR imaging and quantitative thin-section CT for evaluation of clinical treatment. Radiology 2014;273:907–16.

152. Ohno Y, Koyama H, Matsumoto K, et al. Oxygen-enhanced MRI vs. quantitatively assessed thin-section CT: pulmonary functional loss assessment and clinical stage classification of asthmatics. Eur J Radiol 2011;77:85–91.

153. Ohno Y, Nishio M, Koyama H, et al. Oxygen-enhanced MRI for patients with connective tissue diseases: comparison with thin-section CT of

capability for pulmonary functional and disease severity assessment. Eur J Radiol 2014;83:391–7.

154. Fain SB, Gonzalez-Fernandez G, Peterson ET, et al. Evaluation of structure-function relationships in asthma using multidetector CT and hyperpolarized He-3 MRI. Acad Radiol 2008;15:753–62.

155. Tzeng YS, Lutchen K, Albert M. The difference in ventilation heterogeneity between asthmatic and healthy subjects quantified using hyperpolarized 3He MRI. J Appl Physiol 2009;106:813–22.

156. Virgincar RS, Cleveland ZI, Kaushik SS, et al. Quantitative analysis of hyperpolarized 129Xe ventilation imaging in healthy volunteers and subjects with chronic obstructive pulmonary disease. NMR Biomed 2013;26:424–35.

157. Fain SB, Panth SR, Evans MD, et al. Early emphysematous changes in asymptomatic smokers: detection with 3He MR imaging. Radiology 2006; 239:875–83.

158. Ireland RH, Bragg CM, McJury M, et al. Feasibility of image registration and intensity-modulated radiotherapy planning with hyperpolarized helium-3 magnetic resonance imaging for non-small-cell lung cancer. Int J Radiat Oncol Biol Phys 2007; 68:273–81.

159. Bates EL, Bragg CM, Wild JM, et al. Functional image-based radiotherapy planning for non-small cell lung cancer: a simulation study. Radiother Oncol 2009;93:32–6.

160. Hodge CW, Tome WA, Fain SB, et al. On the use of hyperpolarized helium MRI for conformal avoidance lung radiotherapy. Med Dosim 2010;35: 297–303.

161. Mathew L, Gaede S, Wheatley A, et al. Detection of longitudinal lung structural and functional changes after diagnosis of radiation-induced lung injury using hyperpolarized 3He magnetic resonance imaging. Med Phys 2010;37:22–31.

162. Eisenhauer EA, Therasse P, Bogaerts J, et al. New response evaluation criteria in solid tumours: revised RECIST guideline (version 1.1). Eur J Cancer 2009;45:228–47.

163. Ohno Y, Adachi S, Kono M, et al. Predicting the prognosis of non-small cell lung cancer patient treated with conservative therapy using contrast-enhanced MR imaging. Eur Radiol 2000;10: 1770–81.

164. Fujimoto K, Abe T, Muller NL, et al. Small peripheral pulmonary carcinomas evaluated with dynamic MR imaging: correlation with tumor vascularity and prognosis. Radiology 2003;227:786–93.

165. Ohno Y, Nogami M, Higashino T, et al. Prognostic value of dynamic MR imaging for non-small-cell lung cancer patients after chemoradiotherapy. J Magn Reson Imaging 2005;21:775–83.

166. de Langen AJ, van den Boogaart V, Lubberink M, et al. Monitoring response to antiangiogenic therapy in non-small cell lung cancer using imaging markers derived from PET and dynamic contrast-enhanced MRI. J Nucl Med 2011;52:48–55.

167. Huang YS, Chen JL, Hsu FM, et al. Response assessment of stereotactic body radiation therapy using dynamic contrast-enhanced integrated MR-PET in non-small cell lung cancer patients. J Magn Reson Imaging 2017. https://doi.org/10.1002/jmri.25758.

168. Yabuuchi H, Hatakenaka M, Takayama K, et al. Non small cell lung cancer: detection of early response to chemotherapy by using contrast-enhanced dynamic and diffusion-weighted MR imaging. Radiology 2011;261:598–604.

169. Ohno Y, Koyama H, Yoshikawa T, et al. Diffusion weighted MRI versus 18F-FDG PET/CT: performance as predictors of tumor treatment response and patient survival in patients with non-small cell lung cancer receiving chemoradiotherapy. AJR Am J Roentgenol 2012;198:75–82.

170. Chang Q, Wu N, Ouyang H, et al. Diffusion-weighted magnetic resonance imaging of lung cancer at 3.0 T: a preliminary study on monitoring diffusion changes during chemoradiation therapy. Clin Imaging 2012;36:98–103.

171. Weiss E, Ford JC, Olsen KM, et al. Apparent diffusion coefficient (ADC) change on repeated diffusion-weighted magnetic resonance imaging during radiochemotherapy for non-small cell lung cancer: a pilot study. Lung Cancer 2016;96: 113–9.

Lung Cancer
Posttreatment Imaging: Radiation Therapy and Imaging Findings

Marcelo F. Benveniste, MD[a,*], James Welsh, MD[b],
Chitra Viswanathan, MD[a], Girish S. Shroff, MD[a],
Sonia L. Betancourt Cuellar, MD[a], Brett W. Carter, MD[a],
Edith M. Marom, MD[a,c]

KEYWORDS

• Lung cancer • Radiation therapy • Proton therapy • Tumor recurrence

KEY POINTS

• Radiation therapy is important in the treatment of patients with lung cancer and is being used with both palliative and curative intent.
• Imaging findings of radiation-induced lung injury are divided into an acute phase (radiation pneumonitis) and a chronic phase (radiation fibrosis).
• Newer methods of radiation therapy delivery techniques result in nontraditional patterns of radiation changes to the lungs and surrounding organs.
• Knowledge of the radiation treatment plan and technique, and the temporal evolution of radiation-induced lung injury, is important to identify manifestations of radiation-induced lung injury and differentiate them from tumor recurrence or infection.

INTRODUCTION

Radiation therapy (RT) is important in the treatment of patients with lung cancer and is being used with both palliative and curative intent. However, a potential limitation in the delivery of tumorcidal radiation dose is the presence of surrounding radiation-sensitive critical organs. Advances in radiotherapy techniques such as 3-dimensional conformal RT (3D-CRT), intensity-modulated radiotherapy (IMRT), stereotactic body radiotherapy (SBRT), and proton therapy allow for the precise delivery of radiation to the tumor by conforming the radiation dose to the tumor, and have improved locoregional control and survival in patients with non–small cell lung cancer (NSCLC). More sophisticated radiotherapy techniques such as 4-dimensional (4D) computed tomography (CT) imaging, mitigate tumor motion owing to respiration during radiation delivery and ensure accurate and optimal delivery of radiation dose to the tumor.

In this review, we discuss the different radiation delivery techniques available to treat NSCLC, the typical radiologic manifestations of conventional RT, and the different patterns of lung injury and

Conflicts of Interest and Source of Funding: Dr B.W. Carter - Amirsys-Elsevier, Inc: Thoracic content co-lead. Additional authors have no financial relationships to disclose.
[a] Department of Diagnostic Radiology, The University of Texas, MD Anderson Cancer Center, 1515 Holcombe Boulevard, Houston, TX 77030, USA; [b] Department of Radiation Oncology, The University of Texas, MD Anderson Cancer Center, 1515 Holcombe Boulevard, Houston, TX 77030, USA; [c] Department of Diagnostic Imaging, The Chaim Sheba Medical Center, Affiliated with Tel Aviv University, Tel Aviv, 2 Derech Sheba, Ramat Gan 5265601, Israel
* Corresponding author. Department of Diagnostic Radiology, The University of Texas MD Anderson Cancer Center, Unit 1478, 1515 Holcombe Boulevard, Houston, TX 77030.
E-mail address: mfbenveniste@mdanderson.org

Radiol Clin N Am 56 (2018) 471–483
https://doi.org/10.1016/j.rcl.2018.01.011
0033-8389/18/Published by Elsevier Inc.

temporal evolution that can be encountered in clinical practice when the newer radiotherapy techniques are used. Knowledge of the radiation delivery technique used, the completion date of therapy, and the radiologic manifestations of radiation-induced lung injury are important in facilitating appropriate interpretation of imaging studies and preventing misinterpretation of radiation-induced lung injury as infection or recurrence of malignancy.

RADIATION TREATMENT PLANNING TERMINOLOGY

In RT planning for lung cancer, the determination of the target volume is standardized and uses defined concentric target volume delineations on imaging. The gross tumor volume outlines visible malignancy, including any involved nodes. The clinical target volume is an added margin around the gross tumor volume to include potential microscopic disease and the internal target volume is an additional margin added around the clinical target volume to account for tumor movement during treatment as a result of respiratory motion. The planning target volume is the final volume treatment plan and is added around the clinical target volume to account for differences in patient positioning during treatment.

RADIATION DOSE AND FRACTIONATION IN THE TREATMENT OF LUNG CANCER

Increasing the radiation dose and or decreasing the time interval between radiation delivery increases tumor damage. However, this step results in increased injury to adjacent normal tissues. This injury can be mitigated by dividing the overall radiation dose into fractions. Currently, for patients with inoperable stage III NSCLC, the standard treatment is 60 to 66 Gy, given in a single fraction per day (2 Gy/fraction), 5 days a week, over a period of 6 weeks with concurrent chemotherapy.[1] Decreasing the number of fractions, in the appropriate clinical scenario, can be effective in tumor treatment, is well-tolerated, and is convenient for the patient. In this regard, SBRT is an extreme form of hypofractionation and delivers the entire radiation dose in daily fractions over 5 or less days.

RADIOTHERAPY DELIVERY TECHNIQUES

Conventional RT uses a limited number of treatment fields without conformal planning and typically delivers a high radiation dose to a large volume of normal tissue outside the planning target volume. High precision dose techniques such as 3D-CRT, IMRT, SBRT, and intensity-modulated proton therapy enable precise delivery of a larger radiation dose to the target and have improved local tumor control.[2,3] Additionally, the improved ability to conform the radiation dose delivered to the tumor reduces toxicity and facilitates dose escalation whereby target dose is increased while injury to normal tissue is limited.

Three-dimensional CRT, based on a 3D computer planning system of coplanar and noncoplanar beams reconstructed from CT data, delivers a maximal conformed radiation dose to the tumor with relative sparing of normal tissues. IMRT increases the 3D technique by using advanced treatment planning algorithms and multileaf collimators.[4–6] SBRT uses a technique similar to 3D-CRT or IMRT to deliver a hypofractionated high dose (10–34 Gy per fraction) to the tumor in 5 days or less. SBRT has an in-field control rate of approximately 90% and a severe toxicity rate of less than 10%.[7–9] SBRT is currently being used with curative intent in medically inoperable patients with NSCLC manifesting as small peripheral tumors without nodal metastasis, as well as to treat patients with metastases from extrathoracic malignancies.[10–13] Proton therapy uses subatomic particles with a positive electric charge to deliver a therapeutic dose to a precise depth (as defined by the Bragg peak) and reduces or eliminates radiation dose to normal tissues. The reduced lateral scatter and sharp dose drop of the proton beam allows delivery of a high-conformal dose without injury to vital structures such as the spinal cord.[14,15] Furthermore, because proton therapy can be delivered precisely to avoid previously radiated normal tissue, it is used to retreat patients with recurrent NSCLC.[16,17]

FOUR-DIMENSIONAL COMPUTED TOMOGRAPHY TECHNIQUE

The accurate delivery of radiation dose to the primary tumor can be degraded by respiratory motion. To mitigate tumor motion, the RT target volume is usually increased by adding the internal target volume to the treatment plan. However, a personalized assessment of tumor movement owing to respiratory motion is recommended over the use of standard treatment planning margins, because lung tumors can have complex motion patterns. Furthermore, many tumors move less than 1 cm and hence require smaller treatment volumes.[18] The use of respiration-correlated CT or 4D-CT for planning RT in conjunction with 3D-CRT, IMRT, and proton therapy is standard for incorporating tumor motion into treatment planning and further improves the target delineation and effectiveness of radiotherapy delivery. Four-dimensional CT and image-guided RT also address differences in tumor movement between treatment sessions and allow tumor delineation to be changed to account for tumor and anatomic changes that occur during therapy. Four-dimensional CT and image-guided radiotherapy enable precise delivery of radiation dose and have enabled techniques such as SBRT to be effectively used in the treatment of small lung tumors.

RADIATION THERAPY AND IMMUNOTHERAPY

Immunotherapy is increasingly being used to treat oncologic patients and improves survival in patients with advanced lung cancer refractory to chemotherapy.[19–21] Based on preclinical trials and isolated case reports, therapeutic response can improve when immunotherapeutic agents are combined with radiation. Radiation improves the immune system's ability to recognize solid tumors by uncovering or releasing previously hidden antigens and immune-stimulatory compounds in the tumor, and this factor can result in an improved antitumor immune response. In this regard, it has long been recognized that local RT could have systemic affects and cause malignancy distant to a radiated tumor to respond to therapy. Although rare, this phenomenon, called the abscopal effect (ab, away from, and scopus, target), has been described with different tumors, including lung cancer, and is believed to be partly T-cell mediated[22–24] (Fig. 1). Given the ability of radiation to produce immunogenic cells death, there is now significant interest in combining immunotherapy with radiation for lung cancer, both concurrently and in the adjuvant setting. In fact, there are now numerous clinic trials evaluating immunotherapy in combination with RT in patients with NSCLC and, based on the PACIFIC trial (A Global Study to Assess the Effects of MEDI4736 Following Concurrent Chemoradiation in Patients With Stage III Unresectable Non-Small Cell Lung Cancer) data, which showed an improvement in progression-free survival when using anti–programmed death ligand 1 therapy after chemoradiation in stage III NSCLC, this interest is expected to increase.[20,25] Radiation potentiates the immunologic response of programmed death ligand 1 agents by releasing tumor-specific antigen. However, dose and fractionation schemes can interfere with the way radiation and immunotherapy interact. Higher radiation doses more effectively enhance immunogenic activity in radiated tumor cells than do lower doses.[26–28] In addition, multiple studies have shown that the large, hypofractionated

dose regimens used in SBRT are superior to the smaller dose, multifraction regimens in terms of tumor immunogenicity.[29–31] Initial reports indicate that immunotherapy is well-tolerated and without increased toxicity when combined with radiotherapy. Boyer and colleagues[32] found no significant clinical toxicity (grade ≥ 3) in patients with locally advanced NSCLC treated with radiotherapy and neoadjuvant immunotherapy.

RADIATION-INDUCED LUNG INJURY
Risk Factors

The development and severity of radiation-induced lung injury is influenced by patient-specific parameters and the radiation technique used. Old age, heavy smoking history, poor lung physiologic function, poor performance status, concurrent chemoradiotherapy, and previous RT can result in more severe radiation-induced lung injury. The radiation delivery system (photons or protons), volume of lung radiated, dose and fractionation of radiation, and concomitant delivery of radiation with chemotherapy also affect the development and severity of radiation-induced lung injury.[33] In terms of the volume of lung radiated, the volume of lung exposed to a radiation dose of 20 Gy or more (V_{20}) is a standard metric for assessing the risk of radiation-induced lung injury.[34,35] When the lung V_{20} is less than 20% of the radiated lung the likelihood of radiation-induced lung injury is close to 0% and when the V_{20} is greater than 40%, the likelihood is approximately 50%.[36] Fraction size is an important factor that contributes to lung injury. Advances in radiotherapy techniques with more accurate delivery of radiation dose and treatment of small lung volumes enable the delivery of a high dose in a small number of fractions so that treatment is completed in 3 to 4 days rather than 5 to 6 weeks and the likelihood of clinically significant radiation-induced lung injury is low.

Imaging Findings

Imaging findings of radiation-induced lung injury are divided into an acute phase (radiation pneumonitis) and a chronic phase (radiation fibrosis). The manifestations of radiation injury after conventional RT have a typical appearance and temporal evolution. The manifestations of radiation-induced lung injury after high precision RT (3D-CRT, IMRT, SBRT, and proton therapy) tend to be similar to those of conventional RT in the acute and chronic phases. However, these newer radiation delivery techniques can have radiologic manifestations that differ from those of conventional RT.

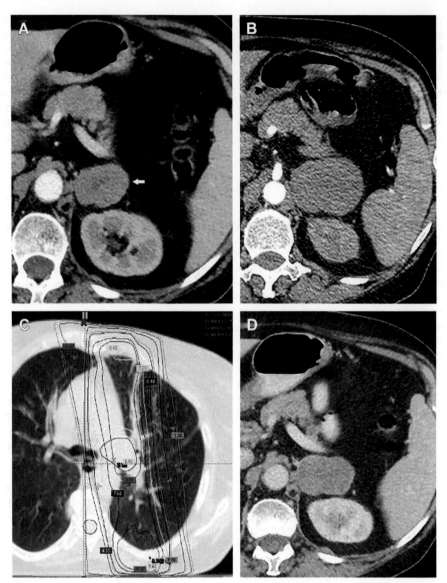

Fig. 1. A 77-year-old man with stage IV left upper lobe squamous cell lung cancer and left adrenal metastasis. (*A*) Contrast-enhanced computed tomography (CT) scan shows the left adrenal gland metastasis (*arrow*) measuring 3.9 × 2.9 cm in diameter. (*B*) Contrast-enhanced CT scan 1 month after immunotherapy initiation shows growth of the left adrenal gland metastasis of more than 50% to 6.2 × 4.6 cm. (*C*) Treatment plan for palliative radiation therapy to the left upper bronchial region owing to local progressive bronchial obstruction and shortness of breath. Treatment was delivered 4 days after image *B*. (*D*) Contrast-enhanced CT scan 1 month after image *B* and 1 month after completion of radiation therapy to the left hilum, while still receiving immunotherapy, shows a decrease in size of the adrenal metastasis to 4.9 × 3.2 cm, a 79% decrease in size, consistent with a partial response. This was considered an abscopal effect of radiation therapy because a follow-up scan revealed gradual progressive disease thereafter.

The imaging manifestations of radiation-induced lung injury usually occur when the total radiation dose exceeds 40 Gy and are uncommon with a radiation dose of less than 30 Gy.[37] Typically, the manifestations are in the radiated lung although rarely pneumonitis outside the radiation treatment plan occurs. In the acute phase, ground glass and consolidative opacities can be visualized on radiographic and CT studies within the radiated lung as early as 1 week after completion of RT, although 3 to 4 weeks may be required to visualize these manifestations radiographically (**Figs. 2** and **3**).[38–41] Additional manifestations that can occur in the evolution of

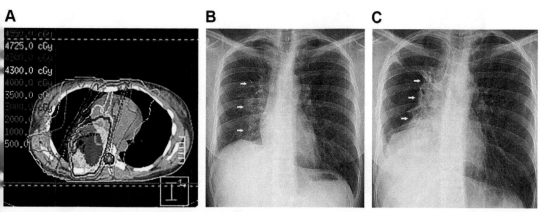

Fig. 2. A 54-year-old woman with metastatic right lower lobe adenocarcinoma. The patient received palliative intensity modulated radiotherapy (IMRT) and systemic chemotherapy. (A) Computed dosimetric axial reconstruction used for IMRT (total dose of 45 Gy in 15 fractions). (B) Frontal chest radiograph 1 month after completion of IMRT shows right lower lobe and perihilar airspace opacities (arrows), consistent with radiation pneumonitis. Note the small right pleural effusion. (C) Frontal chest radiograph 18 months after completion of IMRT shows right lung opacities with geographic border (arrows), volume loss, traction bronchiectasis, and fibrosis typical of the chronic phase of radiation-induced lung injury.

radiation pneumonitis include interstitial septal thickening superimposed on areas of ground glass opacities (crazy paving), areas of consolidation surrounded by ground glass opacities (CT halo sign), ground glass opacities surrounded by a crescentic or circumferential area of consolidation (reversed halo sign), cavitation, and nodular opacities (Fig. 4). Finally, organizing pneumonia and chronic eosinophilic pneumonia occur in the spectrum of radiation-induced lung injury.[42,43] Typically, imaging findings characteristic of organizing pneumonia are poorly

marginated lung opacities outside of the radiation treatment area. Infection should also be considered when acute unilateral or bilateral lung opacities occur before the completion of therapy or are outside the radiation treatment plan (Fig. 5).

In the evolution of radiation pneumonitis, consolidation usually coalesces and has a relatively sharp border that conforms to the radiation treatment plan rather than to anatomic boundaries (see Fig. 3). These opacities can completely resolve when the injury to the lung is limited. However, with more severe lung injury a chronic phase

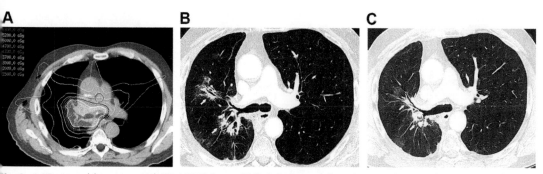

Fig. 3. A 72-year-old woman with T1aN2M0 (stage IIIA) right lower lobe adenocarcinoma. The patient underwent a right lower lobectomy and received postoperative radiotherapy. (A) Computed dosimetric axial reconstruction used in intensity modulated radiotherapy (total dose of 50 Gy in 25 fractions). (B) Axial computed tomography (CT) images 3 months after completion of radiation treatment shows ground glass and consolidative opacities within the radiation treatment plan (arrows) consistent with acute radiation pneumonitis. (C) Axial CT images 6 months after completion of radiation treatment shows atelectatic/consolidative opacities with a sharp margination in the right perihilar region (arrows) typical of radiation-induced lung injury. Note that, in the chronic phase of radiation-induced lung disease, there is fibrosis, traction bronchiectasis, consolidative opacities, and volume loss in the radiated lung.

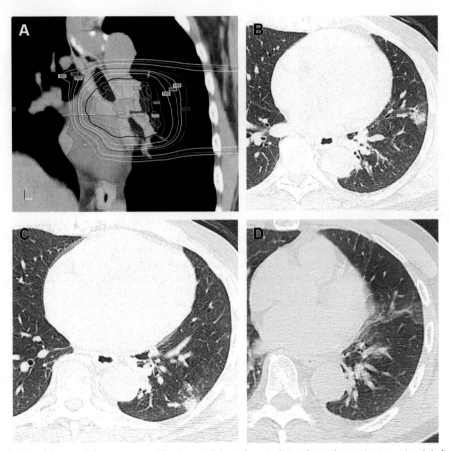

Fig. 4. A 66-year-old man with squamous cell cancer of the left main bronchus. The patient received definitive proton therapy owing to the proximity of the tumor to the spinal cord. (*A*) Computed dosimetric coronal image used for proton therapy (total dose of 80 Gy in 32 fractions). (*B, C*) Axial computed tomography (CT) image 3 months after completion of proton therapy shows ground glass and nodular opacities in the radiated lung (*arrows*). A nodular-like pattern can occur within the radiation treatment plan and should not be misinterpreted as metastatic disease or infection. (*D*) Axial CT image 6 months after the completion of proton therapy shows resolution of left lung nodular opacities. Focal opacities in the lingula are most consistent with postradiation changes.

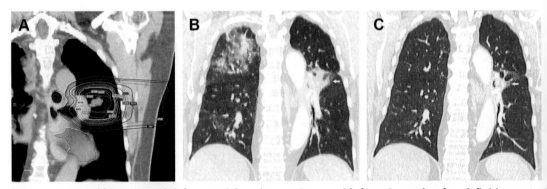

Fig. 5. A 67-year-old woman with left upper lobe adenocarcinoma with fever 9 months after definitive proton therapy. (*A*) Computed dosimetric coronal image for proton therapy (total dose of 87.5 Gy in 35 fractions). (*B*) Coronal computed tomography (CT) image 7 months after completion of proton therapy shows left lung opacities within the within the radiation treatment plan (*arrow*), consistent with radiation-induced lung injury. The right upper lobe opacities are outside of the radiation treatment plan. The patient was presumed to have pneumonia and showed clinical response to antibiotics. Note that correlation with the radiation treatment plan is helpful in the assessment of imaging manifestations after radiation therapy. (*C*) Coronal CT image 15 months after completion of proton therapy shows a decrease in left perihilar opacities, consistent with the evolution of radiation-induced lung injury (*arrow*).

characterized by fibrosis occurs. The typical manifestations of the fibrotic phase are consolidation with a geographic distribution, volume loss, architectural distortion, and traction bronchiectasis in the radiated lung. In addition, cavitation can occur owing to lung necrosis related to RT, although tumor recurrence and infection are also considerations.

Once the chronic manifestations of lung injury have stabilized, the development of a lobulated contour or nodularity, or increased soft tissue within the radiated lung is suspicious for tumor recurrence (Figs. 6 and 7). Additionally, the loss of visualization of bronchi in the radiated lung can denote recurrent tumor, although the differential diagnosis includes superimposed infection and mucoid impaction.

Because the radiation dose delivered by 3D-CRT, IMRT, SBRT, and proton therapy surrounds the tumor, the radiologic manifestations of lung injury usually conform to the shape of the tumor. Accordingly, awareness of the RT technique used and a review of treatment plans with dose distribution lines can be useful in determining whether the opacities detected radiographically or on CT are due to radiation-induced lung injury.[44,45] Importantly, additionally patterns of lung injury have been described after the completion of SBRT that differ from conventional RT. In the acute phase, a decrease in tumor size can occur in the absence of radiologic manifestations of adjacent lung injury. When present, radiologic findings of acute lung injury with SBRT typically manifest later than conventional therapy, that is, more than 3 months after the completion of therapy.[46] Additional manifestations include ground glass or consolidative opacities in the high-dose region of the radiated lung that can be diffuse or nonuniform. The nonuniform appearance is due to ground

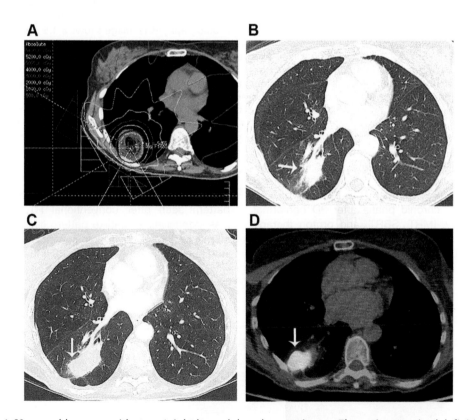

Fig. 6. A 60-year-old woman with stage I right lower lobe adenocarcinoma. The patient received definitive stereotactic body radiotherapy (SBRT). (A) Computed dosimetric axial reconstruction used for SBRT (total dose of 50 Gy in 4 fractions). (B) Axial computed tomography (CT) image 4 years after the completion of radiation therapy shows right lower lobe consolidative opacities (arrow), consistent with sequela of radiation-induced lung injury. (C) Axial CT image 6 months after B shows new convex border along the right lower lobe opacity (arrow). (D) PET-CT image obtained 1 month after C shows focal increased FDG uptake owing to tumor recurrence (arrow).

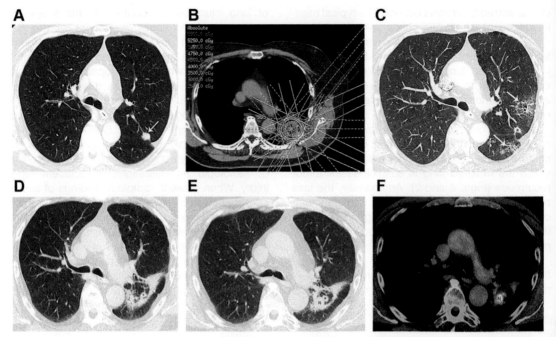

Fig. 7. A 70-year-old man with stage I left upper lobe non–small cell lung cancer treated with definitive stereo-tactic body radiation therapy (SBRT). (*A*) Axial computed tomography (CT) image shows a 1.5-cm left upper lobe primary tumor (*arrow*). (*B*) Computed dosimetric axial reconstruction used for SBRT (total dose of 50 Gy in 4 fractions). (*C*) Axial CT image 4 months after the completion of SBRT shows a decrease in size of the radiated tumor (*asterisk*) and lung opacities within the radiation treatment plan (*arrows*). (*D*) Axial CT image 7 months after completion of SBRT shows residual tumor (*asterisk*) surrounded by radiation changes manifesting as consolidative opacities, volume loss, and architectural distortion within the radiation treatment plan. (*E*) Axial CT image 11 months after the completion of SBRT shows focal increased soft tissue nodule (N) medial to the residual tumor (*asterisk*) suspicious for local tumor recurrence. (*F*) PET-CT shows the soft tissue nodule (N) is avid for 18F-2-deoxy-D-glucose. A biopsy confirmed local tumor recurrence within the radiation treatment plan.

glass or consolidative opacities interspersed with normal lung parenchyma. Patterns of lung injury in the chronic phase after 3D conformal radiotherapy, IMRT, SBRT, and proton therapy can also differ from conventional RT.[47] The chronic phase manifestations include a modified conventional pattern (consolidation, volume loss, and bronchiectasis resembling the fibrotic pattern seen after conventional RT, although less extensive), a scarlike pattern (linear opacity in the region of the original tumor associated with possible volume loss; **Fig. 8**), and a masslike

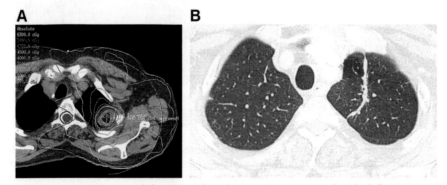

Fig. 8. A 78-year-old man with stage I left upper lobe adenocarcinoma treated with definitive stereotactic body radiation (SBRT). (*A*) Computed dosimetric axial reconstruction used for stereotactic body radiotherapy (total dose of 54 Gy in 3 fractions). (*B*) Axial computed tomography images 18 months after the completion of SBRT shows scarlike opacities within the radiation treatment plan, consistent with radiation-induced lung injury.

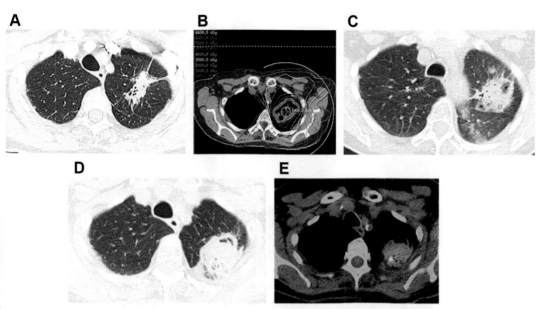

Fig. 9. An 89-year-old woman with T1N0M0 left upper lobe adenocarcinoma. Owing to medical comorbidities, she was not a candidate for surgery and received stereotactic body radiation (SBRT). (*A*) Axial computed tomography (CT) image shows a 2.5-cm lung adenocarcinoma. (*B*) Computed dosimetric axial image used for SBRT (total dose of 50 Gy in 4 fractions). (*C*) Axial CT image 4 months after the completion of SBRT shows radiated tumor and ground glass and consolidative opacities not completely filling the high-dose region (*asterisks*). (*D*) Axial CT image 10 months after the completion of SBRT shows a masslike opacity in the left upper lobe. (*E*) Axial PET-CT shows that the masslike opacity is not avid for 18F-2-deoxy-D-glucose and is consistent with radiation-induced lung injury. This masslike opacity remain unchanged on long-term surveillance. Note the masslike pattern can be misinterpreted as tumor recurrence and awareness of this pattern and correlation with the radiation treatment plan are important to avoid this potential pitfall.

pattern (focal opacity confined to the site of the original tumor; **Fig. 9**).

PET-CT using 18F-2-deoxy-D-glucose (FDG) can improve target delineation during RT planning in patients with NSCLC.[48–54] In this regard, PET-CT helps to differentiate the primary tumor from obstructive atelectatic lung (**Fig. 10**) and decreases planning treatment volumes.[55] Importantly, because the tumor target volume defined on PET-CT is usually smaller than that on CT, radiation dose escalation in RT planning is an option without increasing side effects.[56,57] This step can be performed using a simultaneous integrated boost, in which the inner treatment volume defined by the PET receives an escalated dose and that outer volume receives a lower dose. The detection of unsuspected intrathoracic nodal metastasis by PET-CT can also alter the planning treatment volumes and the more accurate target delineation decreases isolated nodal failures.[56,58,59]

PET-CT can be used to assess treatment failure within the radiated lung and to differentiate locoregional recurrent tumor from focal masslike fibrosis (see **Figs. 6** and **9**).[60] Focal increased FDG uptake within the radiated malignancy in the chronic phase of injury (≥6 months after the completion of therapy) is suggestive of persistent or recurrent tumor. However, after completion of RT there is increased FDG uptake in the radiated lung in the acute phase of lung injury. This increased FDG uptake is due to inflammation and can obscure the treated malignancy, precluding an accurate assessment of the treatment response. Because the increased FDG uptake in the radiated lung diminishes with time, PET-CT is generally performed 6 to 8 weeks or more after completion of RT to assess treatment response. However, there may be a potential role for the earlier use of PET-CT in the assessment of treatment response. Specifically, an RT-induced increased uptake of FDG in the lung can be less confounding when PET is performed during and not after the completion of therapy.[61] Importantly, this assessment may allow early dose escalation during adaptive therapy.

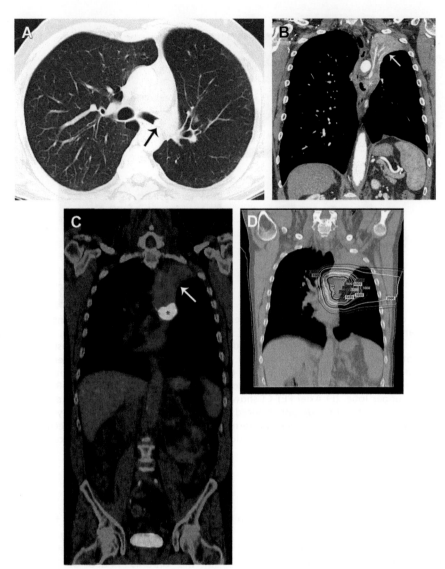

Fig. 10. A 66-year-old man with squamous cell carcinoma of the left upper lobe. The patient was treated with chemotherapy and concurrent proton therapy. (*A*) Axial computed tomography (CT) scan shows a left upper lobe central tumor with endobronchial extension into the left main bronchus (*arrow*). (*B*) A contrast-enhanced coronal CT scan shows left upper lobe atelectasis (*arrow*) owing to central tumor (*asterisk*) with endobronchial extension into the left main bronchus. Note that central obstructing tumors can be difficult to delineate on CT from the adjacent atelectasis. (*C*) Coronal PET-CT image shows clear delineation of the 18F-2-deoxy-D-glucose–avid left upper lobe central tumor (*asterisk*) and adjacent atelectasis (*arrow*). (*D*) Computed dosimetric axial image for proton treatment (total dose of 78 Gy in 30 fractions). For central obstructing tumors with atelectasis, the use of PET-CT in radiation treatment planning allows the planning target volume to be smaller than when performed with CT alone.

SUMMARY

RT using conventional or high precision dose techniques is important in the treatment of patients with lung cancer. Three-dimensional CRT, SBRT, IMRT, and proton therapy allow the optimal radiation dose delivery to the tumor, improve local disease control, and decrease toxicity to adjacent normal tissues. Knowledge of the radiation treatment plan and technique, as well as the temporal evolution of radiation-induced lung injury, is important to correctly identify expected radiologic manifestations of radiation-induced lung injury and differentiate them from tumor recurrence or infection.

REFERENCES

1. Bradley JD, Paulus R, Komaki R, et al. Standard-dose versus high-dose conformal radiotherapy with concurrent and consolidation carboplatin plus pacli-taxel with or without cetuximab for patients with stage IIIA or IIIB non-small-cell lung cancer (RTOG 0617): a randomised, two-by-two factorial phase 3 study. Lancet Oncol 2015;16(2):187–99.

2. Rosenzweig KE, Fox JL, Yorke E, et al. Results of a phase I dose-escalation study using three-dimensional conformal radiotherapy in the treatment of inoperable nonsmall cell lung carcinoma. Cancer 2005;103(10):2118–27.

3. Fang LC, Komaki R, Allen P, et al. Comparison of outcomes for patients with medically inoperable Stage I non-small-cell lung cancer treated with two-dimensional vs. three-dimensional radiotherapy. Int J Radiat Oncol Biol Phys 2006;66(1):108–16.

4. Staffurth J, Radiotherapy Development Board. A review of the clinical evidence for intensity-modulated radiotherapy. Clin Oncol (R Coll Radiol) 2010;22(8):643–57.

5. Murshed HL, Liu HH, Liao Z. Dose and volume reduction for normal lung using intensity-modulated radiotherapy for advanced-stage non-small-cell lung cancer. Int J Radiat Oncol Biol Phys 2004;58(4):1258–67.

6. Jiang ZQ, Yang K, Komaki R, et al. Long-term clinical outcome of intensity-modulated radiotherapy for inoperable non-small cell lung cancer: the MD Anderson experience. Int J Radiat Oncol Biol Phys 2012;83(1):332–9.

7. Ricardi U, Badellino S, Filippi AR. Stereotactic body radiotherapy for early stage lung cancer: history and updated role. Lung Cancer 2015;90(3):388–96.

8. Baumann P, Nyman J, Hoyer M, et al. Stereotactic body radiotherapy for medically inoperable patients with stage I non-small cell lung cancer - a first report of toxicity related to COPD/CVD in a non-randomized prospective phase II study. Radiother Oncol 2008;88(3):359–67.

9. Hoyer M, Roed H, Traberg Hansen A, et al. Phase II study on stereotactic body radiotherapy of colo-rectal metastases. Acta Oncol 2006;45(7):823–30.

10. Onishi H, Shirato H, Nagata Y, et al. Hypofractio-nated stereotactic radiotherapy (HypoFXSRT) for stage I non-small cell lung cancer: updated results of 257 patients in a Japanese multi-institutional study. J Thorac Oncol 2007;2(7 Suppl 3):S94–100.

11. Trovo M, Linda A, El Naqa I, et al. Early and late lung radiographic injury following stereotactic body radiation therapy (SBRT). Lung Cancer 2010;69(1):77–85.

12. Baker S, Dahele M, Lagerwaard FJ, et al. A critical review of recent developments in radiotherapy for non-small cell lung cancer. Radiat Oncol 2016;11(1):115.

13. Kishan AU, Lee P. Radiation therapy for stage I non-operable or medically inoperable lung cancer. Semin Respir Crit Care Med 2016;37(5):716–26.

14. Chang JY, Jabbour SK, De Ruysscher D, et al. Consensus statement on proton therapy in early-stage and locally advanced non-small cell lung cancer. Int J Radiat Oncol Biol Phys 2016;95(1):505–16.

15. Chang JY, Cox JD. Improving radiation conformality in the treatment of non-small cell lung cancer. Semin Radiat Oncol 2010;20(3):171–7.

16. Berman AT, James SS, Rengan R. Proton beam therapy for non-small cell lung cancer: current clinical evidence and future directions. Cancers (Basel) 2015;7(3):1178–90.

17. Plastaras JP, Berman AT, Freedman GM. Special cases for proton beam radiotherapy: re-irradiation, lymphoma, and breast cancer. Semin Oncol 2014;41(6):807–19.

18. Liu HH, Balter P, Tutt T, et al. Assessing respiration-induced tumor motion and internal target volume using four-dimensional computed tomography for radiotherapy of lung cancer. Int J Radiat Oncol Biol Phys 2007;68(2):531–40.

19. Borghaei H, Paz-Ares L, Horn L, et al. Nivolumab versus docetaxel in advanced nonsquamous non-small-cell lung cancer. N Engl J Med 2015;373(17):1627–39.

20. Brahmer J, Reckamp KL, Baas P, et al. Nivolumab versus docetaxel in advanced squamous-cell non-small-cell lung cancer. N Engl J Med 2015;373(2):123–35.

21. Herbst RS, Baas P, Kim DW, et al. Pembrolizumab versus docetaxel for previously treated, PD-L1-positive, advanced non-small-cell lung cancer (KEY-NOTE-010): a randomised controlled trial. Lancet 2016;387(10027):1540–50.

22. Prise KM, O'Sullivan JM. Radiation-induced bystander signalling in cancer therapy. Nat Rev Cancer 2009;9(5):351–60.

23. Brooks ED, Schoenhals JE, Tang C, et al. Stereotac-tic ablative radiation therapy combined with immu-notherapy for solid tumors. Cancer J 2016;22(4):257–66.

24. Golden EB, Demaria S, Schiff PB, et al. An abscopal response to radiation and ipilimumab in a patient with metastatic non-small cell lung cancer. Cancer Immunol Res 2013;1(6):365–72.

25. Lynch TJ, Bondarenko I, Luft A, et al. Ipilimumab in combination with paclitaxel and carboplatin as first-line treatment in stage IIIB/IV non-small-cell lung cancer: results from a randomized, double-blind, multicenter phase II study. J Clin Oncol 2012;30(17):2046–54.

26. Reits EA, Hodge JW, Herberts CA, et al. Radiation modulates the peptide repertoire, enhances MHC

class I expression, and induces successful anti-tumor immunotherapy. J Exp Med 2006;203(5): 1259–71.

27. Garnett CT, Palena C, Chakraborty M, et al. Sublethal irradiation of human tumor cells modulates phenotype resulting in enhanced killing by cytotoxic T lymphocytes. Cancer Res 2004;64(21): 7985–94.

28. Chakraborty M, Abrams SI, Camphausen K, et al. Irradiation of tumor cells up-regulates Fas and enhances CTL lytic activity and CTL adoptive immunotherapy. J Immunol 2003;170(12):6338–47.

29. Schaue D, Ratikan JA, Iwamoto KS, et al. Maximizing tumor immunity with fractionated radiation. Int J Radiat Oncol Biol Phys 2012;83(4):1306–10.

30. Lee Y, Auh SL, Wang Y, et al. Therapeutic effects of ablative radiation on local tumor require CD8+ T cells: changing strategies for cancer treatment. Blood 2009;114(3):589–95.

31. Lugade AA, Moran JP, Gerber SA, et al. Local radiation therapy of B16 melanoma tumors increases the generation of tumor antigen-specific effector cells that traffic to the tumor. J Immunol 2005;174(12): 7516–23.

32. Boyer MJ, Gu L, Wang X, et al. Toxicity of definitive and post-operative radiation following ipilimumab in non-small cell lung cancer. Lung Cancer 2016; 98:76–8.

33. Marks LB. Dosimetric predictors of radiation-induced lung injury. Int J Radiat Oncol Biol Phys 2002;54(2):313–6.

34. Jennings FL, Arden A. Development of radiation pneumonitis. Time and dose factors. Arch Pathol 1962;74:351–60.

35. Wang S, Liao Z, Wei X, et al. Analysis of clinical and dosimetric factors associated with treatment-related pneumonitis (TRP) in patients with non-small-cell lung cancer (NSCLC) treated with concurrent chemotherapy and three-dimensional conformal radiotherapy (3D-CRT). Int J Radiat Oncol Biol Phys 2006;66(5):1399–407.

36. Tsujino K, Hirota S, Endo M, et al. Predictive value of dose-volume histogram parameters for predicting radiation pneumonitis after concurrent chemoradiation for lung cancer. Int J Radiat Oncol Biol Phys 2003;55(1):110–5.

37. Libshitz HI, Southard ME. Complications of radiation therapy: the thorax. Semin Roentgenol 1974;9(1): 41–9.

38. Bennett DE, Million RR, Ackerman LV. Bilateral radiation pneumonitis, a complication of the radiotherapy of bronchogenic carcinoma. (Report and analysis of seven cases with autopsy). Cancer 1969;23(5):1001–18.

39. Ikezoe J, Takashima S, Morimoto S, et al. CT appearance of acute radiation-induced injury in the lung. AJR Am J Roentgenol 1988;150(4):765–70.

40. Nabawi P, Mantravadi R, Breyer D, et al. Computed tomography of radiation-induced lung injuries. J Comput Assist Tomogr 1981;5(4):568–70.

41. Mah K, Poon PY, Van Dyk J, et al. Assessment of acute radiation-induced pulmonary changes using computed tomography. J Comput Assist Tomogr 1986;10(5):736–43.

42. Crestani B, Valeyre D, Roden S, et al. Bronchiolitis obliterans organizing pneumonia syndrome primed by radiation therapy to the breast. The Groupe d'Etudes et de Recherche sur les Maladies Orphelines Pulmonaires (GERM"O"P). Am J Respir Crit Care Med 1998;158(6):1929–35.

43. Cottin V, Frognier R, Monnot H, et al. Chronic eosinophilic pneumonia after radiation therapy for breast cancer. Eur Respir J 2004;23(1):9–13.

44. Libshitz HI, Shuman LS. Radiation-induced pulmonary change: CT findings. J Comput Assist Tomogr 1984;8(1):15–9.

45. Libshitz HI. Radiation changes in the lung. Semin Roentgenol 1993;28:303–20.

46. Linda A, Trovo M, Bradley JD. Radiation injury of the lung after stereotactic body radiation therapy (SBRT) for lung cancer: a timeline and pattern of CT changes. Eur J Radiol 2011;79(1):147–54.

47. Choi YW, Munden RF, Erasmus JJ, et al. Effects of radiation therapy on the lung: radiologic appearances and differential diagnosis. Radiographics 2004;24(4):985–97 [discussion: 998].

48. Bradley J, Thorstad WL, Mutic S, et al. Impact of FDG-PET on radiation therapy volume delineation in non-small-cell lung cancer. Int J Radiat Oncol Biol Phys 2004;59(1):78–86.

49. Fowler JF, Chappell R. Non-small cell lung tumors repopulate rapidly during radiation therapy. Int J Radiat Oncol Biol Phys 2000;46(2):516–7.

50. Lavrenkov K, Partridge M, Cook G, et al. Positron emission tomography for target volume definition in the treatment of non-small cell lung cancer. Radiother Oncol 2005;77(1):1–4.

51. MacManus M, Nestle U, Rosenzweig KE, et al. Use of PET and PET/CT for radiation therapy planning: IAEA expert report 2006-2007. Radiother Oncol 2009;91(1):85–94.

52. Nestle U, Kremp S, Grosu AL. Practical integration of [18F]-FDG-PET and PET-CT in the planning of radiotherapy for non-small cell lung cancer (NSCLC): the technical basis, ICRU-target volumes, problems, perspectives. Radiother Oncol 2006; 81(2):209–25.

53. Nestle U, Kremp S, Schaefer-Schuler A, et al. Comparison of different methods for delineation of 18F-FDG PET-positive tissue for target volume definition in radiotherapy of patients with non-Small cell lung cancer. J Nucl Med 2005;46(8):1342–8.

54. Yu HM, Liu YF, Hou M, et al. Evaluation of gross tumor size using CT, 18F-FDG PET, integrated

18F-FDG PET/CT and pathological analysis in non-small cell lung cancer. Eur J Radiol 2009;72(1): 104–13.

55. Ding X, Li H, Wang Z, et al. A clinical study of shrinking field radiation therapy based on (18)F-FDG PET/CT for stage III non-small cell lung cancer. Technol Cancer Res Treat 2013;12(3):251–7.

56. De Ruysscher D, Wanders S, van Haren E, et al. Selective mediastinal node irradiation based on FDG-PET scan data in patients with non-small-cell lung cancer: a prospective clinical study. Int J Radiat Oncol Biol Phys 2005;62(4):988–94.

57. van Der Wel A, Nijsten S, Hochstenbag M, et al. Increased therapeutic ratio by 18FDG-PET CT planning in patients with clinical CT stage N2-N3M0 non-small-cell lung cancer: a modeling study. Int J Radiat Oncol Biol Phys 2005;61(3): 649–55.

58. Ashamalla H, Rafla S, Parikh K, et al. The contribution of integrated PET/CT to the evolving definition of treatment volumes in radiation treatment planning in lung cancer. Int J Radiat Oncol Biol Phys 2005; 63(4):1016–23.

59. Kitajima K, Doi H, Kanda T, et al. Present and future roles of FDG-PET/CT imaging in the management of lung cancer. Jpn J Radiol 2016; 34(6):387–99.

60. Patz EF Jr, Lowe VJ, Hoffman JM, et al. Persistent or recurrent bronchogenic carcinoma: detection with PET and 2-[F-18]-2-deoxy-D-glucose. Radiology 1994;191(2):379–82.

61. Kong FM, Frey KA, Quint LE, et al. A pilot study of [18F]fluorodeoxyglucose positron emission tomography scans during and after radiation-based therapy in patients with non small-cell lung cancer. J Clin Oncol 2007;25(21):3116–23.

Targeted Therapy and Immunotherapy in the Treatment of Non–Small Cell Lung Cancer

Girish S. Shroff, MD[a], Patricia M. de Groot, MD[a],
Vassiliki A. Papadimitrakopoulou, MD[b],
Mylene T. Truong, MD[a], Brett W. Carter, MD[a],*

KEYWORDS

- Lung cancer • Immunotherapy • Targeted therapy

KEY POINTS

- Targeted therapies for non–small cell lung cancer are directed at the product of specific mutations, such as epidermal growth factor receptor (*EGFR*) and anaplastic lymphoma kinase (ALK).
- Specific oncogenic driver mutations in non–small cell lung cancer tend to result in different patterns of disease on computed tomography (CT) and fludeoxyglucose PET/CT.
- Immunotherapy facilitates the recognition of cancer as foreign by the host immune system, stimulates the immune system, and alleviates the inhibition that allows growth and spread of disease.
- Immune-related adverse effects, such as pneumonitis and colitis, may be encountered on imaging studies performed to evaluate patients treated with immunotherapy; radiologists should understand the appearance of these complications.

INTRODUCTION

The treatment strategy in advanced non–small cell lung cancer (NSCLC) has evolved from the use of empirical chemotherapy to a more personalized approach based on histology and molecular markers.[1] Gene mutations in receptors or protein kinases that result in the uncontrolled growth, proliferation, and survival of tumors (known as oncogenic driver mutations) are found in up to 60% of lung adenocarcinomas and up to 50% to 80% of lung squamous cell carcinomas.[2–4] Targeted therapies are directed at the products of these mutations and come in the form of receptor monoclonal antibodies (mAbs) or tyrosine kinase inhibitors (TKIs). Common targets include mutations of epidermal growth factor receptor (*EGFR*) and anaplastic lymphoma kinase (*ALK*). Targeted therapies have been shown to have significant clinical benefit in patients with advanced lung cancer.[5] Immunotherapy facilitates the recognition of cancer as foreign by the host immune system, stimulates the immune system, and relieves the inhibition that allows growth and spread of disease. In 2015, two immunomodulatory mAbs, nivolumab and pembrolizumab, were the first immunotherapeutic agents approved by the US Food and Drug Administration (FDA) for the treatment of advanced NSCLC.[5,6] Immunotherapy can result in a wide variety of immune-related adverse events, including colitis, hepatitis, and pneumonitis. In this article, the authors describe

[a] Department of Diagnostic Radiology, The University of Texas MD Anderson Cancer Center, 1515 Holcombe Boulevard, Houston, TX 77030, USA; [b] Department of Thoracic/Head and Neck Medical Oncology, The University of Texas MD Anderson Cancer Center, 1515 Holcombe Boulevard, Houston, TX 77030, USA
* Corresponding author. Department of Diagnostic Radiology, The University of Texas MD Anderson Cancer Center, 1515 Holcombe Boulevard, Unit 1478, Houston, TX 77030.
E-mail address: bcarter2@mdanderson.org

Radiol Clin N Am 56 (2018) 485–495
https://doi.org/10.1016/j.rcl.2018.01.012
0033-8389/18/© 2018 Elsevier Inc. All rights reserved.

the role of targeted therapy and immunotherapy in the treatment of NSCLC.

TARGETED THERAPY
Receptor Tyrosine Kinases

Receptor tyrosine kinases (RTKs) are membrane-spanning glycoproteins that, once activated by binding of a ligand, activate numerous intracellular pathways and have an important role in normal processes, such as cell proliferation and differentiation. RTKs also have a critical role in the development and progression of many cancers. Examples of RTKs include receptors for *ALK*, epidermal growth factor (EGF), and vascular endothelial growth factor (VEGF).

Epidermal Growth Factor Receptor–Mutant (Epidermal Growth Factor Receptor–Positive) Non–Small Cell Lung Cancer

Activation of *EGFR* by EGF leads to cellular growth, proliferation, and decreased apoptosis.[7] *EGFR* mutations are more common in lung adenocarcinomas, Asians, females, and never smokers.[4] Patients with *EGFR* mutations, the most common of which are a deletion in exon 19 and a point mutation in exon 21, are usually treated with *EGFR* TKIs, such as erlotinib or gefitinib; these agents enhance apoptosis and inhibit cell growth, angiogenesis, invasion, and metastasis.[7] Several studies have demonstrated the efficacy of *EGFR* TKIs in advanced *EGFR*-mutant lung cancer. The *Iressa Pan-ASia Study* (IPASS) showed that gefitinib was superior to carboplatin-paclitaxel chemotherapy in nonsmokers or former light smokers in East Asia with untreated advanced (stage IIIB or

IV) lung adenocarcinoma.[4,8] In *EGFR*-positive patients, progression-free survival (PFS) was significantly longer with gefitinib than with chemotherapy; in *EGFR*-negative patients, PFS was significantly longer in the chemotherapy group.[8]

Despite the initial response to *EGFR* TKIs, drug resistance invariably develops,[2] most frequently through a secondary acquired *EGFR* mutation called *T790M*. In *T790M*, methionine replaces threonine at position 790 in the tyrosine kinase domain of *EGFR* and decreases the effectiveness of first- (erlotinib, gefitinib) and second-generation (afatinib) *EGFR* TKIs.[2,9–11] Osimertinib is a third-generation *EGFR* TKI that has proven to be effective in *T790M*+ advanced NSCLC (Fig. 1).[11]

Anaplastic Lymphoma Kinase Fusion Oncogene Positive Non–Small Cell Lung Cancer

ALK is another gene that encodes for a receptor tyrosine kinase. In 3% to 7% of patients with NSCLC, the *ALK* gene is fused to the echinoderm microtubule-associated proteinlike 4 (*EML4*) gene yielding the *EML4-ALK* fusion oncogene.[2,12] The *EML4-ALK* fusion oncogene (also referred to as ALK rearrangement) promotes cell growth and proliferation.[13] *ALK* rearrangement (*ALK* positivity) is more likely to be seen in younger patients with adenocarcinoma who are light or never-smokers.[2,4] The *ALK* TKI crizotinib is the treatment of choice for *ALK*-positive NSCLC. Newer-generation *ALK* inhibitors (eg, ceritinib, alectinib, brigatinib) are available for patients who develop resistance to or cannot tolerate crizotinib.

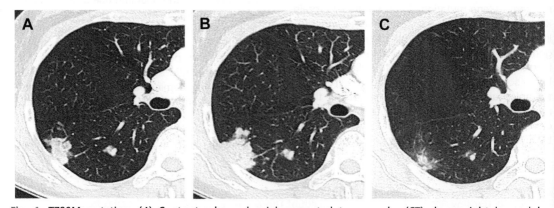

Fig. 1. *T790M* mutation. (*A*) Contrast-enhanced axial computed tomography (CT) shows right lower lobe *EGFR*+ adenocarcinoma and a separate tumor nodule in the same lobe. The patient was being treated with erlotinib. (*B*) Contrast-enhanced axial CT performed 9 months later shows increase in size of the dominant tumor. Biopsy (performed for molecular profiling) revealed *T790M* mutation. Osimertinib therapy was initiated. (*C*) Contrast-enhanced axial CT 3 months later shows response to osimertinib with decrease in size of the primary neoplasm and adjacent tumor nodule.

Kirsten Rat Sarcoma Virus Mutation in Non–Small Cell Lung Cancer

Kirsten rat sarcoma virus (KRAS) is a gene that encodes for rat sarcoma (RAS) proteins, guanosine nucleotide–binding proteins located at the inner surface of the plasma membrane that are involved in the transduction of growth signals from RTKs.[2,14] Although RAS mutations (usually of the KRAS variety) are present in 25% to 40% of NSCLC,[15] targeting has been largely unsuccessful.[2] KRAS mutations are more common in Caucasians and current or former smokers and occur most commonly in lung adenocarcinomas (30%).[2] In terms of genetic alterations, mutations of ALK, EGFR, and KRAS are almost always mutually exclusive.[16]

Angiogenesis Inhibitors

Angiogenesis is a feature of all malignancies and is defined as the formation of new blood vessels from preexisting vessels.[17] VEGFs have an important role in this process. Overexpression of VEGF and/or increased VEGF levels have been found in many cancers, including NSCLC and small cell lung cancer, with adenocarcinomas having the highest degree of VEGF expression.[17,18] The most effective angiogenesis inhibitor is bevacizumab, a monoclonal antibody that binds to and inhibits VEGF-A.[19] Bevacizumab is, however, contraindicated in centrally located squamous cell carcinoma because of the increased risk of life-threatening pulmonary hemorrhage.[20]

Tumoral cavitation is a known response to angiogenesis inhibitors and occurs in up to 24% of patients with lung cancer receiving such therapy (Fig. 2).[21–23] Cavitation can occur during or after completion of therapy and most commonly affects the primary tumor but can also occur in metastatic nodules.[21,22,24]

Imaging Findings of Non–Small Cell Lung Cancer with Oncogenic Driver Mutations

Imaging has a limited role of in the prediction of genetic mutations. However, some imaging features are more commonly associated with certain mutations. For example, ground-glass attenuation and air bronchograms are more common in lung cancers with an EGFR mutation than in those without.[25] In regard to advanced (stages IIIB and IV) adenocarcinomas, EGFR+ tumors are more commonly oval, whereas tumors without EGFR mutation tend to be larger, more irregular, and are more likely to contain calcification.[26] Spiculated margins are more common with EGFR positivity, whereas lobulated margins are more common with ALK positivity.[27] ALK+ status is associated with a central location and large pleural effusions.[28] In terms of metastatic disease, ALK+ tumors are

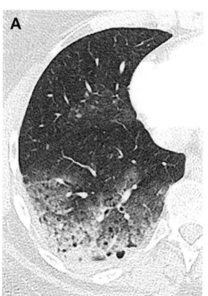
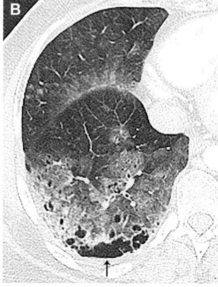

Fig. 2. Bevacizumab-induced cavitation in a 33-year-old woman with stage IV lung adenocarcinoma. (A) Contrast-enhanced axial computed tomography (CT) shows consolidative and ground-glass opacities in the right lower lobe, biopsy-proven to represent adenocarcinoma. (B) Contrast-enhanced axial CT performed after 2 cycles of carboplatin, pemetrexed, and bevacizumab shows new air-fluid level (arrow) in the right lower lobe adenocarcinoma that has cavitated. Tumor cavitation may occur during or after completion of angiogenesis inhibitor therapy.

more likely to be associated with lymphangitic carcinomatosis, advanced (N2-N3) lymphadenopathy, and pleural or pericardial metastases, whereas *EGFR+* tumors have a tendency for hematogenous spread, for example, lung and bone metastases (**Figs. 3** and **4**).[27] *EGFR+* tumors are more frequently associated with the absence of lymphadenopathy than *ALK+* or *KRAS+* tumors.[29] *KRAS* mutations are infrequently associated with metastases to the lungs and pleura.[29]

Because imaging manifestations of tumors with oncogenic driver mutations are nonspecific, tissue sampling is being widely used for genetic profiling. However, computed tomography (CT) texture analysis, an advanced postprocessing method that provides quantitative information about tumor heterogeneity, has shown promise to noninvasively characterize a tumor's molecular features.[30] Additionally, fludeoxyglucose (FDG) PET/CT has been used to study the metabolic characteristics of tumors with driver mutations. FDG uptake of *ALK+* tumors tends to be higher than both *EGFR+* tumors and tumors without *ALK* or *EGFR* mutation (maximum standardized uptake value [SUVmax] of 10.51 ± 6.00, 5.20 ± 4.55, and 6.81 ± 5.19, respectively).[31] *KRAS+* tumors have higher FDG uptake than *EGFR+* tumors and tumors without a *KRAS* or *EGFR* mutation (SUVmax of 13.8 ± 5.9, 8.6 ± 4.2, and 9.9 ± 3.7, respectively) (**Fig. 5**).[32] Investigations into the utility of PET/CT in quantifying the metabolic response to targeted therapies are ongoing.[33] The role of PET/CT in the evaluation of tumors with driver

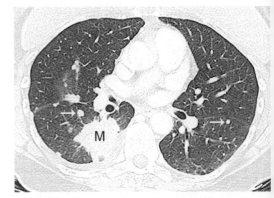

Fig. 4. *EGFR* mutation in a 50-year-old female never-smoker. Contrast-enhanced axial computed tomography shows the right lower lobe mass (M), biopsy-proven *EGFR+* adenocarcinoma, and pulmonary (*arrows*) and pleural metastases along the right interlobar fissures. In terms of metastatic disease, *EGFR+* tumors tend to manifest with hematogenous metastases.

mutations and response assessment to targeted therapies is yet to be clearly established.

Imaging Findings of Drug Toxicity

Pulmonary toxicity is a known complication of targeted agents, including the *EGFR* TKIs gefitinib and erlotinib and the *ALK* TKI crizotinib (**Fig. 6**). Manifestations of pulmonary toxicity include diffuse alveolar damage, organizing pneumonia, acute interstitial pneumonia/pneumonitis, and pulmonary fibrosis.[34] Angiogenesis inhibitors are associated with pulmonary hemorrhage, which may be seen as ground-glass or consolidative opacities with or without interlobular septal thickening (**Fig. 7**). Targeted agents are also associated with gastrointestinal toxicities, for example, colitis and pneumatosis (erlotinib) and bowel perforation (bevacizumab).[35] Complex renal cysts mimicking primary or secondary renal malignancy can develop with crizotinib.[36]

IMMUNOTHERAPY

Immunotherapy is based on the premise that the host immune system plays a critical role in antitumor activity. Cancer cells can avoid detection and the antitumor effects of therapy, and immunotherapy attempts to boost the immune system and allow it to mount a more effective response. Immunotherapy can be classified as active or passive based on its interaction with the host immune system and the response elicited. Active immunotherapy modulates the immune system and can be nonspecific or specific, the former characterized by a general immune response and the latter characterized by the

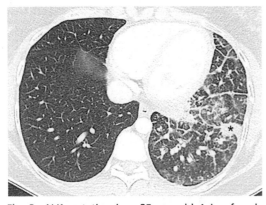

Fig. 3. *ALK* mutation in a 35-year-old Asian female never-smoker who presented with persistent cough. Contrast-enhanced axial computed tomography (CT) demonstrates the left lower lobe tumor (*asterisk*) and lymphangitic carcinomatosis in the left lung. Lymph node, pleural, and brain metastases were also present. Biopsy revealed *ALK* translocation and crizotinib therapy was initiated. In terms of metastatic disease, *ALK+* tumors tend to manifest with lymphangitic carcinomatosis.

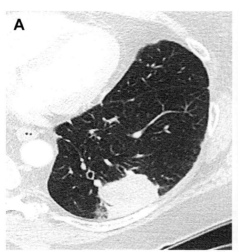
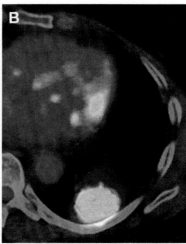

Fig. 5. *KRAS* mutation. (*A*) Contrast-enhanced axial CT shows a left lower lobe tumor. (*B*) Fused axial PET/CT shows FDG-avid tumor with SUVmax 15.2. The patient was treated with carboplatin and pemetrexed. Tumors with *KRAS* mutation typically have higher FDG uptake than those with *EGFR* mutation.

stimulation of humoral and cell-mediated immunity. Recombinant cytokines, biochemotherapy, cancer vaccines, and immunomodulatory monoclonal antibodies are all examples of active immunotherapeutic agents.[37] Immunomodulatory mAbs can be directed against targets, including programmed death protein 1/programmed death receptor ligand 1 (PD-L1) and cytotoxic T-lymphocyte antigen 4. Passive immunotherapy requires no activation of the immune system, and antitumor activity is achieved through the administration of preformed target-specific mAbs that bind to tumor-associated antigens resulting in clearance of cancer cells. Oncolytic viruses and adoptive T-cell therapy are additional examples of passive immunotherapeutic agents.

Immunomodulatory Monoclonal Antibodies

Nivolumab and pembrolizumab, 2 checkpoint inhibitors, have been approved as single agents for second-line treatment of patients with advanced NSCLC. Nivolumab was approved for the treatment of advanced squamous cell lung carcinoma refractory to chemotherapy in 2015 and does not require testing for PD-L1 overexpression. This recommendation was based on the results of several clinical trials, one of which was a phase I expansion trial involving 129 patients with advanced disease who were treated with 3 different doses of nivolumab (1, 3, or 10 mg/kg) every 2 weeks.[38] Response assessments were reported in patients with both squamous and nonsquamous NSCLC. In this trial, the median overall survival was 9.9 months; those receiving a dose of 3 mg/kg had overall survival rates of 56%, 42%, and 27% at 1, 2, and 3 years, respectively. Two phase III clinical trials, the CheckMate 017 and CheckMate 057 trials, confirmed the benefit of nivolumab over docetaxel as a second-line treatment in patients with advanced NSCLC. In the former, the median overall patient survival was 9.2 months with nivolumab compared with 6 months with docetaxel.[39] In the CheckMate 057 trial, the median overall survival was 12.2 months for those patients treated with nivolumab compared with 9.4 months for patients treated with docetaxel; there was higher efficacy in patients with PD-L1–positive primary lung cancers.[40] Based on the results of these clinical trials,

Fig. 6. Erlotinib-induced pneumonitis in a 74-year-old patient with *EGFR*+ adenocarcinoma and progressive shortness of breath. Contrast-enhanced axial CT shows basilar and subpleural predominant consolidative and ground-glass opacities consistent with erlotinib-induced pneumonitis.

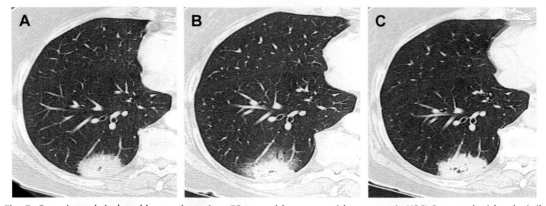

Fig. 7. Bevacizumab-induced hemorrhage in a 78-year-old woman with metastatic NSCLC treated with erlotinib and bevacizumab. (*A*) Contrast-enhanced axial CT before therapy shows a right lower lobe tumor. (*B*) Contrast-enhanced axial CT after 2 cycles of therapy shows new adjacent ground-glass opacities, consistent with hemorrhage. Because of pulmonary hemorrhage, bevacizumab was discontinued. (*C*) Contrast-enhanced axial CT obtained 2 months later shows resolution of hemorrhage but slight enlargement of the lung cancer.

the use of nivolumab has been extended to include other histologic types of NSCLC.

Pembrolizumab is the first immunotherapy approved for the first-line treatment of patients with metastatic NSCLC and, in contrast to nivolumab, requires confirmation of overexpression of PD-L1. The use of pembrolizumab in metastatic NSCLC is supported by the KEYNOTE-010 trial. In this trial, patients with previously treated advanced NSCLC were treated with pembrolizumab 2 mg/kg, 10 mg/kg, or docetaxel 75 mg/m^2 every 3 weeks.[41,42] Overall survival was higher with both doses of pembrolizumab versus docetaxel. Patients with at least 50% of tumor cells expressing PD-L1 had greater survival with pembrolizumab than docetaxel.[41]

Atezolizumab, an anti–PD-L1 agent, was recently approved by the FDA for the treatment of patients with metastatic NSCLC and disease progression during or after first-line platinum-based chemotherapy based on the findings from the OAK and POPLAR clinical trials. Additionally, it can be used for patients with *EGFR* mutations or ALK rearrangements that have progressed while being treated with an FDA-approved targeted therapy. In these trials, patients treated with atezolizumab had greater overall survival compared with patients treated with docetaxel.[43]

Immune-Related Adverse Events

Autoimmune-mediated complications may develop in response to treatment with immunotherapeutic agents and are referred to as immune-related adverse events. These effects are thought to result from either induction of autoimmunity or due to a proinflammatory state.[44] As such adverse events usually resolve with

cessation of therapy, it has been suggested that these complications are likely due to immunologic enhancement.[45]

The clinical presentation of immune-related adverse events is broad and ranges from mild and manageable to severe and life threatening.[46] The most common immune-related adverse events are related to dermatologic toxicity, with other complications, such as enterocolitis, hepatitis, pneumonitis, and endocrinopathies, less frequent.[45,47]

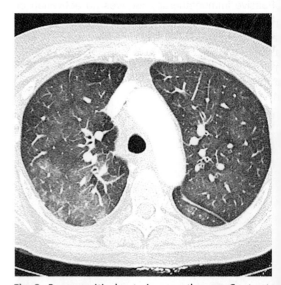

Fig. 8. Pneumonitis due to immunotherapy. Contrast-enhanced axial CT in a 67-year-old woman with lung cancer treated with nivolumab shows diffuse ground-glass opacities in both lungs. Several patterns of pneumonitis due to immunotherapy have been described, including ground-glass opacities, cryptogenic organizing pneumonia–like pattern, interstitial pattern, hypersensitivity pneumonitis-like pattern, and pneumonitis not otherwise specified.

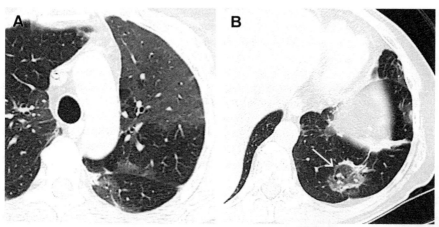

Fig. 9. Two patterns of pneumonitis due to immunotherapy in a 57-year-old woman with lung cancer. Contrast-enhanced axial CT shows (A) ground-glass opacities in the left upper lobe and to a lesser extent the right upper lobe and (B) COP-like appearance of immune-related pneumonitis in the left lower lobe with central ground-glass opacity and surrounding consolidation (*arrow*).

Other effects like sarcoid-like reaction, acute kidney injury, pancreatitis, neurotoxicity, cardiotoxicity, and ophthalmologic toxicity are relatively uncommon. Another potential complication of immunotherapy is opportunistic infection.[48]

Imaging Findings of Adverse Events

Various immune-related adverse events can be identified on CT or PET/CT, and awareness of these imaging manifestations is important to avoid misinterpretation as infection or disease progression and allow appropriate management. Pneumonitis is the most common adverse event in the chest; several different patterns have been described, including (1) ground-glass opacities (**Fig. 8**), (2) cryptogenic

organizing pneumonia (COP)-like (**Fig. 9**), (3) interstitial pattern, (4) hypersensitivity pneumonitis-like, and (5) pneumonitis not otherwise specified.[49] The manifestations of immune-related adverse events can evolve; for instance, patients with a COP-like pattern can develop widespread ground-glass opacities and patients with a ground-glass pattern can develop interstitial abnormalities.[49] Sarcoid-like reaction is a rare adverse event that can manifest as multiple small pulmonary nodules with or without ground-glass opacities and/or mediastinal/hilar lymphadenopathy[50] (**Fig. 10**).

Several cardiovascular abnormalities can occur, such as pericarditis, which typically manifests as a pericardial effusion with or without pericardial thickening/enhancement on CT (**Fig. 11**). Septal

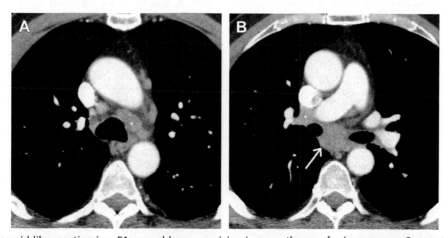

Fig. 10. Sarcoid-like reaction in a 51-year-old man receiving immunotherapy for lung cancer. Contrast-enhanced axial CT shows (A) an enlarged left paratracheal lymph node (*asterisk*) and other prominent but smaller lymph nodes and (B) enlarged right hilar (*asterisk*) and subcarinal (*arrow*) lymph nodes. Lymph node biopsies revealed no evidence of malignancy and inflammatory change consistent with sarcoid-like reaction.

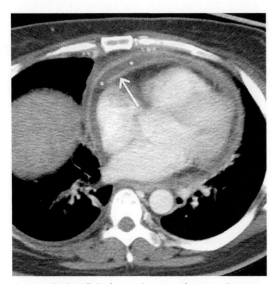

Fig. 11. Pericarditis due to immunotherapy. Contrast-enhanced axial CT of a 36-year-old woman with lung cancer treated with nivolumab shows a small pericardial effusion (*asterisks*) and pericardial thickening and enhancement (*arrow*) consistent with pericarditis.

bounce and respiratory septal shift consistent with ventricular interdependence and constrictive effusive physiology can be identified on echocardiography and MR imaging.[51–53] Thyroiditis is the most common thyroid-related complication of immunotherapy. Although thyroiditis can be diagnosed on iodine-123 thyroid scintigraphy and/or ultrasound, findings can also be identified on CT as enlargement and hypoattenuation of the thyroid gland and diffusely increased FDG uptake on PET/CT (Fig. 12).

The most common immune-related adverse events in the abdomen and pelvis include colitis

and hepatitis, the former of which is associated with the highest mortality of all adverse effects.[54] On CT, findings of immune-related colitis include segmental or diffuse wall thickening, mucosal enhancement, submucosal edema, air-fluid levels, infiltration of the adjacent fat, and ascites (Fig. 13). Findings of hepatitis can be identified on ultrasound and CT and manifest as periportal or portal vein hyperechogenicity on the former and periportal edema and hypoattenuation of the edematous liver parenchyma on the latter.[55,56] Immune-related pancreatitis results in imaging findings similar to that of acute pancreatitis unrelated to immunotherapy, such as pancreatic enlargement and edema with adjacent fat stranding, edema, and fluid on CT[57] and diffusely increased FDG uptake on PET/CT.[58]

Evaluation of Treatment Response

Specific response criteria have been developed for use with immunotherapeutic agents, including immune-related response criteria (irRC), immune-related Response Evaluation Criteria in Solid Tumors (irRECIST), and immune RECIST.[59–61] However, a thorough discussion of these criteria is beyond the scope of this article. Briefly, irRC is a novel set of response criteria adapted from the World Health Organization (WHO) criteria designed to specifically address appropriate imaging follow-up recommendations for patients treated with immunotherapy. irRC differs from WHO and RECIST in several ways. For example, it is recommended that response assessment after the completion of treatment should be made with 2 consecutive follow-up imaging studies at least 4 weeks apart because of a potentially

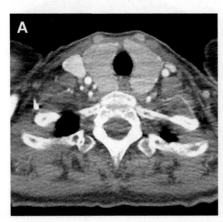
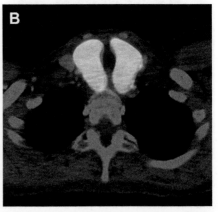

Fig. 12. Thyroiditis due to immunotherapy in a 60-year-old woman with lung cancer. (*A*) Contrast-enhanced axial CT shows diffuse enlargement of the thyroid gland. (*B*) Fused axial PET/CT shows diffuse increased FDG uptake within the thyroid gland. Immune-related thyroid toxicity most commonly manifests as thyroiditis.

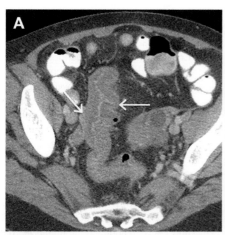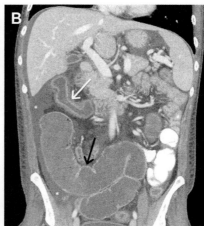

Fig. 13. Colitis due to immunotherapy. (*A*) Contrast-enhanced axial CT in a 67-year-old woman with lung cancer shows focal wall thickening of the sigmoid colon (*arrows*) consistent with colitis. (*B*) Contrast-enhanced coronal CT of a 36-year-old man with lung cancer shows diffuse wall thickening of the proximal transverse colon (*white arrow*), dilated and fluid-filled sigmoid colon (*black arrow*), and ascites (*asterisks*).

delayed response to therapy. Additionally, new lesions are not automatically considered progressive disease, as they can result from immune cell recruitment to sites of microscopic disease, also known as pseudoprogression. Accordingly, progressive disease must be confirmed by repeat imaging at a minimum of 4 weeks later. The application of irRECIST is similar to RECIST 1.1 regarding definitions of measureable and unmeasurable disease and criteria for selecting target and nontarget lesions. Additionally, the thresholds for response are overall aligned with RECIST 1.1. However, in contrast to RECIST 1.1, new lesions are not considered progressive disease. These lesions, if measurable, can be selected as new target lesions and incorporated into the response assessment.

SUMMARY

Targeted therapies are routinely used to treat advanced lung cancers that have specific driver mutations. Commonly targeted mutations include *EGFR* and *ALK*. Each mutation is more likely to be seen in certain populations and have certain imaging characteristics. Angiogenesis inhibitors are another class of targeted therapy and are known to cause tumoral cavitation. Additionally, the use of immunotherapy to treat patients with lung cancer continues to expand. An understanding of the mechanisms underlying the efficacy of targeted therapy and immunotherapy as well as the spectrum of potential adverse events is important in image interpretation and determination of appropriate patient management.

REFERENCES

1. Gadgeel SM. Personalized therapy of non-small cell lung cancer (NSCLC). Adv Exp Med Biol 2016;890: 203–22.
2. Chan BA, Hughes BG. Targeted therapy for non-small cell lung cancer: current standards and the promise of the future. Transl Lung Cancer Res 2015;4:36–54.
3. Alamgeer M, Ganju V, Watkins DN. Novel therapeutic targets in non-small cell lung cancer. Curr Opin Pharmacol 2013;13:394–401.
4. Savas P, Hughes B, Solomon B. Targeted therapy in lung cancer: IPASS and beyond, keeping abreast of the explosion of targeted therapies for lung cancer. J Thorac Dis 2013;5:S579–92.
5. Nivolumab approved for lung cancer. Cancer Discov 2015;5(5):OF1.
6. Lim SH, Sun JM, Lee SH, et al. Pembrolizumab for the treatment of non small cell lung cancer. Expert Opin Biol Ther 2016;16(3):397–406.
7. Pirker R, Filipits M. Targeted therapies in lung cancer. Curr Pharm Des 2009;15:188–206.
8. Mok TS, Wu YL, Thongprasert S, et al. Gefitinib or carboplatin-paclitaxel in pulmonary adenocarcinoma. N Engl J Med 2009;361:947–57.
9. Sequist LV, Waltman BA, Dias-Santagata D, et al. Genotypic and histological evolution of lung cancers acquiring resistance to EGFR inhibitors. Sci Transl Med 2011;3:75ra26.
10. Kobayashi S, Boggon TJ, Dayaram T, et al. EGFR mutation and resistance of non-small-cell lung cancer to gefitinib. N Engl J Med 2005;352:786–92.
11. Mok TS, Wu YL, Ahn MJ, et al. Osimertinib or platinum-pemetrexed in EGFR T790M-positive lung cancer. N Engl J Med 2017;376(7):629–40.

12. Morris SW, Kirstein MN, Valentine MB, et al. Fusion of a kinase gene, ALK, to a nucleolar protein gene, NPM, in non-Hodgkin's lymphoma. Science 1995; 267:316–7.

13. Soda M, Choi YL, Enomoto M, et al. Identification of the transforming EML4-ALK fusion gene in non-small-cell lung cancer. Nature 2007;448:561–6.

14. Suda K, Tomizawa K, Mitsudomi T. Biological and clinical significance of KRAS mutations in lung cancer: an oncogenic driver that contrasts with EGFR mutation. Cancer Metastasis Rev 2010;29:49–60.

15. Guin S, Ru Y, Wynes MW, et al. Contributions of KRAS and RAL in non-small-cell lung cancer growth and progression. J Thorac Oncol 2013;8:1492–501.

16. Gainor JF, Varghese AM, Ou SH, et al. ALK rearrangements are mutually exclusive with mutations in EGFR or KRAS: an analysis of 1,683 patients with non-small cell lung cancer. Clin Cancer Res 2013;19:4273–81.

17. Alevizakos M, Kaltsas S, Syrigos KN. The VEGF pathway in lung cancer. Cancer Chemother Pharmacol 2013;72:1169–81.

18. Bonnesen B, Pappot H, Holmstav J, et al. Vascular endothelial growth factor A and vascular endothelial growth factor receptor 2 expression in non-small cell lung cancer patients: relation to prognosis. Lung Cancer 2009;66:314–8.

19. Chirieac LR, Dacic S. Targeted therapies in lung cancer. Surg Pathol Clin 2010;3:71–82.

20. Johnson DH, Fehrenbacher L, Novotny WF, et al. Randomized phase II trial comparing bevacizumab plus carboplatin and paclitaxel with carboplatin and paclitaxel alone in previously untreated locally advanced or metastatic non-small-cell lung cancer. J Clin Oncol 2004;22:2184–91.

21. Crabb SJ, Patsios D, Sauerbrei E, et al. Tumor cavitation: impact on objective response evaluation in trials of angiogenesis inhibitors in non-small-cell lung cancer. J Clin Oncol 2009;27:404–10.

22. Nishino M, Cryer SK, Okajima Y, et al. Tumoral cavitation in patients with non-small-cell lung cancer treated with antiangiogenic therapy using bevacizumab. Cancer Imaging 2012;12:225–35.

23. Tirumani SH, Fairchild A, Krajewski KM, et al. Anti-VEGF molecular targeted therapies in common solid malignancies: comprehensive update for radiologists. Radiographics 2015;35:455–74.

24. Marom EM, Martinez CH, Truong MT, et al. Tumor cavitation during therapy with antiangiogenesis agents in patients with lung cancer. J Thorac Oncol 2008;3:351–7.

25. Sabri A, Batool M, Xu Z, et al. Predicting EGFR mutation status in lung cancer: proposal for a scoring model using imaging and demographic characteristics. Eur Radiol 2016;26:4141–7.

26. Hsu JS, Huang MS, Chen CY, et al. Correlation between EGFR mutation status and computed tomography features in patients with advanced pulmonary adenocarcinoma. J Thorac Imaging 2014; 29:357–63.

27. Choi CM, Kim MY, Hwang HJ, et al. Advanced adenocarcinoma of the lung: comparison of CT characteristics of patients with anaplastic lymphoma kinase gene rearrangement and those with epidermal growth factor receptor mutation. Radiology 2015;275:272–9.

28. Yamamoto S, Korn RL, Oklu R, et al. ALK molecular phenotype in non-small cell lung cancer: CT radiogenomic characterization. Radiology 2014;272: 568–76.

29. Park J, Kobayashi Y, Urayama KY, et al. Imaging characteristics of driver mutations in EGFR, KRAS, and ALK among treatment-naïve patients with advanced lung adenocarcinoma. PLoS One 2016; 11:e0161081.

30. Weiss GJ, Ganeshan B, Miles KA, et al. Noninvasive image texture analysis differentiates K-ras mutation from pan-wildtype NSCLC and is prognostic. PLoS One 2014;9:e100244.

31. Choi H, Paeng JC, Kim DW, et al. Metabolic and metastatic characteristics of ALK-rearranged lung adenocarcinoma on FDG PET/CT. Lung Cancer 2013;79:242–7.

32. Caicedo C, Garcia-Velloso MJ, Lozano MD, et al. Role of [^{18}F]FDG PET in prediction of KRAS and EGFR mutation status in patients with advanced non-small-cell lung cancer. Eur J Nucl Med Mol Imaging 2014;41:2058–65.

33. Nishino M, Hatabu H, Johnson BE, et al. State of the art: response assessment in lung cancer in the era of genomic medicine. Radiology 2014;271:6–27.

34. Souza FF, Smith A, Araujo C, et al. New targeted molecular therapies for cancer: radiological response in intrathoracic malignancies and cardiopulmonary toxicity: what the radiologist needs to know. Cancer Imaging 2014;14:26.

35. Thornton E, Howard SA, Jagannathan J, et al. Imaging features of bowel toxicities in the setting of molecular targeted therapies in cancer patients. Br J Radiol 2012;85(1018):1420–6.

36. Howard SA, Rosenthal MH, Jagannathan JP, et al. Beyond the vascular endothelial growth factor axis: update on role of imaging in nonantiangiogenic molecular targeted therapies in oncology. AJR Am J Roentgenol 2015;204:919–32.

37. Bhatia S, Tykodi SS, Thompson JA. Treatment of metastatic melanoma: an overview. Oncology (Williston Park) 2009;23(6):488–96.

38. Gettinger SN, Horn L, Gandhi L, et al. Overall survival and long-term safety of nivolumab (anti-programmed death 1 antibody, BMS-936558, ONO-4538) in patients with previously treated advanced non-small-cell lung cancer. J Clin Oncol 2015;33(18):2004–12.

39. Brahmer J, Reckamp KL, Baas P, et al. Nivolumab versus docetaxel in advanced squamous-cell non-small-cell lung cancer. N Engl J Med 2015;373(2): 123–35.

40. Borghaei H, Paz-Ares L, Horn L, et al. Nivolumab versus docetaxel in advanced nonsquamous non-small-cell lung cancer. N Engl J Med 2015;373(17): 1627–39.

41. Herbst RS, Baas P, Kim DW, et al. Pembrolizumab versus docetaxel for previously treated, PD-L1-positive, advanced non-small-cell lung cancer (KEYNOTE-010): a randomised controlled trial. Lancet 2016;387(10027):1540–50.

42. Rittmeyer A, Barlesi F, Waterkamp D, et al. Atezolizumab versus docetaxel in patients with previously treated non-small-cell lung cancer (OAK): a phase 3, open-label, multicentre randomised controlled trial. Lancet 2017;389(10066):255–65.

43. Fehrenbacher L, Spira A, Ballinger M, et al. Atezolizumab versus docetaxel for patients with previously treated non-small-cell lung cancer (POPLAR): a multicentre, open-label, phase 2 randomised controlled trial. Lancet 2016;387(10030):1837–46.

44. Kaufman HL, Kirkwood JM, Hodi FS, et al. The Society for Immunotherapy of Cancer consensus statement on tumour immunotherapy for the treatment of cutaneous melanoma. Nat Rev Clin Oncol 2013; 10(10):588–98.

45. Postow MA, Wolchok JD. Ipilimumab: developmental history, clinical considerations and future perspectives. The Melanoma Letter 2012;30(1):1–4.

46. Voskens CJ, Goldinger SM, Loquai C, et al. The price of tumor control: an analysis of rare side effects of anti-CTLA-4 therapy in metastatic melanoma from the ipilimumab network. PLoS One 2013;8: e53745.

47. Nishino M, Tirumani SH, Ramaiya NH, et al. Cancer immunotherapy and immune-related response assessment: the role of radiologists in the new arena of cancer treatment. Eur J Radiol 2015;84(7): 1259–68.

48. Kyi C, Hellmann MD, Wolchok JD, et al. Opportunistic infections in patients treated with immunotherapy for cancer. J Immunother Cancer 2014;2:19.

49. Naidoo J, Wang X, Woo KM, et al. Pneumonitis in patients treated with anti-programmed death-1/programmed death ligand 1 therapy. J Clin Oncol 2017;35(7):709–17.

50. Prieto PA, Yang JC, Sherry RM, et al. CTLA-4 blockade with ipilimumab: long-term follow-up of 177 patients with metastatic melanoma. Clin Cancer Res 2012;18(7):2039–47.

51. Yun S, Vincelette ND, Mansour I, et al. Late onset ipilimumab-induced pericarditis and pericardial effusion: a rare but life threatening complication. Case Rep Oncol Med 2015;2015:794842.

52. Kolla BC, Patel MR. Recurrent pleural effusions and cardiac tamponade as possible manifestations of pseudoprogression associated with nivolumab therapy- a report of two cases. J Immunother Cancer 2016;4:80.

53. Johnson DB, Balko JM, Compton ML, et al. Fulminant myocarditis with combination immune checkpoint blockade. N Engl J Med 2016;375(18): 1749–55.

54. Kim KW, Ramaiya NH, Krajewski KM, et al. Ipilimumab associated colitis: CT findings. AJR Am J Roentgenol 2013;200(5):W468–74.

55. O'Regan KN, Jagannathan JP, Ramaiya N, et al. Radiologic aspects of immune-related tumor response criteria and patterns of immune-related adverse events in patients undergoing ipilimumab therapy. AJR Am J Roentgenol 2011;197(2): W241–6.

56. Kim KW, Ramaiya NH, Krajewski KM, et al. Ipilimumab associated hepatitis: imaging and clinicopathologic findings. Invest New Drugs 2013;31(4):1071–7.

57. Bronstein Y, Ng CS, Hwu P, et al. Radiologic manifestations of immune-related adverse events in patients with metastatic melanoma undergoing anti-CTLA-4 antibody therapy. AJR Am J Roentgenol 2011;197(6):W992–1000.

58. Alabed YZ, Aghayev A, Sakellis C, et al. Pancreatitis secondary to anti-programmed death receptor 1 immunotherapy diagnosed by FDG PET/CT. Clin Nucl Med 2015;40(11):e528–9.

59. Wolchok JD, Hoos A, Bohnsack O, et al. Guidelines for the evaluation of immune therapy activity in solid tumors: immune-related response criteria. Clin Cancer Res 2009;15:7412–20.

60. Nishino M, Giobbie-Hurder A, Gargano M, et al. Developing a common language for tumor response to immunotherapy: immune-related response criteria using unidimensional measurements. Clin Cancer Res 2013;19:3936–43.

61. Seymour L, Bogaerts J, Perrone A, et al. iRECIST: guidelines for response criteria for use in trials testing immunotherapeutics. Lancet Oncol 2017; 18(3):e143–52.

Moving?

Make sure your subscription moves with you!

To notify us of your new address, find your **Clinics Account Number** (located on your mailing label above your name), and contact customer service at:

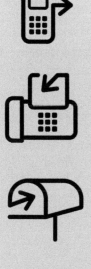

Email: journalscustomerservice-usa@elsevier.com

800-654-2452 (subscribers in the U.S. & Canada)
314-447-8871 (subscribers outside of the U.S. & Canada)

Fax number: 314-447-8029

Elsevier Health Sciences Division
Subscription Customer Service
3251 Riverport Lane
Maryland Heights, MO 63043

*To ensure uninterrupted delivery of your subscription, please notify us at least 4 weeks in advance of move.

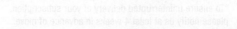

Printed and bound by CPI Group (UK) Ltd, Croydon, CR0 4YY

08/05/2025

01864711-0008